DATE DUE

PAIN:

THE FIFTH

VITAL SIGN

PAIN:

THE FIFTH

VITAL SIGN

Marni Jackson

Crown
Publishers
New York

Published by Crown Publishers, New York, New York.
Member of the Crown Publishing Group, a division of Random House, Inc.
www.randomhouse.com

CROWN is a trademark and the Crown colophon is a registered trademark of Random House, Inc.

Excerpts from *Naked Lunch* by William S. Burroughs. Reprinted by permission of Grove/ Atlantic.

Excerpts from *The Pain Journal* by Bob Flanagan and the manifesto "Why" by Bob Flanagan reprinted with permission of Semiotext(e) Press and Sheree Rose.

Poems "650" and "967" and excerpts from poem "341" from *The Poems of Emily Dickinson* by Emily Dickinson, edited by Thomas H. Johnson. (Cambridge, Mass.: The Belknap Press of Harvard University Press). Copyright © 1951, 1955, 1979 by the President and Fellows of Harvard College. Reprinted by permission of Harvard University Press and the Trustees of Amherst College.

Lyrics from the songs "Closing Time" and "The Future" by Leonard Cohen and the epigraph taken from the poem "The Drawer's Condition on Nov. 28, 1961" used with gracious permission of the author.

Lyrics from "Night Nurse" words and music by Gregory Isaacs and Sylvester Weise. Copyright © 1982 by Charisma Music Publishing Co. Ltd. and Splash Down Music. All rights for Charisma Music Publishing Co. Ltd. in the U.S. and Canada controlled and administered by EMI April Music Inc. All rights reserved. International copyright secured. Reprinted by permission of EMI April Music Inc.

Lyrics from "You're a Big Girl Now" by Bob Dylan. Copyright © 1974, 1975 by Ram's Horn Music. All rights reserved. International copyright secured. Reprinted by permission of Ram's Horn Music.

The author gratefully acknowledges using excerpts from "Oral History Interview with Ronald Melzack, 16 October 1993 (Ms. Coll. No. 127.3) and "Oral History Interview with Cicely Saunders, 11 August 1993 (Ms. Coll. No. 127.23), as well as material from the William K. Livingston Papers, in the John C. Liebeskind History of Pain Collection, History & Special Collections Divisions, Louise M. Darling Biomedical Library, University of California, Los Angeles.

Printed in the United States of America

DESIGN BY BARBARA STURMAN

Library of Congress Cataloging-in-Publication Data
Jackson, Marni.
      Pain—the fifth vital sign : the science and culture of why we hurt / Marni Jackson. (HC)
      1. Pain—Popular works. I. Title.
      RB 127 .J24   2002
      616'.0472—dc21   2002024150

ISBN 0-609-60375-2

10 9 8 7 6 5 4 3 2 1

First Edition

For Brian

ACKNOWLEDGMENTS

I began this expedition with one or two intuitions that I hoped to test as I went about educating myself about pain. All I had to do was acquire a working knowledge of physiology, neurology, psychology, philosophy, pharmacotherapy, Chinese medicine, molecular biology, and acupuncture while browsing through the canon of Western literature. In practice, what this has meant is that I have depended on the expertise and generosity of many experts and authors who have devoted their lives to such matters.

For their patience in dealing with a civilian, I would like to thank the following scientists, physicians, dentists, clinicians, and therapists: Frank Adams, Angela Mailis, V. S. Ramachandran, Harold Merskey, Allan Basbaum, Joel Katz, John Dostroevsky, Karen Davis, Paul Kelly, Simon Vulfsons, Sydney Brenner, Patrick Wall, Kathleen Foley, Nikolai Bogduk, Chris Wells, Chris Mains, Maureen Dwight, Laura Dempster, Marion Harris, Rosa Spricer, Xiaolan Zhoa, Miriam Erlichman, Paula Nieustratten, Robin Conway, John Loeser, Mike Salter, Jeff Mogil, Ron Melzack, Wendy Simmons, Gordon Waddell, Mark Sullivan, Ned Block, Ellen Thompson, Patricia McGrath, Allen Finley, and the members of the Comprehensive Pain Program unit at the Toronto Hospital.

Two books in particular persuaded me that this was indeed a rich subject and not a chimera: The first was *The Body in Pain: The Making and Unmaking of the World*, by Elaine Scarry, a work that eloquently addresses the silence surrounding this subject. The second was *The Culture of Pain*, by David B. Morris, a book that I was too apprehensive to open for the first two years of my research. I am glad I waited. It is a work of stunning scholarship, both broad and deep, written with unusual grace. If I had encountered it earlier, it might have convinced me that I had nothing to add on the subject. As it turns out, although our paths are convergent, our missions are quite distinct. But *The Culture of Pain* set the ropes on this route almost ten years ago.

Two institutions have been indispensable to my education: the International Association for the Study of Pain, and the Louise M. Darling Biomedical Library at UCLA in Los Angeles, home of the John C. Liebeskind History of Pain Collection. The IASP has done a tremendous job of promoting pain awareness and research, and I have relied on their newsletters, publications, and conferences to gain some grounding in the science of pain. President Barry Sessle was especially helpful in steering me to individuals. I am also indebted to Kathleen Donahue, archivist Russell Johnson, the late John C. Liebeskind, and medical historian Marcia Meldrum for their help and guidance during my visit to the History of Pain Collection. The portraits of Silas Weir Mitchell, William Livingston, and Cicely Saunders included here are based on extensive interviews conducted by John Liebeskind and Marcia Meldrum, as well as personal papers in the archives. I have relied on research collected by Martin Booth and Barbara Hodgson in their respective books on opium in the chapter "Smoke and Pills."

I didn't have to look far for pain stories: they are everywhere. Invisible courage surrounds us. I owe respect and thanks to the following for sharing this most private experience: Lori Biduke, David and Anna Kelly, Teresa Stephens, Debbie Dyja, Eileen Whitfield, Sandy Kybartis, Barry Arsenault, Heather, Zoe Yanovsky, Ramiro Puerta, Carole Corbeil and Layne Coleman, Jori Morrison, Olive and Clyde Jackson, Alice van Wart, Reverend Ken Martin, and Cathleen Hoskins. Thanks as well to "Chuck G." for helpful hints from the "Torture Garden," and to Bob Dylan and Leonard Cohen for all their fieldwork.

Pain moves around, and so did I. For their generosity in offering writing refuges, I thank Jill Frayne, Barbara Gowdy, Sue Swan, Anne Nicholson and Arne Moore, and Doug Bell. In particular, Jill's house set my compass in the right direction. I made liberal use of their bookshelves as well.

If pain is solitary, I made sure that writing about it wasn't. Many thanks to the following friends for their support, advice, and timely edits: Anne Mackenzie, Beret Borsos, Barbara Gowdy, Judith Timson, Jane O'Hara, Ian Brown, Jill Frayne, and Brian Johnson.

Thanks to Kirsten Hansen for her helpful manuscript suggestions. A version of the chapter on Dr. Angela Mailis appeared in *Toronto Life* magazine, with the invaluable editing of Angie Gardos. A portion of my interview with Dr. Paul Kelly appeared in *Maclean's* magazine. In the matter of the great title debate, special thanks to Michael Ondaatje and Linda Spalding, David Reed, Robert Ramsey and Jean Marmoreo, Anne Mackenzie and Zalman Yanovsky ("Mein Kramp") for their thoughts. Naming pain isn't easy.

My interest in the intertidal zones of science and art is a direct result of conversations around the dinner table, with my quasi-medical, scientifically adventurous family. My mother and father, Olive and Clyde Jackson, remain terribly curious, about everything. My brother Bruce, an early pain initiate, and his wife, Kathy, helped me with the biochemistry of it all. I have also learned much about graceful strength from my sister Jori, and Lola Johnson.

Once again, my editor and publisher, Anne Collins, imagined that I could do this, and gamely waded through the swamps and bogs with me. No Anne, no book. Her rare combination of intelligence, integrity, and giddiness is something I continue to cherish. I was also aided and calmed by Pam Robertson at Random House. My agent, Anne McDermid, never once blanched at the idea of selling a lovely book about pain; I thank her and Ann Patty for their early enthusiasm for the project. To Doug Pepper at Crown I offer thanks for editorial steadiness during a shaky time in New York. I am grateful as well for the care and engagement of production editor Pam Stinson-Bell.

Now, do you know what it is like to be married to or mothered by someone who is writing a book about the nature of pain? For years? Who wants to talk about shingles or stump pain over dinner? Luckily, I had two discerning writers under the same roof who understood this chronic state—my husband, Brian Johnson, and my son, Casey. I leaned on their good judgment and support. Not only were they patient through the troughs of gloom that come with such enterprises, but they *stayed interested*. Amazing. Above all, my love and gratitude to Brian for never letting me lose sight of the pleasure principle.

CONTENTS

PAIN:

THE FIFTH

VITAL SIGN

INTRODUCTION: THE STING

I was riding a bike in the Rockies, near Banff, Alberta, when a bee flew into my mouth. At first I thought I'd been hit by a flying cork (as if champagne bottles are always popping off in the woods). Then I felt a slim, unambiguous lance of pain, like a splinter of glass. The feeling of the sting crystallized everything about the morning so far— my impatience to catch up to the others, the chill of the mountain air on my arms, a small worry about having taken the wrong road.

My husband and son eventually noticed my absence and circled back. We stood around waiting to see if I would topple over, a not unheard-of event on our family vacations. I've had little dying spells before, anaphylactic reactions to this or that, although never to bee venom. But as a well-read hypochondriac, I knew that a sting at the back of the throat can cause the airway to swell up and close. A bee could, in other words, lead me to literally strangle myself on this flat stretch of pavement . . . or so my thoughts ran. (Pain experts have a word for this: *catastrophizing*.)

The strange thing about my random bee sting was that it immediately sprouted a narrative. I knew it wasn't just bad luck that a bee had stumbled into me. It made perfect sense. I saw the sting as punishment for biking "the wrong way"—too fast, all in a lather, panting with open mouth. My husband and fourteen-year-old son were hoping for hills and off-road trails, but I wanted mountains, shade, and pavement, so we had struck a compromise that thrilled no one. I was churning away on my bike, pretending to have fun, when the bee came along and rinsed the morning clear of small deceptions.

The three of us made our way to a golf course, where the groundskeeper offered to drive me into town to get some antihistamines, just in case. I was now puffy-lipped but fine. I persuaded my family (easily, as it turned out) to bike on and rode into town as the groundskeeper regaled me with stories of golfers who had died on the green, from just such a bee sting as mine. A doctor at the local clinic examined me and said there was nothing to worry about. She plucked the stinger out of my mouth, gave me some Advils and anti-histamines, and told me to call her later, "if things got weird."

But apart from developing fabulous Angelina Jolie lips, the only consequence was an afternoon spent in manageable, medium-intensity, finite pain. Which got me thinking.

The first thing I noticed was that pain lacks a language of its own and must recruit metaphors or similes: knifelike, killing, burning. The experience feels just beyond our grasp, like a tape run backward that tantalizes with garbled, half-recognizable inflections. It's a place bereft of words. Pain arrives as a fusion of sensation, emotion, nerve, and memory, as irreducible and vivid as a poem. No wonder the study of pain has eluded the prose of science so successfully.

Science is objective, looking for measurable events, whereas pain is always subjective. You can never cut the "I" out of pain. At the same time that it fuses mind and body, it splits us, too. We enter a dialogue with ourselves whenever we're in pain. Consciousness divides into Siamese twins of subject and object, joined at the spot where we hurt. It turns us into observers—scientists, even—of our own pain.

I WENT BACK TO our hotel and climbed into bed with a book, grateful at first for an excuse to retreat from the world for an afternoon. Pain focuses the self. But the ache in my jaw kept blossoming, and it wouldn't let me read. Annoyed to be derailed by something so trivial, I did my best to dismiss the feeling. But pain won't be slighted. ("To kindness, to knowledge, we make promises only," Proust wrote. "Pain we obey.") So I occupied myself by going further into the feeling, touring the contours of this cave, aware that it couldn't really hurt me. It wasn't the bone pain of cancer, after all, or the warning squeeze of angina. It was just an accidental, transient spasm with no meaning—a very modern pain.

For a brief afternoon I joined the ranks of one of the world's biggest invisible subcultures—everyone who lives with some form of daily pain. This includes both the whiners and moaners as well as the ones who say "never mind" and push themselves through the day. Pain affects one in three families; more than 50 million Americans experience chronic forms of it, at a staggering economic cost to society. Back pain is the most common, followed by headache and migraine, arthritis, and on down through the misunderstood agonies of conditions like trigeminal neuralgia, fibromyalgia, and phantom limb pain. (Bee stings, I believe, are close to the bottom.)

My own relationship to pain is nothing out of the ordinary. I get migraines, make the odd trek to the suburbs of depression, and have experienced the interesting, carcass-rending pain of unmedicated childbirth. Nevertheless, it struck me that the relationship we all have with pain runs deeper and is much more entangled than we imagine.

I noticed how my awareness immediately shrank to the size of the pain, and how it became the new frame of my world. Then I began to wonder if I was cowardly or brave. How much pain *was* I feeling, anyway? Hardly any? A great deal? Compared to whom? The sensation in my mouth seemed custom-made to my ability to handle it. Next I became aware how pain alters time, too, amputating any sense of before or after. (As Emily Dickinson wrote, "Pain—has an element of blank / It cannot recollect / When it began—or if there were / A day when it was not.") My Afternoon of Venom also made me realize that the little pain I inhabited had taken the vague bruises of the past few years and transformed them into something clean and clear, with boundaries. Now I was stung in a way I couldn't ignore. It was as if physical pain is always historical, tapping into the body's Rolodex of past traumas. Pretty soon I was lying there reliving a gory scene from thirty years earlier, when I discovered my boyfriend in bed with someone else.

But what did the effects of bee venom have to do with a long-buried heartache? It seemed that small injuries can open up deeper channels of pain that have been lying in wait. Perhaps pain is like a river, I thought, not only running underground in our own lives, but flowing into us from previous generations as well. Each current unique.

In my room I lay watching the changeable sky, scrolling fast through mountain weather, as all sorts of old emotions came up, like little fish, to feed on the surface.

But pain also had its compensations. It made me feel more coherent and whole, anchored in my body. By midafternoon, all the wispy anxieties and milling concerns of my day had contracted to one bright point—this little tête-à-tête between me and pain. The sense of being in such intimate, uneasy dialogue with the self began to feel vaguely familiar. Ah yes, I realized, it was like writing (no wonder so many writers self-medicate).

My husband called to ask how I was. Well, it hurts, I said, but I'm fine. What was the point of trying to convey to him the baroque sprawl of thoughts and feelings I had been lost in? Silence surrounds pain. But like a taciturn cowboy, this silence has a certain appeal. So much sensation, which we seem to be so intent on killing: $3 billion a year spent on Advil, Tylenol, and all the rest. A big investment in not feeling.

The two of them came back to the hotel sunburned and solicitous. I roused myself to go out to dinner with them, even though I was now beginning to feel rather ill and dizzy. But pain always arrives with this corollary of shame, as if we're responsible for our own suffering, regardless of the origin. One must soldier on! I forced myself to sit in a Japanese restaurant and stare at the menu, while longing to be back in bed. A mild allergic reaction had set in. I felt weird and anxious. Soon I was observing my husband and son, laughing and eating sushi, as if through the wrong end of binoculars. This will pass, I said to myself, a trick that middle age perfects. And it did. But I had a brief glimpse of how isolating it must feel to be held hostage to pain and the anxiety that accompanies it.

I LIKE TO READ explorers' journals. My shelves are full of books about polar expeditions, sagas of frostbite and heroism and hardship that could be subtitled the Literature of Pain. The subject of pain is a kind of Antarctica, too, a vast, inhospitable, and largely unexplored terrain. Despite the tremendous progress that science has made in its understanding of it over the past fifty years or so, pain remains for the most part a *terra incognita* on the map of consciousness. We imagine there's not much there, but it's our own blind spot that prevents us from reading the landscape properly. I was curious to go more deeply into that blank white space.

The morning after the bee episode, big-lipped but back to normal, I found that the person who had toured the Casbah of pain had disappeared. I began to doubt my insights. Pain no longer seemed a rather rakish companion, but a bully and a bore, someone best forgotten. This is part of pain, too—our disloyalty to it. This is what refreshes pain's power. No sooner are you free of it than you suppress the memory, along with whatever illuminations it brought, until the next ambush. It's too intense a place to stay for long.

Back home in Toronto, I kept puzzling over certain questions. Why do we persist in this distinction between mental and physical pain when pain is always an emotional experience? What explains the fact that something as universal as pain is so poorly understood, especially in a century of self-scrutiny? Has nobody noticed the embarrassing fact that science is about to clone a human being, but it still can't cure the pain of a bad back? Americans consume four tons of aspirin a year, while chronic pain is on the rise. It's almost as if pain flourishes on our diet of analgesics.

Many medical students receive no more than one hour of instruction in pain management. Some schools don't even have pain on the curriculum, even though pain is the number one reason that sends people to their GPs. Most doctors know more about cosmetic chemical peels than cancer pain. It's not the fault of physicians—this is how we teach them.

Why are we, the most medicalized of societies, a culture in pain?

During the past four years that I've spent doing research into these questions, people often ask why I would want to spend my time on such a depressing subject. While I've "caught" more than one pain syndrome in the course of writing this (shingles has been my greatest somatic achievement), it has turned out to be the most fascinating subject I can imagine. My last book was about the myths and silences that surround motherhood—another realm of feeling that resists articulation, and a not unrelated topic. I wrote it because no one was talking about the experience of being a mother the way

I felt going through it myself. I have the same sense of exasperation toward the subject of pain: Neither science nor medicine seems to be telling the whole story, and literature, our other great storehouse of knowledge about pain, has largely lost touch with the specialized grammar of science. I thought it might be possible to zigzag back and forth between the perceptions of writers and poets, people suffering pain, doctors and pain experts, to create a portrait that would be . . . more like pain itself. Right now, we tend to characterize pain as either a physical injury or some (more suspect) psychic affliction. But this is not how pain feels. We all understand that pain is an experience at once private and public, cell-deep and world-sized. The political events of the past year have taught us that private pain quickly moves out in a shock wave, to embrace a much wider circle. The news hurts. To imagine that pain is merely an event in the nerves of the body is to overlook an experience that is cultural and historical as well.

So my goal here has been to describe pain in the round, from as many sides as possible. As someone who is neither a doctor nor a scientist, this has occasionally struck me as a ridiculous endeavor, like trying to inscribe the history of love on a grain of rice. But the problem with most scientific approaches to the elucidation of pain is that they narrow down just when they should open out. Being a writer, an expert in nothing, has at least allowed me to integrate and synthesize—the one thing that pain insists we do.

For a writer, the wordlessness surrounding pain is, on good days, like having a desert island all to yourself. So much horizon! Not a soul in sight! On bad days, however, writing about pain is like trying to nail a bead of mercury. The more you try to pin down pain, the more it shatters into ungraspable fragments.

The book is structured around my own fairly impulsive, divining-rod forays into the pain world. It is by no means comprehensive. I went back into the history of our ideas about pain and forward into the possibilities of pain genetics. I talked to people who live with tic douloureux and neuropathic pain. When my mother broke her shoulder, I watched the home-care nurses, in order to learn how to move someone in pain. My sister herniated a disk in her back and discovered what the world's experts in back pain already know—there is an entire industry of surgeries and gadgets and treatments out there that can't do a thing to hasten recovery. I spent some time in a Toronto multidisciplinary pain clinic run by a woman with a black belt in Tae Kwon Do. I took a meditation workshop led by a former director of a pain clinic who now teaches a Buddhist approach to pain. I went to Vienna to attend the Ninth World Congress of the International Association for the Study of Pain, where I watched the jousting of international scientists at the top of their game. I talked to both Patrick Wall and Ronald Melzack, whose gate-control theory revolutionized the way science understands pain. Of the many books I consulted, I returned again and again to two classics: Melzack and Wall's *The Challenge of Pain* and David Morris's brilliant, humane study *The Culture of Pain*. And at the History of Pain Project at UCLA, I encountered the work of some of the maverick thinkers from the last two centuries of pain research.

There's something about this field that attracts wrestlers, writers, and other eccentric polymaths—the anesthetist John Bonica, the Civil War physician Silas Weir Mitchell, and the surgeon William Livingston. I learned how Cecily Saunders, the founder of the hospice movement, began her work as a nurse, many of whom have been on the front lines of pain research. I came upon case studies that read like novels, written by nineteenth-century doctors who were men of literature as well as medicine.

My investigations led to further questions: Why doesn't contemporary science draw more on literature? Why is it easier for a heroin addict to buy narcotics on the street than it is for someone with chronic, nonmalignant pain to get a prescription for morphine? Why do we spend $2 billion a year putting drug offenders in jail while denying opiates to the hospitalized elderly, half of whom die in pain? What is this love-hate relationship we have with drugs?

To explore this, I tell the story of a fifteen-year-old girl, a heroin addict with her own particular relationship to pain and drugs, and compare it to the role narcotics plays in the death of a friend from cancer. People in the intermediate stages of cancer continue to be undertreated for pain or are given high doses of "milder" drugs, anti-inflammatories that can lead to more damaging consequences. Somehow, we have encouraged a culture of addiction while still withholding relief from people in pain. Doctors have always had the legal option to treat pain in their patients, or to take a pass. Many choose to take a pass. But in 2000 in Oregon, the first malpractice suit was brought against a doctor for failure to treat a patient in pain.

Right now, the strict regulations surrounding the prescription of narcotics discourage doctors from taking on chronic pain cases. There is alarm as well over the diversion of drugs like OxyContin to the streets. Doctors fear investigation and reprisal if they prescribe too many opiates: Dr. Frank Adams, a Houston pain specialist, had his Canadian license suspended as a result of prescribing high dosages of opiates to patients with unrelenting pain. Dr. Adams gave me his side of the story. In the case of cancer pain, I bring in the work of Dr. Kathleen Foley, former head of pain services at Memorial Sloan-Kettering Cancer Center in New York City. Dr. Foley, perhaps America's preeminent authority on pain, has been working hard for many years to change the legislation regarding pain treatment and palliative care service in North America.

It's a slow business, educating doctors about pain and changing our attitudes toward it. If we knew more about pain treatment, would Robert Latimer, a Saskatchewan farmer, have felt he had no other recourse but to kill his severely disabled daughter, who suffered daily pain? Reports claimed that Tracy, a twelve-year-old girl with severe cerebral palsy, couldn't be treated with the usual analgesics because of the anticonvulsive medication she was on. At least one pain specialist I spoke to disagreed with this explanation. Perhaps this case and others like it have a misplaced focus. They have led to intense public debate about the rights of the disabled and the ethics of taking someone else's life, when a more useful starting point might be: Could the pain have been relieved if we knew more about how to treat it? These are heartbreaking stories that a better understanding of pain might have prevented.

So what can pain teach us? That pain is what the patient says it is. This idea has begun to radically change the relationship between physician and patient. The growing popularity in the West of

Buddhist approaches to pain is also a response to everything medicine has shut itself away from. In the same way that we're coming to accept death as part of the continuum of life, pain has to be reintegrated into our idea of health. We lack compassion for ourselves.

Other changes are under way. One of the things Bill Clinton saw to before his term as president was over was the signing of a congressional bill that declared the first ten years of this century the "Decade of Pain Awareness and Research." This is only the second official "medical decade," after the 1990s were designated the "Decade of the Brain"—which it was. The neurosciences went wild. And after the brain comes pain.

In America, there has also been a recent campaign to treat pain as the fifth vital sign. This idea was launched in 1995 by James Campbell, the president of the American Pain Society. Just as the four traditional vital signs, temperature, respiration, pulse, and blood pressure, must be charted, American hospitals are now obliged to assess pain in their patients, too. It's not a perfect system—vital signs are only taken every eight hours, but pain should probably be measured only when it's present, and then more frequently—but this approach helps make pain more visible. The other encouraging trend is the spread of the multidisciplinary pain clinic, where the issue of pain is the main focus rather than a frustrating side issue for doctors. Pain clinics, drawing on the expertise of psychologists, neurologists, chiropractors, social workers, and others, acknowledge the complexity of pain.

Our magic-bullet mentality would prefer a simpler solution, or one big pain pill. But as science has discovered, our experience of pain has no fixed center, no miracle neuron that controls it all. Doctors have to look beyond isolated symptoms to the story under or around it. Pain always arrives with a hidden narrative. Science prefers the same thing to happen, in the same way, over and over, but pain is subjective, invisible, multifaceted, and individual. This is why science and pain have been uneasy bedfellows, whereas the shifting valence of suffering is a central theme in literature.

I have left out a number of important topics here—the new discoveries in pain treatment for children and the issue of pain in animals. I only touch on the immeasurable role that the pharmaceutical corporations play in shaping the way we think about pain. But the field of pain studies is littered with the carcasses of unfinished or abandoned books, undertaken by people who know much more about it than I do. I could sit in my room for thirty more years and still feel there was more to write. This book is intended to reflect an ordinary sense of confusion in the face of pain and to explore the new paths that open up when you go looking for answers. It's for company, in pain's solitude.

I made the decision to write in my own voice because pain is personal, and I include a few of my own pain sagas for the same reason. But I also wanted to link up the views of science and medicine with the voices of philosophers, writers, and other storytellers. Pain is a biochemical event, as well as an expression of who we are and who we have been. How we define pain also shifts according to the dominant ideas of the time—as I would find out when I went back in history to find some earlier answers to my original question: When we're in pain, where do we go?

1

A MICROHISTORY OF PAIN

I have given a name to my pain, and call it "dog."

FRIEDRICH NIETZSCHE, *The Gay Science*

PAIN IS THE SASQUATCH OF SCIENCE, NEVER witnessed, only endlessly speculated on. We can't even agree on the species. Man or beast? A sensation or an idea? It doesn't help that *ideas* about the meanings of pain are double-barreled abstractions that soon drift away from the experience itself into an epistemological fog.

Our efforts to describe pain soon confront us with another small problem: How do we define the self? What particular nexus of mind, body, and soul is this modern "I" who feels the strange brew of modern pain?

I've been ruthlessly selective in this chapter, skipping over many names and entire centuries, to avoid disappearing down philosophical cul-de-sacs. But as I began to investigate the earliest ideas of pain, what struck me was that philosophy, medicine, and drama were once much closer in the way they viewed pain. It wasn't until Descartes came along in the seventeenth century with "proof" of the mind-body split, followed by the age of Enlightenment, that pain began to shed its emotional and social dimensions. One of the earliest definitions of tragedy, for instance, was human pain—as our exile into something that can be witnessed and pitied, but never shared.

Philoctetes, a play written by Sophocles in 409 B.C., is a story that pivots around the physical pain of its main character, who suffers from a wound that began as a snake bite. "Terrible it is, beyond words' reach" is how Philoctetes describes his condition. This inviolate, unspeakable aspect of human pain is what the drama tries to voice. "*Philoctetes* makes us feel the power of pain to reduce a life to utter emptiness and misery," author David Morris writes in *The Culture of Pain.* "It unweaves the self until the self is nothing but pain. The body in tragedy is not just something we possess like an identifying birthmark or robe or kingdom," Morris argues, "but what we *are.* It both defines us, and, fatally, limits us."

Aristotle was another astute observer of human dramas, including pain, and his writings on the subject turn out to have a rather modern flair. He defined pain as an emotion rather than a mechanical sensation. He characterized both pain and pleasure as "appetites" that drive us toward the objects of our desires and away from the things that hurt us. For Aristotle, pain was not only a sensory event in the body, but a subjective state, like longing and fear. He saw the human cost of pain, how it "upsets and destroys the nature of the person who feels it." Aristotle may not have understood physiology, but he accepted the idea that pain is an expression of who we are.

Our uncertainty about the province of pain is conveyed by the roots of the words we use for it. *Pain* is probably derived from the Latin word *poena,* meaning punishment, and the English word tends to connote physical pain. But the French word *douleur,* from the Latin *dolor,* refers to both physical and mental pain. The French word *peine* suggests punishment, but it can mean sorrow as well. Oddly enough, the Italian language has no word for *ache,* despite the fact that studies of pain expression in different cultures report that Italian women in labor are louder than women from other countries.

The concept of pain as punishment turns up most vividly in the biblical story of Job, a wealthy, upright man whose faith in God is tested by Satan in a series of terrible afflictions. First he loses his wealth, then he becomes an outcast from his community. Finally Satan pulls out all the stops and inflicts a "plague of boils" on Job. "He slashes open my kidneys and does not spare," says Job, describing Satan's work. "He pours out my gall on the ground." William Blake's illustration of this scene shows the figure of Job writhing on the ground, his hands arched back in pain, as a naked, burly Satan stands over him like a TV wrestler in triumph. Job's test of faith is the first example of the theme of bloody martyrdom that runs throughout Christianity. Pain is inseparable from faith and "the central Christian mystery of a being who suffers pain in order to redeem others," as Morris writes. It was the pain that Jesus Christ suffered on the cross that proved to us that God's son was human, too. Suffering pain is how faith is forged; transcending pain is a mark of sainthood. The image of St. Sebastian pierced with arrows, with upturned eyes, carries the message that a belief in a life beyond the body has the power to undo pain. The idea of pain as spiritual punishment is still deeply entrenched in our attitude that physical pain arrives as a kind of moral test of character and should be toughed out. The price of admission for being human, the story of Job reminds us, is this: Expect boils.

Fast-forward to the Middle Ages, a time when it was hell to have a toothache, even though laudanum, a preparation of opium, was readily dispensed. One of the opiophiles of the era was the enlightened sixteenth-century practitioner Paracelsus. He was the original patient-centered physician. "Every physician must be rich in knowledge," he wrote in *Man and His Body*, "and not only of that which is written in books; his patients should be his book, they will never mislead him . . . and by them he will never be deceived. But he who is content with mere letters is like a dead man; and he is like a dead physician." We may be overdue for a Paracelsus revival.

The man most responsible for our modern misconception of "mental pain" versus "physical pain," however, was the seventeenth-century philosopher and scientist René Descartes. Although he is often blamed for the mind-body split that came to characterize Western thinking, in other ways, Descartes's investigation into pain was farsighted. In the treatise *De l'homme,* his hypothesis about pain pathways and the "delicate threads" that conduct pain signals, for instance, turned out to be a crude but correct notion of nerve fibers and neurotransmitters. But it was his theory of the transmission of pain signals that led to what is known as the "specificity theory" of pain—the notion of pain as one fixed pathway or center. This idea dominated the study of pain until the last thirty or forty years.

Descartes's theory was accompanied by a famous illustration of a rather hunchbacked naked man, eyes a-bulge, who appears to be stepping into a campfire. His foot is in the flame. "If for example fire comes near the foot," he wrote in 1640, "minute particles of this fire, which you know move at great velocity, have the power to set in motion the spot of skin on the foot which they touch, and by this means pulling on the delicate thread which is attached to the spot of the skin, they open up at the same instant the pore against which the delicate thread ends, just as by pulling on one end of a rope one makes to strike at the same instant a bell which hangs at the end."

Descartes has helpfully labeled the diagram. The sensation of pain (A) is perceived in the foot and then travels up to the "common sense center" (F) in the pineal gland, which interprets the signal as pain. This same stimulus-response model still defines our popular understanding of pain: The coffee table hits your toe, a sensation in the nerves then tugs at the bell-rope of the brain, which interprets this event as pain. No coffee table, no pain. But even in his time, Descartes had to defend this theory against critics. When it was pointed out to him that some amputees still feel pain in their missing limbs—phantom limb pain—he nimbly responded that the brain was just being tricked by false signals. But he still characterized the mind as a passive central switchboard instead of as a coauthor of pain.

In Descartes's mechanistic view, pain is something that happens to the body, a sensation which is then promoted to the status of a concept in the brain. A worker-CEO arrangement, you could say, except that the goods flow only one way. Although the brain is the boss, it is a passive decoder, and pain only runs along one track, with its own special apparatus, impervious to emotions or environmental factors.

After Descartes, the race for pain's Northwest Passage—the path it takes in the body—was under way, and for the next three hundred years science pursued this mysterious trail. Pain began to lose its multiple meanings, as a visionary experience in religion, or as an expressive element of tragedy. Instead, pain became the property of science and medicine, even though they didn't quite know what to make of it. The focus shifted from exploring the questions of identity, consciousness, and grace that pain raises to describing its mechanisms in the body and brain. The pharmaceutical age began near the end of the nineteenth century. Cutting pain out of the body, cutting nerves, and killing pain became the new goals.

A time line of some of the landmarks of pain science and treatment over the past two centuries might look like this:

1803	Morphine is synthesized from opium
1846	The discovery of anesthesia
1853	The invention of the hypodermic needle
1853	Acetylsalicylic acid, predecessor to aspirin, is developed
1914	The Harrison Act in the United States sets restrictions on narcotic drugs
1943	*Pain Mechanisms* published by William Livingston
1946	Henry Beecher's work on the power of the placebo
1965	The gate-control theory of pain published by Melzack and Wall in the journal *Science*
1965	First multidisciplinary pain clinic
1966	The first hospice, St. Christopher's, opens in the United Kingdom
1973	International Association for the Study of Pain holds its first congress
1975	The McGill Pain Questionnaire (first measurement of pain intensity)

1976	Discovery of endorphins
1986	The World Health Organization publishes *The Analgesic Ladder: Guidelines to Cancer Pain Relief*
1995	The American Pain Society endorses the designation of pain as "the fifth vital sign"
2000	The U.S. Congress declares the next ten years the "Decade of Pain Control and Research"

The distinction between "mental pain" and "physical pain" has led to a punishing skepticism about "real" pain versus "invented" pain. The specificity theory describes pain as an event in the periphery of the body that is open to interpretation, and distortion, by the mind; pain that couldn't be connected to an injury or some sort of organic cause was "psychological" and therefore suspect. This theory doesn't account for why one person can be more sensitive to pain than another, and it led to the belief that the intensity of pain is always in direct proportion to the intensity of the stimulus. But the lightest breath of air on the skin can cause severe pain for someone suffering the neuropathic pain known as reflex sympathetic dystrophy (RSD). Long after recovery from an injury, people with RSD can suffer chronic pain, to the exasperation of their doctors. The specificity theory made it possible to blame people for their own pain. Descartes could be called the father of malingering.

We now know that even the pain of a minor accident can sensitize the central nervous system in some people, as if the "on" switch for pain works, but the "off" switch is broken. People with phantom limb pain can suffer vivid, detailed pain in a hand or leg that no longer exists. Descartes was right about the fact that nerves in the periphery of the body carry signals to the brain, but what science has discovered since then is that the spinal cord and central nervous system play major roles in pain perception. Descending messages from the brain can block or modify the sensory information coming in. As pain researchers Ron Melzack and Patrick Wall would demonstrate, pain is the result of a complex feedback loop.

Above all, pain is in the brain—not Descartes's passive, traffic-cop model, but one in which pain lights up multiple areas at once, a fluid, dynamic event responding to information from the senses at the same time that it alters and shapes that response. The brain doesn't just react to the foot in the flame. The body and the mind create a neural narrative together.

As neuroscience maps the brain in more detail, the gap between mind and body begins to narrow and to show itself for what it is—a false construct. The body begins to look much smarter and more soulful (flesh as "spirit thickened," as surgeon and author Richard Selzer has written) at the same time that the mind incarnates itself, as a biochemical event. Descartes's "bell" now includes not just skin, nerves, and sensation, but also memory, thoughts, and feelings.

In the nineteenth century, Silas Weir Mitchell, the father of neurology, collected case studies of nerve injuries in soldiers with gunshot wounds. His description of the mysterious burning pain of "causalgia" was part of the gradual shift away from this equation of injury to pain. What Mitchell described was a very real agony that had no obvious connection to tissue damage at all. Mitchell (to whom I will return later) also had some curious notions about women, hysteria, and pain, but he was an outstanding example of a departed nineteenth-century figure—a doctor who published both fiction and poetry, who worked both in the field and in the lab. Mitchell understood the relationship between pain, personal history and environment fifty years before the rest of science.

In the middle of the nineteenth century, the invention of anesthesia brought a measure of control over pain and enabled surgeons to do more complicated, lifesaving operations. We began to live longer as a result. Before anesthesia, surgery was a horrific cut-and-grab procedure that was performed as fast as possible by barbers. Anesthesiologists have been in the forefront of pain studies ever since. (The International Association for the Study of Pain, an organization of professionals in the pain field, was founded in 1973 by an anesthetist, John Bonica.) But the arrival of anesthesia also put the focus on erasing pain rather than exploring its role in health and disease. Anesthesiology doesn't target pain; it puts the patient in a twilight state—a kind of mock death, actually, with machines taking over the patient's vital functions. This demonstrates one of the most obvious qualities of pain: It requires a consciousness to feel it. What the unconscious patient feels as the knife cuts into him is unknown, but it's not what we call pain.

The idea of being "put to sleep" was greeted with some suspicion at first. Despite the fact that Queen Victoria gave birth to two of her children under the painkilling influence of ether, there was a cadre of obstetricians who violently opposed its use in labor. Pain was considered a necessary and natural part of giving birth, not to mention part of Eve's punishment for disobeying God.

The idea of pain as a fixed, mechanical system in the body began to give way to the modern view of pain as an individual subjective experience around the middle of last century. This is when pain became a separate field of study, instead of being pushed to the margins of medicine as an annoying but non-life-threatening symptom. Now, many scientists consider pain a disease in itself, one that can rob a person of sleep and energy, undermine the immune system, and reorganize the central nervous system. To ignore pain, as a doctor or a patient, can have serious health consequences.

The medicalization of pain has its upside and its downside, however. Calling pain a disease helps give it status and visibility in our pathology-smitten culture, but it separates pain from the social, economic, and political aspects that shape our experience of pain as well. And it can bring out the lurking Descartes in pain researchers, too. For instance, studies on the imaging of "pain cells" in the brain are thriving, even though they may be more futile attempts to locate the ever-elusive "pain center."

In fact, the increase in chronic pain has been partly the result of science's brilliant accomplishments in other areas, eliminating such scourges as smallpox and polio. Scientific progress has also extended the lives of people with some forms of cancer. As a result, we've been granted the privilege of longer lives—which has increased the number of people living with the pain of arthritis, osteoporosis, and assorted cancers. Now science has to address suffering itself, and this is beginning to happen. Medicine is slowly turning from a focus on crisis-management, disease and cure, to include wellness, prevention, and palliative care. These two developments have exposed more doctors to people in different kinds of pain—an education currently overlooked in medical schools. But faced with pain they can't fix, doctors understandably become frustrated or burned out. GPs don't want to be bothered with chronic pain patients. Treating them takes time, and the financial rewards are slim compared with specializing in something else—say, cosmetic surgery. The pain field tends to attract the mavericks who crave intellectual challenge and don't mind sacrificing the money and status that go along with hotter fields.

Some of these pioneers (whom I write about in detail later in the book) include William Livingston, a Seattle surgeon who challenged the fixed-pathway notion of pain and wrote about it—personally and engagingly—as an "evolving idea" instead; Cecily Saunders, the English founder of the hospice movement, a brilliant polymath, and the first to institute the regular giving of morphine to help the suffering of the terminally ill; Dr. Kathleen Foley, former director of pain services at Memorial Sloan-Kettering Cancer Center in New York City, who has taken forward Saunders's philosophy of palliative care; and the two scientists who forever changed the way science understood pain, Ronald Melzack and Patrick Wall.

Patrick Wall was an Oxford-trained physiologist, an expert in the spinal cord, and a provocative mix—a pure scientist who was nevertheless attuned to the social and political aspects of pain. Melzack, the product of a Jewish family in Montreal, now professor emeritus in the psychology department of McGill University, is an expert in pain and pain perception in animals and humans with an interest in language as well. These two gifted scientists met up in the 1950s and put their two areas of expertise together to arrive at a new theory of how pain works. It was the beginning of the end of the Cartesian view of pain.

Basically, Melzack and Wall took the focus off the pain source and put it on the brain and the central nervous system instead. According to their theory, pain arrives in two sorts of volleys, via two different kinds of nerve fibers. The immediate, sharp sort of pain, when you twist an ankle, travels along particular nerves known as A fibers, zipping up to the brain quickly and directly. If you burn your hand on a hot stove, you instantly snatch it away without mulling over the decision. But when that first acute pain fades, another, slower pain—burning, aching, or throbbing—sets in, traveling along slow-conducting C fibers to enter a butterfly-shaped region of the spinal cord known as the dorsal horn. This is where the "gate controls" come in. Triggered by cell changes launched by these C fibers, the brain sends descending messages that alter the sensory input, turning the volume of pain up or down. Pain isn't pain until it reaches the brain.

The simplest demonstration of the gate-control theory is this: When I run into the rowing machine in the middle of the night, I curse, hop around, and rub the place that hurts. The extra stimulus of rubbing then interrupts the pain signal. Fear and anxiety, on the other hand, can make the pain more intense. In other words, pain is a highly negotiable, variable, individual experience.

This view of pain helped make sense of such mysterious conditions as phantom limb pain. It also broke down the old stimuli-to-sensation equation. As Melzack put it, "You don't need a body to feel pain." And by making our feelings, attitudes, and memory part of the perception of pain, the gate-control theory also factors in culture—or at least culture as defined as "higher cortical activity."

The new field of pain really began to open up in the 1960s and '70s. In 1965, the same year that Melzack and Wall published their new theory, the Washington anesthestist John Bonica organized the first multidisciplinary pain clinic. He saw that specialization in medicine had resulted in a tragic oversight: No one was addressing the central problem of suffering in patients. Bonica also founded the International Association for the Study of Pain, which held its first international symposium in 1973, at Issaquah, Washington. Along with other groups like the American Pain Society, the IASP, with more than seven thousand members around the world, has been crucial in raising pain awareness and fostering new research. One of the first things the IASP addressed was the fact that no one could agree on what pain means. In 1977, a committee headed by Dr. Harold Merskey, a London, Ontario, psychiatrist and pain specialist, developed a definition that has gained wide acceptance: Pain is "an unpleasant sensory and emotional experience associated with actual or potential tissue damage, or described in terms of such damage." (The IASP is now working on an addendum to avoid the possible suggestion that patients who can't articulate their pain—babies, or people with dementia, for instance—don't suffer pain.)

But even if you can scientifically define pain, how do you measure it? In 1975, Ronald Melzack published the McGill Pain Questionnaire, a list of seventy-eight descriptive words and a zero-to-five pain-intensity scale. The MPQ is now used worldwide for measuring pain. The mid-1970s were also when scientists explored the role of endorphins, the body's own painkilling resources, and the placebo effect. The focus was shifting from surgery and anesthesia to a deeper understanding of pain processes and how the body heals itself.

Medicine now distinguishes between two sorts of pain. Acute pain is the kind you feel after surgery or when you break a leg. It tends to be immediate, severe, and short-lived. Pain that extends beyond the normal recovery time, is cyclical, like migraine, or lasts longer than six months is called chronic. This includes lower back pain, fibromyalgia, arthritis, diabetic neuropathy, and phantom limb pain, to name just a few. Neuropathic pain, such as the kind associated with a phantom limb, is related to damaged nerves. This affects the central nervous system and can be the most difficult pain of all to diagnose and treat.

But pain is not just about the body. Pain is something we also share in reaction to catastrophic events, such as the terrorist attacks on the United States that took place on September 11, 2001. The loss of lives involved and the unerasable imagery carried by the media had a profound and visceral effect that is still being felt. North America's nervous system changed overnight. The devastation unleashed a twenty-first-century sort of psychic pain, for which there is no simple treatment.

Among the volunteers who arrived on the scene in the ruins of lower Manhattan was Stan Mattox, a thirty-four-year-old carpenter who lost five friends in the collapse of the World Trade Center. A reporter spoke to him. "This thing hurts," Mr. Mattox said as he helped clear the wreckage, "it hurts really bad."

A new wound has been invented.

NOW THE DECADE DEVOTED to pain control and research has just begun. Perhaps we will discover as much about pain in the next ten years as we have learned about the brain in the past decade. There are hopeful signs already. For the terminally ill and for cancer patients, pain management has become more enlightened. Drugs for arthritis have improved. Integrative medicine is drawing on the wisdom of Chinese medicine and other older approaches to suffering. But for the millions who live with chronic pain, there is still a gap between what science understands about pain and the way doctors treat it. "We know a lot more now, but we're not using what we know" is how one physician summed it up at the Ninth World Congress of Pain Studies in 1998.

The future of pain science is moving in the same direction as other fields—toward molecular biology and genetics. Genetic research has already discovered that a predisposition to some pain conditions, such as migraine or fibromyalgia, can be inherited and that each person has a unique response to pain. It turns out that we are fossils of ourselves, inscribed with our own history. Pain may be bred in the bone, too.

2

MAJOR HEADACHES

PAIN LACKS A PERFECT HISTORY, HOWEVER, because we love, *love,* to forget it. Conjuring up a bout of physical misery is like trying to describe what it felt like to be a baby before language. The only thing that can convey the nature of pain is the story that grows up around it, like a tree trunk or a scar.

My first migraine took hold in my late twenties and was easily the most painful thing I had ever experienced. I was on a long cycling expedition in South America with my boyfriend. He was riding his bicycle from Ottawa to Peru, an insane agenda that took him about two and a half years. He hooked up with a National Geographic expedition that was on its way from Alaska to Tierra del Fuego, and I joined them for the loop through southern Mexico and Guatemala. Then Tom and I headed into South America on our own for three more months.

The Pan-American Highway in Ecuador often devolves to a cow path, and the road to Baños, east of Quito, was particularly rough. On the map it appeared to be an appealing downhill switchback, which would land us in a town famous for its mineral springs. I was looking forward to immersing my tired biker's body in hot sulfurous baths.

One morning, we began our descent. The road, such as it was, was under construction. There was a steady, hot head wind that carried the dust and sand into our faces from the unpaved road and from the roadwork going on ahead of us. The ride turned out to be one daylong sandblasting, coating our teeth, filling our eyebrows, and needling our skin. Tom took a picture of me on this descent. I'm wearing the red wool poncho I bought in Otavalo, my bike is bungeed about with gear and bags, and I'm zooming down an empty mountain road. What the picture doesn't reveal is the fist of pain behind my right eye. Triggered by the steady needling sensation of the sand on the skin, it's one of twenty-one kinds of head pain distinguished by the National Headache Foundation, and it's known as a "wind in the face" migraine.

By the time we reached Baños and had found a room in a cheap hotel, the pain in my face and head was so bad I thought I had some exotic form of meningitis. I had never experienced a migraine before. All I knew was that I couldn't bear being touched, and Tom had to hang blankets over the windows. Light was excruciating, and even having my pillows adjusted was unbearable. Every movement caused waves of nausea. My long-suffering partner went out to find a *farmacia* that was still open. If I had known what it was, I would have just gone into hibernation and waited it out, something I learned to do in later years. But as far as I was concerned, I was dying of brain fever in a small town on the edge of the Amazon jungle.

The migraine lasted three days. Tom nursed me and cooked soup on our tiny camp stove, on our tiny balcony. Bit by bit, my eyeballs agreed to entertain daylight again. The curtains were opened. Years later, I read about how certain factors—wind on the face being only one of many—can help unleash the vascular mayhem and whole-body nausea of a migraine. The condition affects three times as many women as men; 18 percent of women get migraines, compared with 6 percent of men—25 million "migraineurs" in the United States. Children get them, too. Migraines tend to peak in the thirties and forties, and then taper off. There are even some forms of "abdominal" migraines, various forms of digestive misery, that don't involve pain in the head at all. Not all scientists subscribe to the trigger theory, but the Baños experience left me forever leery of head winds. Whenever I'm in a canoe, a steady wind in the face will spook me like a horse that smells smoke in the barn.

The word *migraine* is a corruption of "hemicranial," or "half the head," because the headaches tend to affect one side or the other, near the front. They aren't especially connected to muscular tension, which usually affects the back of the neck. (Hypochondriacs, please note: Brain tumors usually cause pain that radiates to the top of the head.) The pain used to be blamed on dilating and constricting blood vessels, but it doesn't start there. Nobody is sure how migraines originate, but it seems to have something to do with the hormone serotonin and how it affects receptors on the trigeminal nerve that runs up the neck and the side of the head. When something—a food allergy, a stressful event, a strobing light—alters serotonin production in the brain, the arteries in the neck and head first constrict. Then, in a response to this blood starvation, the arteries rapidly expand, which causes the unbearable sense of pulsing pressure that characterizes a migraine. The slightest movement, even pounding of the heart, can set off a sickening throb. Once a migraine locks in, all you want to do is shut yourself away and lie low, like the sick animal you are.

Hormones definitely play a role, and the "menstrual migraine" is one well-known variation; this mercifully tapers off in women after menopause. (Men, however, can boast of the excruciating agony of cluster headaches, another form of headache that tends to afflict older males and lasts for days.) Triggers that are sometimes blamed for bringing on migraine include everything from red wine, aged cheese, chocolate, citrus, and beans to sudden shifts in barometric pressure, a change in sleep patterns, and a down period after stress ("the weekend migraine"). Other researchers claim that environmental triggers are irrelevant, and that migraines originate with a "wave of activity" from the brain stem. (What are we to make of a "wave of activity"?)

Even if we don't know what causes it, the consequences are very clear. Migraines make you put your life under a microscope in order to understand what might contribute to them. The first thing every sufferer learns is that unless you treat the pain early, you're in for the whole ride. Once a migraine locks in, it's very hard to catch up to it with analgesics, no matter how strong they are. Lots of migraine sufferers simply do what I did and take to their beds, with the blinds closed and a basin handy.

There is an upside, however—when it stops. The first hour or two after a migraine recedes is a unique form of bliss. The world seems unusually present, and the senses feel refreshed. Things have a halo of newness. A migraine can even act as a sort of spiritual Drano, providing an opportunity to retreat from the world and get a little psychic housecleaning done.

When that first headache lifted, I tottered out of our hotel and went to the baths, which turned out to be an old quarry of stone vaults, streaked with livid mineral deposits. We soaked in the hot springs. Then we packed up and pedaled on. By the time we reached the Atacama Desert in northern Peru, I was ready to throw in the towel. The Atacama is more than a thousand miles long, and I was really, really tired of the sun and the sand. We ended up tying our bikes on top of a local *colectivo,* a shared taxi, for the seven-hundred-mile trip to Peru. It was the best and longest cab ride of my life.

After I came back home, migraines became a fact of my life. One comforting aspect about migraines is this: They go up, peak, and then recede. On the way up, it's excruciating. But when the turnaround point comes, you know it's just a matter of time before you can once again rejoin the human race. Since there's no fighting a migraine, you learn to treat it as a grace period of sorts. Biologically speaking, they may even play a protective role, forcing the migraineur to retreat and recoup in the face of too much stress.

I've learned that I'm more likely to develop a headache coming off a deadline than going into one. They strike whenever I begin to relax (which tends to make them rare). Sometimes I get the classic premigraine auras, which in my case is a pixilated disk of light that dances in my vision after I've been in strong sunlight or stared too long into the computer screen.

But when the migraines lift, you feel so great! The world sparkles, and you feel returned to yourself in a such a lucid way. I often wonder if the body's natural painkillers go into overdrive when you have a migraine—then, as the headache recedes, you're left with a swarming surplus of endorphins, which delivers the post-migraine high.

I have one particular sensitivity. Just as strobe lights can cause an epileptic seizure in some people, they can bring on a migraine in me in a matter of seconds. I've missed every disco scene ever filmed, because when the strobe light starts going in a movie I have to cover my eyes. My family is also used to the sight of me wearing my hat over my face in the car whenever we drive through the countryside late in the afternoon—the sunlight flashing through the trees flips the migraine switch, too. Sometimes I will walk into a room and feel uneasy without knowing why. Then I look up and see an overhead fan turning; the light and dark intervals in the corner of my vision are enough to give me premigraine angst. Jet lag—light when there should be darkness—will do it as well. I seem to need a steady diet of darkness.

Over the years I've learned to control my migraines, for the most part. In fact, they were my first lessons in this business of working with the body instead of against it. I realized I didn't have to give in and endure them, for starters. The best defense against the pain of a migraine is to recognize the warning signs early enough to take a big whacking dose of painkillers—one doctor learned that a gram of acetaminophen at the earliest possible hint would ward off his migraines. A gram is a lot. Some people feel they should fight the pain as long as possible before giving in and taking medication. But once the migraine blooms, you're sunk.

There are various medications that help. The ergot drugs, such as Migranal, constrict the blood vessels, and in the last decade, a class of drugs known as triptans has become popular in the treatment of migraines. (Imitrex is the best known of this category; Zomig is another.) And they do help. But they are expensive and come with hefty side effects that can be dangerous for people with heart trouble or vascular disease. Sumatriptan will, however, arrest a migraine in midcourse, whereas ordinary analgesics won't.

My coping strategy has always been to stop whatever was setting the scene for the headache in the first place—which could be anything from going too long between meals, to weird sleep patterns, to overwork. Then I would take an Advil or extra-strength Tylenol and retreat, ideally to bed, with a bag of frozen peas on the back of my head, or into a hot bath laced with chamomile oil. My theory was that I had to get the blood out of my head and back down into my body where it belonged. I would "think" my hands warm. This kindergarten biofeedback technique worked remarkably well—as long as I had immediate access to chamomile, a bath, and frozen peas.

The most important rule, in my experience, is to "honor thy migraine." Be alert to its earliest symptoms and attend to them humbly. (The descent into pain, and our struggle to deny it, is perfectly described in Virginia Woolf's novel *The Voyage Out,* in which the heroine suffers from terrible headaches.) Pain in the head arrives as a more dreadful, intimate sort of misery than the pain of a broken toe or a wrenched knee. And according to the diligent scientists who like to arrange pain on a scale of intensity from merely annoying to soul-scalding, one of the worst pains anyone can experience is another kind of pain in the head—tic douloureux, or more commonly, trigeminal neuralgia.

TERESA STEPHENS IS AN elementary school teacher, with two small children at home. Like many people who live with chronic pain, she's become something of an expert on her version of it, trigeminal neuralgia (TN). "I've read a lot about it, and been in touch with the Trigeminal Neuralgia Association in New Jersey," she told me. "Apparently four percent of people who suffer trigeminal pain have ophthalmic pain, which is what I have. It affects both my eyes, which is rare—usually, it's only one side. It's not a headache, but shooting pains and a tightening in my head—it's as if all my nerves are being pulled tight and stretched."

Although it affects the fifth cranial nerve that runs up the side of the face, nobody knows what causes TN. The pain leaves no tracks. It strikes sporadically and can be triggered by the mildest things—brushing the teeth, even putting on blusher. Sometimes surgery will temporarily relieve compressed nerves—but in most cases the pain will come back. The fact that anticonvulsive drugs like Tegretol sometimes help suggests that TN has more to do with the brain stem than nerve fibers in the face—but nobody knows for sure. People who have it look fine. They just have this blinding, inexplicable pain.

As somebody who teaches all day and comes home to a family, stress must surely affect it, I said.

"Actually, with stress the pain seems to disappear," Teresa said. "That's why I try to keep myself busy. I used to be quite an introspective person—I used to love to be alone and read. But now I must go out, I have to see people. I take ballroom dancing, I keep busy. Otherwise, the pain would drive me crazy."

Trigeminal neuralgia causes periods of intense, electric-shock-like pain, which one woman with TN referred to as a "frying sensation." The pain is usually on one side, where the three main branches of this nerve fan out around the lips, nose, eyes, forehead, and jaw. Tic douloureux, as it was originally known, was a term coined by an eighteenth-century surgeon, Nicolaus Andre, although the condition has been around for centuries. It is described as a "lancinating" sensation, a series of white-hot, dentist-drill jolts often compared to lightning in the head. (The logo of the Trigeminal Neuralgia Association is a face in profile, with a very impressive lightning bolt stabbing away in the cheek and jaw.) It affects more women than men, by a ratio of two to one. It usually sets in after fifty, and like migraine, it may be related to hormonal fluctuations. Sometimes it causes pressure on the nerve from blood vessels, in which case surgery can offer relief. Antidepressants can help the depression that often accompanies something as unpredictable and inexplicable as TN; drugs like Elavil and Effexor also raise the serotonin level, which directly influences pain perception.

The ferocity of TN pain sets up a special kind of dread about when it will strike next. Smiling can bring it on. Nobody dies from trigeminal neuralgia, though. They just suffer unimaginable pain.

When I first talked to Teresa on the phone, I was struck by the vigor of her voice—not the wan tone of someone in constant pain. It's as if good copers have figured out how to be as big a presence— or bigger—than their pain. "Before I knew what this was," said Teresa, "I was an emotional wreck. I thought it was a brain tumor. I went to a neurologist and got a CAT scan, but it showed nothing. They thought it might also be the beginning of MS, which frightened me. Finally, the neurologist told me it was trigeminal neuralgia, and that nobody knows what causes it, or how to treat it. They keep talking about an operation that wraps a piece of Teflon around the nerve, but that's not for me! I don't even like taking painkillers, and I certainly didn't want to delve into brain surgery.

"Instead, I go to a psychologist, who has helped me learn to live with the pain. The mind plays such an important part. But the pain has changed my whole way of thinking, and who I am. I used to plan a lot, but now I don't think about the future. I just try to live in the present. I try not to think too much."

She laughed. "And I'm trying to be frivolous, to just have fun. I have to be distracted."

I asked her to describe the sort of pain she had. "At times it's like an electric shock, like a storm on one side. It feels as if someone is pulling on the top of my scalp. Sometimes in the shower, if I hold my hand over my head, I can feel something like an electrical current. It's wild.

"It can be excruciating; other times it's just there, a constant, daily pain. I've had it for more than a year now, and lately it's been getting better. Maybe it's because of the homeopathic treatments I'm getting. Or maybe it's just resolving in time, I don't know.

"I have been very, very depressed with it, but I'm okay now.

The doctors and psychologists I saw at first were not helpful, since they assumed it was all in my head." Another half-laugh, since that is true, technically. "I also fit the so-called trigeminal profile: I get upset easily, and I'm a controller. But the person who helped me the most was a social worker, someone a friend put me in touch with. She taught me some self-hypnosis strategies. And I've learned to think of the pain differently—there's a certain pain that I get on one side that I love! It's a nice pain, and I love to touch my head when I have it. You simply have to make friends with the pain, otherwise you're resisting, and you'll go crazy with it.

"Now I can function. I know this is as good as it's going to get. As long as I stop thinking about when the pain will go away, I'm all right."

I asked her if religious faith was a factor in handling it. "I'm Catholic, and yes, I do say prayers to my friends, and novenas to St. Jude, the patron saint of hopeless cases—which includes me. I keep a daily journal of how I feel, and a scale of its intensity. It all helps. But I see no pattern about why or when the pain comes—sometimes eye movements will make it worse, but really, I can't put my finger on why it happens. It's unpredictable.

"It runs in the family, too. My mother has it, although she hates going to doctors. When I got mine, she said, 'Ignore it, learn to live with it.' Hah, I thought. Some people think pain is given to you to make you grow. But honestly, I don't need any more character, I have enough!"

Microvascular decompression, a surgical procedure, does often work for TN. But as many as 40 percent of patients will mysteriously end up with a recurrence of the pain over the next decade. Anticonvulsive drugs like carbamazepine can quiet it, too, but they're hard on the liver. The problem with chronic pain like TN is that even when it begins as something mechanical, it can transform itself into what is called "central pain"—pain that originates and is controlled in the central nervous system. It's not about cutting nerves or fooling around with the periphery of the body any longer. It's pain that has taken root.

"I have dark days," Teresa said. "There are times when all I do is think about this pain, this pain, this pain. But I've learned that suffering doesn't necessarily eliminate joy. You can go on living, even with the pain. And I do. I used to think I couldn't bear one more day of this. Now I think, What's a year?"

3

CATCHING PAIN

READING THE MCGILL PAIN QUESTIONNAIRE (MPQ), which measures pain intensity, is a bit like reading a novel with the plot neatly filleted out: "flickering, quivering, pulsing, throbbing, beating, pounding, jumping, flashing," and so on, down through "nauseating" and "dreadful," to "wretched" and "blinding." The words leap out of any medical texts where they appear like a flash of humanity.

A pain scale like the MPQ helps make pain visible. But ranking pain conditions in terms of their dreadfulness is rather pointless, since each person's response is different. Pain is relative. Most specialists would agree, though, that the pain conditions listed below, in no special order, would make most top ten lists.

> Childbirth (unmedicated)
> Burn pain and the process of
>   debridement (removing
>   dead skin)
> Shingles

Cancer pain (bone pain in particular)
Cluster headaches and trigeminal neuralgia
Kidney stones
Rheumatoid arthritis
Migraine
Depression
Fibromyalgia

Depression isn't normally included in a list like this. But the psychic pain of depression is a form of suffering that can be as chronic, debilitating, and soul-devouring as the worst sort of bodily pain. Depression often accompanies chronic pain, in part because chronic pain can make life restricted and joyless. But there is a deeper intimacy between pain and depression that is demonstrated by the fact that antidepressants will sometimes act as a pain reliever, even when there is no mood disorder involved. Many experts believe that chronic pain ends up affecting not just mood but memory and concentration as well. It also leaves a stain on everyone who lives with or comes into regular contact with someone who copes with chronic pain. There is a contagious quality to pain—even to thinking too much about it—which I discovered when I took myself off to the library again. I wanted to learn more about shingles.

It was pretty vivid reading. By now I had been immersed in pain stories for a number of months. My friends were also beginning to tell me all about their trick backs and erupting cysts and hammertoes. I was browsing through photos of people with great red swaths of shingle blisters on their torsos, when I idly scratched my arm. Scratched again, and looked down. An odd, pea-shaped little . . . blister had risen on my skin. It began to tingle. Could I have caught shingles from reading? Could I be that suggestible, that porous? It seems I could.

To be a candidate for shingles, I read, you must have had chicken pox (check). The same virus that causes chicken pox, the varicella zoster virus, can remain alive but dormant in the nerve ganglia of the spine, and then leap out and become active again during some temporary dip in immunity. This usually happens after the age of fifty (check), and your chances of suffering shingles increase with age. It begins with a tingling or itching (!) on one side of the body, often on the back or on the skin over the ribs, but it can occur anywhere, including the head. This prodrome period, similar to the kind that comes with herpes simplex viruses, is followed by a rash of little blisters, not unlike Job's boils: painful, pea-shaped, with a "tense surface teeming with the virus." Charming! This stage lasts a few weeks or a month. The blisters eventually erupt, and sometimes that's all it amounts to. But others are in for the really unpleasant part—the nasty pain of postherpetic neuralgia, as shingles is also known.

Shingles is a virus that follows the nerve pathways like a line of fire, leaving damaged, vulnerable nerves. Postherpetic pain can last for months or up to a year. It can vary from a patch of vague sensitivity on the skin or a mild burning sensation to the worst sort of agony, where the touch of a sheet on the skin is intolerable. Nerve pain is an exasperating affliction—especially since it doesn't come with a body cast to announce it.

The condition can be treated or at least muted, but you have to catch it early and treat it with antiviral agents like acyclovir. Some people also use topical creams with capsaicin, too, which contain a natural pepperlike substance that depletes a certain chemical (substance P) involved in pain transmission.

Now officially a Person with Shingles, I left the library, bought flowers, and had a chocolate bar. Why, I thought, was I not writing the history of Belgian chocolate instead? My miniature, free-sample, library-induced case of shingles eventually amounted to two blisters, one on my arm, another on my ribs. They lasted a week, followed by a few days of flulike aches and that weird skin sensitivity down one side. I could feel the nerve path, like a frayed cord, from shoulder to hand. Then it vanished.

Psychosomatic? But of course. I include this as my little scrap of evidence concerning the power of imagery and the imagination to alter the immune system. Pain is contagious. Who knows what lurks in the ganglia of the spine, waiting for the wrong paragraph to come along. Do not read books on shingles, unless you already have it and need to know more.

FACED WITH SOMEONE suffering, unable to help, it's hard not to flinch or feel the urge to run away. No wonder so many doctors are uneasy in the presence of pain. If they can't fix it, they would prefer to fax it somewhere else. We do the same thing with shocking news in the paper, about children bombed to bits in an Israeli pizzeria. There is a deep need to take in the pain of strangers, to turn it into a story—and then to pass it on. We need to pass it on. Nobody wants to be left holding the hot potato of pain.

Early in my research, I read an essay in the newspaper about the folly of high-speed police chases, which had cost half a dozen lives so far that year. The piece was written by a United Church minister who had been involved in a car accident thirty-seven years ago that was the result of a high-speed police chase. The accident left him in chronic pain from a neck injury and took the life of a young woman. It was a passionate piece with a lot of pain between the lines. I arranged to interview him, not knowing quite what I was in for.

I made my way along the shore of Lake Ontario to a town of twelve thousand souls and five churches. By the time I drove by each of the churches looking for the right one, I was a little late. When I arrived at Trinity United, I sped down several halls, past the choir room, the church office, the neat cloakroom, as memories of Sunday school at my own United Church in Burlington rose up, and found Ken Martin's name on the door of the corner office. I knocked and a dog barked.

A rather bearish, dark-browed man, wearing glasses, rose to greet me. He banished his sheltie collie, Lassie, explaining that the dog is actually one of his pain strategies. "It helps to have to care for the dog and take her out for walks." When he goes on visits to nursing homes, he takes the collie along, too. "She really is a pastoral dog in training," said the Reverend Mr. Martin, who was wearing a tie with a sheltie on it.

Despite his injury, Martin gave the impression of a robust man, with thick, wavy black and white hair. His head seemed screwed tightly onto his body—the result of not one but two serious car accidents that damaged his vertebrae. Arthritic spurs on the disks have made things worse, and the anguish of surviving an accident that claimed someone else's life, a mother of two children, is another incalculable factor.

Martin had made reservations for lunch at a restaurant a few blocks away. The place had brightly painted chairs and a patio with hanging pots of nasturtiums and impatiens. It was all a little more charming than I had anticipated in this Loyalist-stock town with its glum lakeside parkette. I also expected a minister to be more conservative and less adventurous, intellectually and otherwise, than I was discovering Ken Martin to be.

Before he became a minister, Martin earned four degrees, wrote a thesis on "corporate grief," and taught psychology. But what he really likes to do, he said, stiffly swiveling his head my way, is to scuba dive. Anywhere, but preferably in warm water, which eases his pain. Off Cuba, or the Yucatán, near Cozumel. He would like to go to the Grand Caymans next. He has done some serious traveling, up into the Blue Mountains of Jamaica, down into wrecks on the bottom of Lake Huron—often with his son, one of three grown children. His son had just gone off to school in British Columbia, and he missed him. Now he and Beverley, his wife of forty years, live on their own in the country north of Cobourg. As we talked, Martin's talent for creating shapely stories, as in a sermon, came into play.

He told me about a night dive in the ocean off Mexico, how his light failed, and he lost track of the boat above, carrying his son and the others who were diving with them. He was submerged in blackness with no idea whether he was heading up or drifting farther down into an ocean trough.

"Then I remembered that if you hold your bare hand over the air vent, you can feel the bubbles rising—and that way is up," he said. So he slowly ascended, judging his speed. He was wearing a buoyancy jacket that can be inflated into a life preserver, and when he surfaced he broke open an emergency flare. In more darkness he floated on top of the ocean, waiting to be rescued.

The sky was marvelous, he told me. He had never seen the stars like that. A fishing boat responded to the flare, and in hours he was reunited with his shell-shocked son, who had assumed his father was dead. "It was quite a moment when I got back to the boat," he said dryly. I was wondering why he was telling me this, since it didn't seem to bear on pain. But it did make the point that one can come back from a hopeless place.

After lunch we went back to his office, where he asked his secretary not to let any calls through. The two of us sat in a pair of lugubrious pink velour chairs and he told me his pain story. One day in 1961, after a church function in a small southern Ontario town, Martin offered a lift home to a woman with two children and to a second mother with her baby. It was a Sunday evening, on a rural road. They were on their way when a car came speeding toward them in the other lane and struck them. The driver, a teenage boy who had been drinking, was being chased by a police car at a high speed. The mother of the two children, a friend of Martin's, was killed. Everyone else survived.

Our conversation had been light, if not sprightly, but now his face darkened. I asked him to describe the pain in his neck, and he compared it to living with a bad toothache all the time—out of ten "maybe a seven." It had been worse lately, for some reason, he said. He had been trying cortisone treatments at the Sunnybrook Hospital Pain Unit in Toronto, and sometimes the needle itself seemed to bring on a headache. He pointed to his neck, as if gesturing to someone else. "There's something wrong in there."

I didn't need to ask many questions. This was a story he had shaped himself and needed to tell. His anguish was not just physical, but emotional and spiritual. The accident had shaken his faith in God absolutely. As soon as Martin recovered, he left the ministry and spent the next six years "wrestling with demons," unwilling to serve a god who would allow a young mother to die for no reason. He lived in Vancouver and spent a lot of his time walking by the sea, which helped.

Was there a particular moment that turned him back toward the church? Yes, there was. He was in the hospital again, ill with hepatitis. He had had his gallbladder removed, and then had kidney stones—more excruciating pain. Coincidentally, his roommate on the ward was another United Church minister, who tried to help him. "Don't talk to me about God," Martin said and turned his back. But one night, Martin became dangerously ill. His fever spiked, and the nursing staff was overworked. His roommate, gravely sick himself and hooked up to an IV stand, took over. Bathed him to bring down the temperature. Helped him to the bathroom. Cared for him. The next day Martin said, "Now you can talk to me about God."

At this point in the story, Martin's eyes filled with tears. So did mine. Pain was loose in the room. My shoulders were up, my back ached, and I wanted nothing more than to have a cup of tea. But in for a penny, in for a pound, when someone passes on their pain story. He went on to tell me that the roommate became a friend who led him back to the church. Martin became a partner in a congregation, but his spiritual ambivalence remained. He refused to take money for his first year of ministry. At the same time, he was teaching university psychology, which he had assumed would be his new post-theological career. But gradually he allowed his faith to creep back. He decided that God doesn't inflict suffering— "He suffers, too."

Martin also said that at certain crucial moments in his ordeal, angels appeared. There have been people who have met him at moments of crisis, looked at his face, and wordlessly embraced him, sensing his despair. As he told me this, he positively radiated anguish. I felt both helpless and guilty, unable to pluck him out of his torment. Was he hoping for more angels? Perhaps I should close my little notebook, leap out of my velour chair, and massage his rigid neck.

I felt a little cornered. Maybe, I wondered, I couldn't sit in the same room with such torment. Here was someone pushed to the edge, who spent his days at funerals or comforting people who were dying and many of his evenings in board meetings with church bureaucrats, all the time with a claw of pain in his neck. I began to experience what many people feel when confronted with the inconsolable: I wanted to leave.

On the drive home, I stopped at a coffee shop to decompress and organize my notes. To my horror, I discovered that my tape recorder had been set to the wrong speed and the interview was nearly inaudible. I scribbled down what I could remember, but even though I could reconstruct most of the details, the center of the story still felt lost. But, I doubt that a perfect recording would have solved this. It seemed to me that the pain was not to be found in a certain spot in his neck or in the facts of his history. The pain was what had passed between us in the room.

My first instinct, I admit, was to doubt. Surely he was hanging on to his pain as a way to arouse sympathy in strangers like me. Or was a permanently painful neck the price he had decided to pay for the guilt of not being able to save his friend? Whatever the explanation, I didn't want to accept the disembodied darkness that psychologist William Fordyce has called "transdermal pain."

Once I got home, I had an urge to call someone whom I spoke to only once in a blue moon. Her voice on the phone was low and strained. Cathleen, I said, we're overdue for a visit. Oh, it can't be tonight, Cathleen said, my daughter has just had her wisdom teeth extracted, and she's in terrible pain. On top of that, someone she was close to died last week, and we're all a wreck.

"Did they give you a prescription for Tylenol Threes or Percocets?" I asked.

"Yes, but we're waiting until it gets really bad to take them."

"Don't wait until it gets really bad," I said, "the earlier you do something about it the better." We hung up.

Several hours later, she called back to thank me for being so bossy. The painkillers had helped. I told her about my trip to Cobourg and that I had been spooked about my sudden compulsion to get in touch with her. Maybe being around people in grievous pain attunes you to it in other places. No wonder medicine prefers to avoid the issue altogether.

I called Reverend Martin months later to check my tape-garbled details, and to ask how he was faring. "Things have improved, although it's always there," he said. "What has made the greatest difference has been regular massage. I go to a registered massage therapist once a week, and it has really helped. I also go to the Y every morning for an hour and a half. I've lost thirty-five pounds."

So my instinct to get my hands on his neck hadn't been so misguided after all. I was happy to hear that he had switched from getting needles in the neck to something more comforting. But my urge to either get in closer or to run away made me wonder how people in the line of fire stay open to pain in others without being overwhelmed by it.

How do doctors cope with this kind of daily irradiation by pain coming from patients they treat? Now I understand why pain clinics prefer the team approach: It not only reflects the multiple dimensions of pain but also helps break down the professional intensity and isolation of treating it. It's time, I thought, to see how the experts handle pain.

4

VARIOUS SORTS OF LIVING HELL

MY FIRST CONTACT WITH DR. ANGELA Mailis is her voice on the phone, returning my call. The accent is crisp and Greek, and the tone says, "I am a serious female scientist trying to do my job—who are you?" When I tell her I am a journalist and I want to interview her about pain, she makes an exasperated sound.

"Well! That will be very difficult, because my schedule is quite impossible. I have six hundred patients on the waiting list, and I'm not sure how I can help you."

"I understand you're very busy." I hang on the phone. "It's just that people keep telling me to talk to you." Dr. Mailis runs a multidisciplinary pain clinic in the Western Division of the Toronto Hospital. There are nibbling keyboard sounds on the other end.

"Okay. I can give you exactly half an hour on April twenty-third at eleven-thirty A.M.," she says. The date is one month away.

"Fine!" I say. "I'll see you then—" But her phone has already crashed into its cradle. By the time our appointment rolls around,

I've learned that the fifty-two-year-old doctor was trained in physiatry (an area of medicine concerned with rehabilitation) and is an expert in neuropathic pain. She also does research, especially on the placebo response. Her Comprehensive Pain Program is a fourteen-member unit that takes a team approach to the diagnosis and treatment of pain. The toughest cases come to them, usually after multiple consultations with other doctors and lots and lots of waiting—for appointments, for tests, and for hospital elevators, which tend to be as slow as dray horses.

On the designated day, I arrive early to deal with the elevator factor. When I reach the fourth floor of the hospital, Anna, her assistant, warns me that Dr. Mailis has been called upstairs for an emergency. I am to wait in a chair outside her office. Twenty minutes elapse. I begin to think about the full cup of coffee I abandoned on a ledge in the lobby. On my way to the elevators I see a rather glamorous woman in a little black dress and a tiger-striped jacket bending over some files in Anna's office.

"Miss Jackson," says the bent-over figure, "I will see you shortly, but we must be finished by twelve noon." The tiger-lady straightens up and looks at me balefully through large, slightly smoky glasses. She wears dangly gold earrings, her long dark hair is caught up in a comb, and her skirt is very much above her knees. Although Greek, Angela Mailis reminds me of an actress in a Fellini movie—womanly, larger than life, and unapologetic. Her expression says, Another day already shot to hell, and now this writer person.

I nip downstairs, retrieve my coffee, and return to my post in the hall. Dr. Mailis is at her desk; the door is open, and she is talking loudly and indignantly on the phone. She is speaking to an unlucky sales representative about her broken cell phone.

"But this is a disaster!" she cries. "I cannot use my phone unless you find those parts." It's not too late, I think, to just slink away.

"Now, Miss Jackson," her voice raps out, "come in and we will see what we can do."

Her office, the size of two hospital rooms, seems to be arrested in midrenovation. There are unusual works of art on the wall—gifts, it turns out, from former patients. One is a painting of a tight-faced bellhop in a red hat waiting for an elevator. It was done by an artist whose legs were injured in a car accident, and it is the "face of pain," Dr. Mailis says. Anxious and burdened, but still hopeful that the doors in front of him will open.

Her desk is buried under teetering ziggurats of file folders, and her daily schedule is up on her computer, with each line full. She points a long red fingernail at the screen. "You see, something at noon, another meeting at one-thirty, this morning we have emergencies, now you're here . . . and this is how it goes, always." A staff member pops in with a scheduling crisis. Mailis smites her brow, sorts it out, and does a mock collapse into her arms. Dr. Mailis seems to move in a permanent and energetic state of indignation—a suitable attitude for someone faced with the kind of pain she sees day in and day out. She also gets angry at how other doctors treat pain.

"There are basically three games that people in my profession play when they are dealing with pain," she says, ticking them off on her fingers.

"One: the whole-enchilada game. They use one big diagnosis to explain everything. Two: the ostrich routine. They stick their heads in the sand and hope the pain will go away. You can't measure pain, you can't palpate it or auscultate it—therefore, for these doctors, it doesn't exist. And three: They play the blind men with the elephant game. One man feels the tail and says, 'This is a snake.' Another feels the leg and says, 'This is without a doubt a tree.' A third feels the trunk and says, 'It's nothing but a rope.' With pain, if you don't work hard to connect up all the different parts of the picture, you won't get an accurate portrait of the beast."

But the time is finally ripe, Dr. Mailis says, for public pain awareness. A Centre for the Study of Pain is already in the process of being established at the University of Toronto. "Mark my words," says Dr. Mailis, "in two or three years, Toronto will become the mecca for pain."

I refrain from saying the obvious—that Toronto has been a big pain center for some time now—and concentrate on the gush of facts that Mailis delivers. Ask her one question, and she will talk for twenty minutes straight, throwing out data like one of those automatic serving machines on a tennis court.

"Oh, I have a problem with this!" she admits. "With pain, you must always talk about so many things at once, the social, the economic, the psychological—not just the sore knee or the bad back. But people are not used to this approach. I was preparing to give a seminar at a pain conference once, and a colleague took me aside. 'Angela, for God's sake, don't present a hundred thousand pieces of information, people can't absorb it. When someone's thirsty, they can't drink from a fire hose.' "

As she talks, with two manicured fingers she tweezes her dark panty hose up her leg, eliminating sag. Even after twenty-three years in Canada, her body language is uninhibited. And that little quasi-cocktail dress she is wearing—is she headed for a function later on? No, no, she says, with a flap of her jacket, she hasn't worn a lab coat for fifteen years. ("I don't believe in symbolic crap like that.") Mailis is a bit of a warrior on and off the job. She has a black belt in Tae Kwon Do, which she practices twice a week. Today she wore dark stockings, she explains, to hide her bruised knees.

"You know, in our unit here, we have eighteen research projects on the go, we have reviewed twenty-three thousand patients—nobody else does this volume of work! But without a good team, it would be impossible. If you try to deal with pain alone, you burn out. You fry. You need the support of your colleagues and the excitement of the academic work to keep you going. I always say, to go into academia, you must be a freak, but in a good sense.

"My approach is, I'm not the healer, I'm the partner. The power to heal has to come from within, or it's hopeless. The person who says, 'Help me cope with my pain' is very different from the person who says, 'Cure me.'

"Our clinic sees the hardest cases, and doctors refer patients to us for three reasons." (She loves enumerating.) "One—we can't help this patient, so let's get rid of him. Two—despair: God, I have no idea what to do; he's a whiner and has taken a huge amount of medication and I don't know how to help. And three—expertise. Very often, surgeons will send patients to me before they cut and say,

'What do you think?' And I will often say, 'Don't cut.' I believe every modality—drugs, physiological, psychological, surgical—has a role in pain treatment. But you've got to make sure you have the proper diagnosis first. For that, you need the old bedside skills—a thorough, proper history. No technology can take the place of that. I always say that pain is a time-consuming, labor-intensive, unsexy field." And then it is noon: She points a nail at her computer screen as if it were a small, demanding person, and I get up to leave. She wheels out with me, high heels rapping down the hall, talking on, stopping in another office to find me a recent résumé, seventeen pages and still counting. She grabs my hand.

"We will talk again."

Chutzpah. The woman has truckloads.

On the way home, I feel overwhelmed by my ignorance of this serpentine topic. I know nothing about pain. Dr. Mailis, on the other hand, is a woman who has armored herself in her medical and scientific training. A pain warrior. But I see a glint of warmth behind the doctor's smoky aviator glasses, and she has agreed to let me sit in on one of the clinic's weekly team conferences. I start boning up.

IN AN ARTICLE FOR the journal *Humane Medicine,* Dr. Mailis summed up the current situation regarding pain treatment with her customary bluntness: "Despite the fact that 11 to 14% of all Canadians suffer chronic pain," she writes, "we misdiagnose, under-diagnose, maltreat and undertreat pain. We plague patients with unnecessary narcotics when there are better alternatives or we deny medications when they are needed. We try to determine the underlying physical disease . . . but ignore illness behavior, and on the other hand, we miss significant organic causes and send the patient to a psychiatrist or psychologist." And for doctors who treat it "sincerely," she adds, pain can be frustrating and demoralizing.

Canadians spend $2 billion on headache remedies alone, and in the province of Ontario, the Ministry of Social Services spends $6 billion yearly on medical welfare, of which perhaps 10 percent represents people disabled by pain. When no-fault insurance was adopted in 1990, it led to a Wild West boom in private pain-assessment clinics—more than three hundred at last count, none of them regulated. Then there are the individual therapies—acupuncture, nerve blocks, shiatsu, chiropractic, Feldenkrais, meditation groups. Pain patients schlepp from one to another, looking for answers and languishing on waiting lists. The average wait for Dr. Mailis's program is eight months to a year.

Created in 1982, Dr. Mailis's Comprehensive Pain Program is the only multidisciplinary inpatient facility of its kind in North America (even though it has only two beds). Although there are other hospital pain clinics in Toronto, this one is the court of last resort. Most people here have been in pain for more than five years and have seen at least fifteen doctors before they find their way to the fourth floor of Toronto Western.

Not many doctors choose to specialize in pain. It's low-tech. Nobody is sewing baboon organs into human chests. It's more about broad-based medical knowledge than miracle cures. "You have to spend three to four hours taking a patient's history," says Dr. Mailis, "and you don't earn money that way."

Dr. Mailis is simultaneously involved in research, education, administration, teaching, and consultation. She does it all, partly because she can—and partly because in order to treat pain properly, you have to have a finger in many pies. When a patient walks into a clinic complaining of a nine-year history of chronic back pain with no obvious physical cause, the doctor has to look closely at everything—anatomy, neurology, psychology, family background, the work situation. Long-term pain also alters the neurochemistry of the brain; scientists know that now. This can end up hardwiring chronic pain in certain people. Dr. Mailis's specialty is in this difficult-to-treat, invisible pain.

Sometimes simple injuries can result in what is known as reflex sympathetic dystrophy. The nerves remain oversensitized, locked into a feedback loop that can keep people in ongoing agony. Pain research is discovering what many therapists already accept: The body never forgets. The distinction between "mental pain" and "physical pain" has become a meaningless one. By bringing physicians together with psychologists and pain experts from other fields, the multidisciplinary clinic reflects this new model of pain.

Although the Comprehensive Pain Program at Toronto Western lacks a cognitive-behavioral arm, it has come a long way toward dragging pain treatment away from the symptom-based mechanical approach to one that looks at the whole patient, without sacrificing science. Indeed, it is so rigorously scientific that it sometimes gives the impression of enlisting its patients in research, rather than the other way around, as I learned when I sat in on one of the team's weekly conferences. (Some identifying details of the cases have been changed.)

THE MEETINGS TAKE PLACE in an overheated beige space with the curtain tracks still on the ceiling from when it was used for patients. I walk into a room with seven or eight people waiting for Dr. Mailis. This week's discussion includes three psychologists, a psychiatrist, the clinic fellow, and a chiropractor. The chiropractor sleeps through much of the meeting, like the dormouse at Alice's tea party.

Dr. Mailis sails in, carrying a box of Greek pastries.

"These must go, so eat them," she says, putting them on a table and taking her chair. Today she's wearing ankle boots with frilly socks and a dark blue pantsuit. She sits in her chair with her legs apart like a boxer and the meeting commences.

"Okay, first let me tell you a little about what will happen next week," she begins. "We're only seeing one patient, and it is a very sad story. He is a Hungarian man, fifty-six, who was hit by a snow-removal truck in a parking lot and dragged one hundred meters underneath. He was skinned, he has lost his memory, and now he is like a vegetable, except that he cries constantly, has vivid nightmares of the accident, and is in terrible pain. It appears to be a conversion type of deficit, and he has been cared for by his wife for four years. He didn't get a penny from the accident."

"This would come under the heading of 'catastrophic,' " someone interjects. No one objects to that.

"Are we talking about retrograde amnesia?" asks one of the psychologists, with a slight eye-rolling gesture, as in, Please, not more retrograde amnesia.

"It would seem to be a kind of pseudodementia . . ." says another.

"This man cannot lift his arm, cannot speak," Dr. Mailis continues. "It is really very sad. Now this may be a case in which electroshock therapy could take some of the pain away—it is clearly a post-traumatic stress reaction. . . ."

The chiropractor comes to life. "I would like to try homeopathic therapy on this patient." Dr. Mailis murmurs her consent, and the case is dismissed until the following week.

Then an overhead TV is turned on, rolling a videotape of the second patient, whom I will call Miss R.

Miss R. has been in pain for seven years, ever since she had surgery to remove fibroids. She is currently on morphine, "doped and zombied" in Dr. Mailis's words, and has been in the hospital for seven weeks in agony.

With Miss R.'s consent, the clinic's team did their customary diagnostic experiment—a double-blind procedure involving two injections: one a barbiturate, the other a saline solution. Then Dr. Mailis did some tests on the patient to measure pain responses and mobility. Over half will show an improvement when given a placebo—a typical placebo response. This process helps distinguish "inorganic" from "organic" pain, Dr. Mailis claims, although it sounds suspiciously like giving someone a lie detector test. But the response to the barbiturates sometimes reveals that a pain that was considered inorganic actually has an underlying physiological cause. So it swings both ways: The diagnostic test can unmask pain that owes more to depression than tissue damage, and it can detect a neurobiological basis for pain that other doctors have dismissed as "all in the head."

With the saline injection, Dr. Mailis reports, Miss R.'s pain levels fell from a four to a three on a scale of ten. Her MRI results were normal. She is on a high dose of morphine. She had a reported ten out of ten pain intensity for four months. But when she went home from the hospital to a family celebration, Dr. Mailis added, her pain dramatically lessened. Once she was back in the hospital, her pain levels shot up again.

A psychologist speaks up. He fills in the woman's family history, which is troubled, and holds up various psychological profiles of the patient. The only phrase that makes sense to me is that she has a "high dependency spike."

"She's someone who strikes you as being very, very organic," he says, meaning that her pain seems to have a physiological basis, "but then there is the matter that her pain went down to zero on saline and rose on the barbiturates."

When the team learns that the woman has also had the "yuppie flu," there are skeptical noises around the room. The psychiatrist says, "She makes a good impression, although she's a bit driven." Then he points out that no true neuropathy would go from bedridden status to functioning just like that.

Their conclusion? Inorganic pain, mistreated by her doctors. She should have had more counseling and fewer drugs.

"They should not have loaded her up with morphine like that," says Dr. Mailis. "She was on amitriptyline, Tegretol, Valium . . . first she gets better, then six to eight weeks later, she gets worse. My feeling is that the pain took care of itself by itself."

Things are moving along briskly. I'm not sure I would want to be injected with "truth serum" and then videotaped for research purposes. The group moves on to their next patient, Sara, a blackjack dealer from Nova Scotia who has chronic pain in her arms. The video we're watching is so underlit it's hard to decipher. But it's clear that Sara is a very pretty red-haired woman who never smiles. Her pain has been treated with nerve blocks, three times a week, since January.

Several people make disapproving noises. Nerve blocks, the mainstay of many private pain clinics, involve deep injections of analgesics. They are painful in themselves, and, although effective, they only provide a few hours of relief. They do nothing to address any underlying condition.

Dr. Mailis describes Sara as a defensive, hostile individual who doesn't like her job, or anything, for that matter. She notes that the only times Sara smiled were when they gave her the barbiturate injection, and when Dr. Mailis arm-wrestled with her. (Mailis won. "She couldn't take me," she says, laughing.)

There is some indication of thoracic outlet syndrome (a compression of nerves in the neck), Dr. Mailis continues, and Sara's job as a dealer has exacerbated this.

"But three blocks a week that last six hours each—nobody in their sane mind would do this!" says Dr. Mailis.

Sara's doctor had her on a barbiturate—80 milligrams a day. "In every possible way, this is medical mismanagement," exclaims Dr. Mailis. "We have a crazy doctor here, doing crazy things."

The psychiatrist describes the antagonism between Sara and her employer, a man who yells at her and "runs her ass off." It also comes out that an old boyfriend has been stalking her. She says that her whole life revolves around pain and this stalker. The police don't take her seriously, he adds.

One of the psychologists adds that Sara was abused physically as a child; the Children's Aid Society was called at one point. He holds up charts that indicate "extreme elevation in the narcissistic and paranoiac indices."

"Is this a personality disorder?" Dr. Mailis asks.

Nods of agreement all around.

"The one person she had affection for was her brother, who died two years ago. Normally she was very stiff, but her whole body relaxed when she talked about him," Dr. Mailis notes. "She clearly needs one-to-one therapy, but I need to serve it to her in a way she can accept. Unless she has therapy, I'm afraid that she has no hope in hell. It's like those wrist-slashers, you know. They try to get away from all their psychological pain by having physical pain. She needs a kindly therapist, most of all."

This particular meeting was starting to make people in chronic pain sound like psychiatric cases, which is misleading. But by the time many people make it to a clinic like this, the effects of months or years of pain, depression, and fruitless therapy have become so entangled that it's impossible to unravel them. This is why Mailis stresses the importance of dealing with pain early, before it sends down roots deep and wide.

The fourth case of the morning is a man who has had full-blown AIDS for several years. He is wheelchair-bound, and reports terrible pain in his feet, although no underlying cause can be found. He's on assorted drug cocktails. But one of the psychologists reports that he is "jolly as all get-out, which is weird, considering his situation, and he is probably in denial. He's focused away from the AIDS and on the pain in his feet."

The group spends a few moments talking about the man's situation. When did he stop work? Where is his family? Are there any friends in the picture? A partner? The man seems utterly alone. "He appears to have given up," the psychiatrist says. A brief silence falls. The group seems genuinely touched by each case. But when pain is your job, you must economize your emotions, and they move on.

"Are we agreed that this is some sort of conversion reaction?" asks Dr. Mailis.

"This is a sad story," says the psychiatrist.

"A very, very sad story," echoes Dr. Mailis.

Her assistant clicks the monitor off. Dr. Mailis hurries out. The pastries on the table are mostly eaten, and the meeting adjourns.

Needless to say, Dr. Mailis has her fans and her detractors among her colleagues (for a while she had a sign on her office door—a hand with a prominently raised middle finger). Pain science is as competitive and political as any other turf, and her big mouth can get her in trouble. She's controversial. Dr. Mailis is also a director of the Workmen's Safety Insurance Board and furnishes the board with pain assessments of her own patients—one too many hats to wear, perhaps. But many of her patients have great respect and affection for her. And neuropathic pain, her specialty, is one of the most mysterious challenges in the field of pain studies.

I went to talk to one of her patients, David Kelly. He lives with a neuropathic pain problem in his back and leg and another sort of chronic misery: his struggles with the province's Workplace Safety Insurance Board to receive compensation. In theory, the

WSIB's policy of "a safe and early return to work" sounds enlightened, but in practice it can end up punishing people trying to live with chronic pain.

WHEN I FIRST REACH him on the phone, Kelly is at home recovering from a back operation for a ruptured disk (his third such operation, in addition to fourteen outpatient surgeries). I can hear his son, Daniel, playing in the background. Kelly's voice is warm and deep—an FM sort of voice. And he still has a sense of humor, despite being in constant, ten-Percocet-a-day pain since he hurt himself on the job in 1992. When Kelly was getting out of a tractor-trailer he fell several meters and injured his arm, shoulder, left leg, and back. The damage left him with a numb left foot, which led to another back injury when he tried to go back to work too soon. Then he developed disk trouble, and his pain problems snowballed—all of it, according to Dr. Mailis, related to that first injury and to the pressure from the Workplace Safety and Insurance Board to get him back on the job, pain or no pain.

Before his injury, Kelly skydived, boxed, played hockey, drove a Corvette, and took home $125,000. Now it's a big deal for him to ride the bus.

I drive out to the Kellys' bungalow in Mississauga, a suburb of Toronto. It's February, and the Christmas decorations are still on the lawn—one more chore that Kelly can't do on his own. I go inside and meet his wife, Anna, a manager in a chemical distribution company. A thick sheaf of prescriptions is tacked on the bulletin board, over the oilcloth-covered kitchen table. Vacuum-cleaner stripes are visible on the living room rug, and Anna has lit a few candles around the room—everything neat and orderly, in the face of the living hell they've been through in the past few years. She describes the way her husband's day proceeds.

"It's a four-hour cycle. He starts off in the morning like this," she says, crouching over and hobbling around the room. "Then the painkillers kick in, and he can straighten up and take on the day. Three hours later, he starts to curve over again—you can see the pain come back in his face and his body."

I can see it as Kelly comes down the stairs, leaning on a cane, and then gingerly lowers himself into a rocking chair. But to most people, and especially to insurance companies, chronic pain like this is invisible, hard to clearly diagnose, and therefore suspect. If you're an injured worker with a leg in a big plaster cast, you will be quickly compensated, but if you're a worker disabled by pain that lasts "too long," or is hard to visualize, it becomes the opinion of the board's medical advisers (often "nurse-managers" who do not actually examine the applicants) against the opinion of your own doctor.

Kelly experiences both deep pain in his lumbar region and total numbness from the left thigh down, a rare disorder officially called maladaptive neuropathy.

"The way I understand it," says Kelly, "one, I have nerve damage from my injury, so the signals are kind of jumbled anyhow, and secondly, the maladaptive thing is the way my brain has reacted to the constant pain signals—by just shutting down. Here, I'll show you."

He takes his wooden cane and whacks his left leg hard, many times. It sounds like a bad beating. Dr. Mailis also has videotapes of Kelly hitting his shin almost to the point of bruising. This numbness affects his balance, and yet doesn't touch the deep pain he also experiences. He's had two ruptured disks, but the WSIB doesn't consider these related to his original injury—an opinion not shared by his neurosurgeon and Dr. Mailis.

Dr. Mailis sees the wisdom of rehabilitating injured workers rather than letting them languish on compensation. (There is a concept in the pain-science world known as "secondary gain" from pain, and disability pay is one example.) At the same time, it drives Dr. Mailis crazy when she knows her patients are suffering and the WSIB rejects diagnoses by experts in pain regarding patients the board hasn't even met, interviewed, or examined. It was years before the WSIB even got the nature of Kelly's injury straight, referring to it as "shoulder pain."

In January 1998, a new bill was introduced in Ontario that shifted the focus from long-term compensation to rehabilitation and a speedy return to work. This was intended to deal with the horrendous economic toll of compensation and to prevent "malingerers" from abusing the system. No one could argue with these aims. But the "board assessors" are not pain experts and don't necessarily accept the diagnoses of the experts they consult. Workers trying to qualify for compensation must make their way through a Kafkaesque tangle of bureaucracy and appointments. It's a process that a healthy person would find taxing and humiliating, let alone someone already dealing with pain or illness.

The chronic pain policy of the WSIB is currently under revision, but in the meantime, pain patients like Kelly keep running into surprises. They may go to the drugstore to get a prescription filled and learn that their coverage has been abruptly suspended without notice, or that their board evaluators have been switched. (Kelly estimates that he has dealt with more than twenty-five evaluators over the years.) This runaround wears down all but the most stubborn or desperate. But Kelly is not only stubborn, but also methodical, motivated, and infuriated by how he has been treated.

"It's not that I don't want to work," Kelly says. "I would give anything to be able to work. I spent nine months taking a computer training program, and I aced it. But the WSIB thought that once I graduated from the business course, my condition would be magically healed. Training doesn't end the pain."

In the journal *Pain Management and Research,* I came across an article with the mischievous title "Improvement Means Deterioration," by Dr. Harold Merskey. Merskey is the pain expert who hammered out the most widely accepted scientific definition of pain. He had a suspicion that the "improved" pain policies of the WSIB were in fact eroding the rights of patients in pain, and he went about documenting this. He followed the experiences of thirty-one patients who suffered chronic pain. Ten of them, he learned, had had the experience of walking into the drugstore to discover that their drug coverage had been withdrawn without notice or explanation. The WSIB policy regarding pain treatment appears to be a version of cold turkey.

"By the time I got to see Dr. Mailis," says Kelly, describing a process that took him through two years and numerous doctors, "I thought I was losing my marbles. What was happening to me made no sense—my left leg was numb, but my back was still in all this pain. Dr. Mailis was the first doctor to figure out what was wrong with me, and what I was going through." She put him on pain medication, sent him to a neurologist, and began collecting medical evidence to convince the WSIB that Kelly was indeed in pain and unfit to work.

After Kelly hands me a wad of documentation concerning his case, I leave. Sometime later, I check in with him to see how he is faring. He says the pain is "gradually improving." His $700-a-month medication bill is still being covered by the WSIB. He is down to two Percocets a day and has just had a "spinal stimulator" surgically implanted in his body. This device operates on the gate-control theory that competing stimuli to the spine can alter the pain signals. In Kelly's case, it seems to be helping so far. But their luck sure needs some rehabilitation: Anna Kelly has just been involved in a serious car accident; she was hit by someone driving with a suspended license. She is now unable to work as well. "Otherwise," says Kelly, "we're pretty good."

UNFORTUNATELY, DAVID KELLY CAN'T get pregnant. It was the hormonal shift of pregnancy and breast-feeding that brought the most sustained pain relief to another one of Dr. Mailis's chronic pain patients, Lori Biduke. Lori was home taking care of her first child, a nine-week-old son, when I came to visit her. She looks like the sort of good-natured, pretty, practical woman who might never have had a down day in her life.

Twelve years earlier, when she was twenty-four, Lori was at her job in a retail store, with her arms full of clothes, when she tripped over a box and landed hard on her right knee. It become swollen and painful.

"I tried to ice it and sort of left it for a couple of days as I hobbled around. I was never the type to run to the doctor. But after two days, I couldn't even get my shoe on, there was so much swelling throughout my whole leg, and I was in so much pain. I went to a clinic and they said, 'Oh, ruptured tendons and ligaments, take anti-inflammatories, stay off your feet.' I did that for a weekend, then went back to work on crutches."

The knee eventually healed, but the pain got worse. After Lori spent nearly a year making the rounds of doctors, her GP referred her to Dr. Mailis, who diagnosed her with reflex sympathetic dystrophy. (This is also known, equally unmemorably, as complex regional pain syndrome, or CRPS.) Lori has been in pain ever since her injury.

"It never feels chronic in the sense of low-grade," she said. "It still feels acute. Basically, the nerves go into a frenzy and stay that way."

This is the condition Silas Weir Mitchell called "causalgia" in the nineteenth century. He described it as persistent, severe pain that is characterized by burning, a change of temperature in the affected extremity, and sometimes swelling and discoloration of the skin. Lori's leg became blue and cold. The area can also become so sensitive that a puff of air or a drop of water is agonizing (a state known as allodynia). Mitchell had one patient who found it so painful to expose his affected hand to the air that he walked around with it submerged in a bucket of water all the time.

Lori Biduke has learned how to manage her life around the pain in her knee, which affects her back as well, but the months it took to get a diagnosis and the years of fiddling with drugs and futile treatments were hell.

"I've done it all," she said, "everything invasive you can imagine, as well as all the alternative stuff. I resisted pain medication for a long time, because I don't respond well to drugs. Then I tried epidurals and nerve blocks. I once spent ten days in a hospital on a continual epidural. Drugs were the last resort, but they ended up helping enormously."

Dr. Mailis, she said, was "really quick to get things happening for me. She was just like a bulldog. She'd call me from her home at eight P.M. to check on me. And a lot of the symptoms I had I couldn't describe, or I would dismiss, because I didn't know how they fit into the picture. Also, I didn't want to look like a whiner. But Mailis would say, 'Are you having that tingle?' and I would say, 'Yes, it's driving me crazy.' She was clear about the disease. She didn't cure the problem, but she helped me manage the pain. For a long time, I didn't have any hope—and I began to question myself, too. You can't help it."

Not everything they tried worked. Dr. Mailis referred Lori to a neurosurgeon, who recommended the same operation Kelly had opted for—an implanted spinal electrostimulating device. "It worked well in the hospital," said Lori, "but when I got home and went about my day, odd things would happen. I would reach up and get this sudden rush from the device—it was awful. Or if I sneezed, it was like getting electrocuted. And my leg was getting more irritated. I found the device harder to handle than the pain itself."

Dr. Mailis told her to forget the implant and to go the medication route, which Biduke resisted at first. "A doctor had said to me, 'Be careful, or you'll get addicted.' So I was scared. The last thing I wanted to deal with was addiction." It took nine months of throwing everything up, but she finally responded to Demerol. "Even then I had to take a lot of Gravol to tolerate it. It took me a year to get over the side effects."

"I didn't want to tell people I was on Demerol, either. I was concerned about people's reaction, that they might think I was taking it to get high, although I never felt high, ever. It ended up working for me."

Lori adds that she had to learn about breakthrough pains, too. These are spikes of sporadic, intense pain, for which doctors prescribe additional "rescue doses" of painkiller. She resisted those as well. "That was just my mentality, to wait until the pain was really bad before I took something."

We were talking in her living room, where her baby was in his basket, making small squawking noises in his sleep. She seemed a most relaxed new mother.

"The pain was often, like, a ten. A ten plus. I had zero functionality. You don't sleep. Your whole day and night just blend into each other, and you lose control of your life. I'm sure there was depression, even though I'm not a depressed person at all. And people would totally minimize it. Oh, they'd say, you can't be in that much pain. You just need some distraction.

"Then I got pregnant, and gradually, the pain improved. Breast-feeding has really helped, too. Something hormonal must have happened. And people would say, you see, you just needed a distraction. That is so diminishing! I have to say, I wasn't the most sympathetic person to pain before my injury. Until you go through it, you don't know what it's like.

"I kept saying to myself, This is going to be over, I just have to go through this next bit . . . and lo and behold, ten years went by and I was exactly the same."

The baby woke up, and Lori moved carefully from the couch to pick him up.

"One of the big things has been to learn my limitations and not take on too much. If I'm going to do groceries today, I'm not going to meet a friend for lunch. That was a really hard lesson. It's funny, my husband is better at recognizing when I'm going to hit the wall than I am. He'll come up to me at a party, when I'm standing up—nobody talks to you when you're sitting down—and he'll come by and draw up a chair for me. I used to shoot dirty looks at him, because I didn't want the attention, you know, but after a few evenings like that I would come home and be in tears from the pain. Luckily, he's a very sensitive, compassionate man. The problem is that I try and push the pain out of my head as much as possible so that it's not the focus of my life. But it does catch up with you. The other thing that amazes me is how tiring it is—it's really draining. Rainy days are bad days for me, and so are cold days. It's exhausting, to fight it all the time. Often, I just need quiet time. I think that's one thing that has changed. . . . I'm probably not quite as social. Sometimes I can't deal with it.

"And people doubt it. They doubt that I can be in that much pain. I work really hard, I fight, not to look like I'm wounded, I really do. Maybe my life would be easier if I let people see me when I'm down, but I don't. I don't want to accept myself as that, either."

5

TAKING THE SUFFERING
OUT OF PAIN

Our resistance and fear, our dread of the unpleasant, magnify pain. It is like closing your hand around a burning ember. The tighter you squeeze, the deeper you are seared.

STEPHEN LEVINE, *How We Die*

RIGHT INSIDE THE DOOR OF DR. PAUL Kelly's waiting room is a big horseshoe of books—shelves of philosophy and literature, not just neuroscience textbooks. In another corner is one of those plug-in water sculptures, trickling away. Dr. Kelly, a psychologist who teaches meditation techniques to people in chronic pain, came out of his inner office to meet me, and I shook hands with a tall middle-aged man, slightly stiff in his body (it turns out he has a bad back), with gray hair cut in a short, soft fuzz.

Like Angela Mailis, Kelly once ran a hospital pain clinic. But his approach is quite different. Although he knows a great deal about the brain, over the years his interest has been shifting downward to include the heart as well. In his view, the most important element in addressing chronic pain may not be drugs or the "technology" of a particular treatment, but the compassionate presence of the therapist. After much reading, schooling, and experience with thousands of suffering patients, Dr. Kelly's approach is simple: Breathe. Don't try to block pain out; tune in to it instead.

Dr. Kelly spent eleven years as the director of a "stress, pain, and chronic-disease clinic" at the Toronto Hospital, where he taught meditation strategies to help patients cope with their pain. But in 1997, budget cuts axed the program, and Kelly opened his own practice. He works with individuals or small groups, covering twenty-two hours of instruction in the Zen practice of mindfulness meditation. Unlike most North Americans these days, he is not a recent convert, having studied Zen Buddhism for the past thirty-two years.

While medicine works at subverting or numbing discomfort, meditation allows a person "to get intimate with the pain" instead of trying to run from it. The ultimate goal, according to Shinzen Young, a Buddhist monk whose teachings Dr. Kelly draws on, is "to try to take the suffering out of pain." This approach also recognizes the med-school concept of three levels of pain: sensory, cognitive, and affective or emotional. Meditation helps a person feel the distinction between these three and gain some control over the anguish and fear of loss of control that accompanies chronic pain.

We went into his consultation room, where I spied a rolled-up yoga mat in the corner. One advantage of being on the twenty-third floor of an unappetizing office tower was the view of the city glittering gold to the north. It was almost sunset when we spoke. Dr. Kelly made himself comfortable in his chair, one of those ergonomic numbers with several levers under the seat. To relieve his back, he had a habit of briskly gearing his chair up and down every now and then, using it as a form of punctuation.

"I try to give the person some sort of stable ground on which to meet the pain," said Kelly. "That way he knows that there is more to him than the pain, and that he doesn't have to be overwhelmed or helpless in relation to it. People who have to live with pain often end up wanting to flee themselves; pain has put them on the outside of their bodies. What meditation does is help them reclaim their bodies and tolerate the pain itself, so they don't feel like victims of it.

"But you know, I basically agree with Ursula Le Guin," he said, referring to the science fiction writer and adapter of the *Tao Te Ching,* "that the best government is the government in which nothing happens. There is this whole heroic tradition in psychoanalytical literature, but when you actually look at the research, the therapies that are most effective work because the patients do the work." The main job of a therapist is simple, he added—to be fully there in the room with the patient and to tune in.

Kelly gave the impression of being a mind-driven man who might have sequestered himself in academia, and he admitted that he had started out in university as a "bit of an intellectual, disembodied chap." Since then he seems to have embodied himself quite nicely. I had the feeling of being with a focused presence and a discriminating listener.

"It helps that I have the good fortune to have had a back problem," he said cheerfully, "which has given me more insight into my patients." After suffering a prolapsed disk, Kelly was encouraged by the progress he made doing the Feldenkrais Method, a body-based therapy that uses a system of exercises to help reintegrate mind and body.

"I used to be the sort of person who had trouble relating to my own body. I thought if I read enough books, I could solve my problems. And I actually *did* read a lot of books; scholarly pursuits are important to me. But my focus has shifted somewhat over the years, from the intellect to the emotions—to the cultivation of compassion. The first question therapists should ask themselves is this: Do they really like humans?"

Kelly, who grew up in a small northern Ontario town in an Irish-Catholic family, began practicing meditation and looking into Zen Buddhism at the same time as he undertook classical university training in psychology. He incorporated both in his Toronto Hospital clinic work in 1988, when he started to run meditation programs for

HIV/AIDS patients. He found this approach worked as well as traditional talk therapy. He sees meditation as a "kind of manual," a very practical tool.

What Kelly has concluded is that the relationship between therapist and patient is at least as important as the type of therapy undertaken. His own published studies have shown that "technique" accounts for 15 percent of a successful outcome—but the relation of therapist to patient accounts for 30 percent. In other words, "you have to be able to be present in the room with someone. To do that, you must be present to yourself." He paused.

Psychologists often have a certain conversational tic. When you ask them a question, they will pause, avert their gaze, and appear to think. In Kelly's case, he does think; this is part of the "technology." Psychologists, after all, don't do surgery or insert people into MRI machines. Their job is to talk, listen . . . and think. In contrast to what he calls "exhortative therapy," a period of silence lets things happen in the room. It's quite effective.

Kelly treats a lot of car accident victims, people injured on the job, and patients with fibromyalgia. When I asked him what he thought caused fibromyalgia—not a very fair question, since no one seems to know the answer—he looked a tiny bit troubled and entered another long, rich pause. Finally, he ventured a reply. "It seems to be the way a certain autoimmune dysfunction manifests itself in some people." When I wondered if a diagnostic label was good or bad, he acknowledged that this was a very delicate problem. People in pain need the validation of a diagnosis, he understands, but sometimes a label can freeze the condition and make it something they don't want to leave behind—precisely because it does legitimize how they feel.

"In my practice we shift from the idea of solving the pain to exploring the experience of it. It's about nonjudgmental awareness. With my patients I try to find something that they enjoy and might pursue. It doesn't have to be a big thing. One of my patients, for instance, always wanted to write mysteries. So she began to do that. And you can build on these things. The important thing is that they have to find some way of beginning to feel some control over their lives, no matter how hopeless or desperate their situation. Many come in here angry and furious that no one has rescued them. But if they can focus on *how* they feel, instead of who did this to them, they can start to find ways to live with their pain in less anguish. The thing is, I don't have to offer them a way to fix their pain—it isn't going to happen. These are chronic cases. My goal is to help them have a better life, regardless of the pain."

The sun was going down. Kelly struck me as a bit like the Tin Man who went off in search of a heart—a rationalist with a "profound respect for natural science" who has nevertheless seen the limits of his profession. As an an all-too-timely gold light filled the room, we talked about the books he regularly refers to, starting with *Full Catastrophe Living,* the popular purge-your-lifestyle manual by Jon Kabat-Zinn, and the Buddhist classic *A Path with Heart,* by Jack Kornfield. He also uses audiotapes by Shinzen Young and Stephen Levine in his sessions.

"Shinzen teaches that we can learn to experience the sensation of pain without having the mind add further commentary," Kelly said. Yes, well, try telling that to a writer, I thought.

I asked him what took him into the pain field. After an even longer pause than usual, he said, "I would probably answer the same as Thomas Merton, when he said that the reasons he became a monk were not the same as the reasons he remained one." Which is very much in line with what the master Suzuki Roshi said when asked to summarize twenty-five hundred years of Buddhism: "Everything changes."

"I grew up in a village where everyone had a place, whether they were smart, or handicapped, or whatever. They belonged. A cohesive community has a stabilizing influence. People sometimes seek out a therapist as a replacement for that. Their real problem is, they're lonely guys."

This is what the traditional medical approach—even the enlightened version practiced by Dr. Mailis's team—has trouble exercising: empathy. It's not taught in medical school and it doesn't necessarily come naturally. You could (if necessary) call empathy a technology, too, one that takes training and practice to use well.

Sometime after my conversation with Dr. Kelly was over, I received a flyer in the mail for a special weekend workshop he was leading, intended for therapists and professionals who dealt with people in pain. I signed up.

THE WORKSHOP WAS CALLED "The Loving-Kindness Meditation Retreat." I do have a hard time with titles like that. But if the Heidegger-reading Dr. Kelly could embrace a therapeutic tool with this particular handle, then surely I could spend a Sunday investigating it. I just wished it didn't sound like a skin cream.

Buddhism is overtaking Freud in the therapeutic world, as more mainstream professionals respond to the fact that Buddhism tackles the whole of the psyche, in a structured scrutiny of the self that is quite a bit older than psychoanalysis. The irony of psychoanalytic thinking is that we can now clearly diagnose narcissism, but we still don't know what to do about it.

Freud's famous goal was to transform neurotic misery into ordinary unhappiness. This involved an expansive concept of self-awareness that would equip the ego for dealing with a world full of hidden agendas. It is, by definition, "self"-centered. But for the Buddhists, neurotic misery arises from our attempts to erect a self that tries to block out sadness, pain, death, and suffering. In the Buddhist view, joy is inseparable from suffering. One can only be cured of the concept of a cure. Psychoanalysis, for all its useful peeling away of the defenses, still seems profoundly uneasy about what's underneath. Buddhism doesn't try to resolve conflicts; it embraces contradiction. (This can be rather maddening, like the smiling taciturn patience of a very old person.) Buddhism doesn't see suffering as a failure of happiness. "If you haven't cried a number of times, your meditation hasn't really begun," said author Achaan Chah. But Buddhism still seems . . . bleakly optimistic about what is at the core of human nature. Pain is not the price of joy, it coexists with it. And Buddhism offers a simple solution for the modern narcissistic dilemma: "No self, no problem."

Our group was small—four women and a man who joined us later in the morning. He had a goatee and sad, sloping shoulders, and seemed to be in a delicate condition. Except for me, the pain amateur, the women were therapists or counselors of one sort or another—middle-aged, professional, well-workshopped, and sturdy. Dr. Kelly said a few words about how the day would proceed and began with meditation. We counted our breaths—in, out, one to ten, then back to one. Forty minutes. The time passed quickly, as debris bobbed to the surface of my mind. It was a bit like cleaning out the fridge. My mind was like the vegetable crisper: It doesn't matter how fresh the food is, if it's too crowded in there, things will rot. Or, as the Buddhists prefer to put it, "Keep that don't-know mind!"

Meditation was not new for me. I did some in my weekly yoga classes, and years ago I dabbled in Kundalini yoga. I had had an alarming experience with it, in fact. One day in a farmhouse in Wales, as I sat fire-breathing and meditating with a group of more advanced yoga types, I felt a stream of energy power up my spine and across the back of my head, like the proverbial fountain of light. It was a case of premature spiritual ejaculation, just as it's described in *Autobiography of a Yogi* by Paramhansa Yogananda. It scared me, and I broke off the moment. I had made the mistake of powering up my consciousness without having the appropriate scaffolding in place. But it left me with a considerable respect for the potential of meditation.

Sitting at the front of the group, Dr. Kelly didn't say a great deal, and he wasn't charismatic. But every once in a while he would emit a surprising little laugh—*hee hee hee!* (Laughing seems to be a Buddhist thing.) He led us through a second meditation in which we concentrated on the heart, and on "a feeling of openness and kindness there." It was odd to meditate on the heart as if it were literally some sort of emotional pantry. Western medicine looks upon the heart as a large muscle and a well-engineered pump. But this is a relatively recent notion. Aristotle believed that all sensations, including pain, originated in the heart. It was only in the seventeenth century that we began to assemble the modern model of the body as a kind of elaborate forklift truck run by the mind.

We sat in the large, sunny studio, with its lone potted plant, and focused on our hearts and our breath. It's one way to get our sense of "I" out of the head. Paying attention to the breath is a reminder that we aren't just consciousness inside the armor of our skulls; our bodies are also linked by the flow of air in and out to the rest of the world.

Our next task was to extend compassion to ourselves—a rusty practice. Normally, under the mantle of self-improvement, we live inside a circle of anxious, bossy thoughts: Don't eat that, slow down, work harder, lighten up, get in shape. In the eyes of Christianity, or in our various secular mirrors, we're always falling short of the mark and chastising ourselves. We confuse compassion for ourselves with self-absorption, I think. But they belong to two different spheres: Self-absorption is usually defensive, isolating, and judgmental; compassion for the self opens us up.

Buddhism is tough, the toughest, but it sees no need for spiritual correction. It does not want to impose new ideas of the self, or to layer on improvements—its goal is to strip away false selves and misleading notions of identity to reveal our true nature, which is already perfect. Buddhism is not about progress and moving on, but about going deeper and becoming still.

Like many people who grew up in a vaguely Christian framework, I always assumed that self-denial was something of a virtue, and that moral progress is just a matter of suppressing the bad parts of ourselves. Sin is our nature, the teaching goes. This is the sort of divide-and-conquer mentality that causes so much misery in the first place, and it's part of the rhetoric of conquest that suffuses Western scientific thought. Buddhism understands that the joy of living is impossible without accepting suffering and sorrow, and the contradictions of our nature. Pain denied becomes pain amplified. In our painkilling culture, the resistance to suffering has become a source of suffering in itself.

Pain is only part of us, the part saying "pay attention." Like a mother who creates a tantrum in a two-year-old by tuning out what the child is trying to tell her, we bring on more unhappiness by turning our back on the pain in our lives. Instead of expending so much energy on our efforts to fend off pain and sadness, Buddhism asks us to simply be aware of what we are feeling and thinking. And as soon as we tentatively enter the sensation of pain, it loses some of its power.

But people reflexively blame themselves for their own pain, literally adding insult to injury. The next meditation in the session concentrated on forgiveness, especially for ourselves. Like doing a set of ab crunches, I went to work on toning up my forgiveness. I found I had a list of matters large and small to practice on.

Although it felt faintly ridiculous at first, after a while this meditation began to subtly shift my view of people in my life. If I could be a candidate for forgiveness, then they must be forgivable, too. It was a surprising sensation to conjure up the faces of people I knew, suspend my judgment for a change, and just extend acceptance to them, whether or not they had earned it. No harm in that.

Then Kelly asked us to meditate with someone we loved in mind. As we breathed in and out, we were to imagine this person happy and calm. Interesting. I discovered that I spend so much time measuring and weighing my relationships—how are we doing? how am I doing in it? what are the problems?—that ordinary well-wishing gets neglected. It felt much lighter to forget about who deserved my kind thoughts and who didn't, and to send blessings anyway. The whole business of being "right" about someone began to seem a bit irrelevant.

The more simpleminded the workshop became, in fact, the more I enjoyed it. Freeing up the mind in this way was like playing some orchestral instrument strictly for fun.

Our next assignment was to conjure up forgiveness for someone we were neutral toward. Neutral was tricky. Everyone I thought of, I had a screaming opinion on. Finally, I settled on a bland acquaintance and lobbed peace and calmness his way. He became a bit more interesting as I did this, I noticed—more particular, even dear. Then we were to do the same with someone we actively disliked. I violently repressed a few excellent candidates. I found that I wanted to address the tough side of people I loved instead. As with pain, resistance to people only generates more resistance. You can't force hatred away any more than you can command compassion or love. But by becoming aware of the feeling, allowing it some room, you can change its texture. Hatred becomes something other than the hard, heavy absolute we imagine it to be. It becomes flexible.

The intimacy of being in a room with a few strangers in such a concentrated silent way was comforting. But then Dr. Kelly asked us to pair off, and I got nervous. I felt I was already paired off on my own. The next exercise was an eyeball-to-eyeball session in gazing. I ended up partnered with Dr. Kelly. Right away, I became worried about being "good" at gazing. What would my gaze reveal? For one thing, it's neither natural nor relaxing to stare into someone's eyes for ten minutes; it has the primal feel of a biological threat. But since Dr. Kelly was an old hand at this, he could set the gazing standards.

We sat opposite each other and let our eyes meet. His face was impassive, and his eyes conveyed nothing at all. It was a little unnerving: He was both present and absent. There was a slight twitch at one corner of his mouth. After a while, one of his eyes seemed to come forward, as the other receded, and he took on a bit of a Cyclops look. His gaze was steady but transparent—I could look through his eyes to . . . nothing at all. His eye had become The Eye. The embarrassment of two egos tangled up in eye beams didn't come into it. I felt I was climbing up through him as if he were a tree, a good, strong climbing tree. It had a mischievous tinge, a playful sense of lobbing the shuttlecock of consciousness back and forth.

Then, without breaking his gaze, he asked us not just to feel the balance of energy between us but to actively extend kindness to our partners. I sent my thoughts down into his chest and his spine. His bad back. I felt a shift, a softening of his gaze, and a subtle warmth in my chest. Tears came briefly to my eyes. Whether it was his thoughts or my own expectations affecting me, it was a palpable current. It made me wonder about the power of negative thoughts—of voodoo. How many of us are in the grip of our own self-generated voodoo, of bearing the weight of our own curses?

I'm sure thought shapes us, in the same way that wind patterns shape sand.

Then people got tired. When Dr. Kelly asked us what we had learned, Bette, a psychologist and veteran of monasteries, said, "I learned that if I meditate lying down, I want to fall asleep." We cruised through the last half hour and called it a day.

In six hours, my intellectual security system had been temporarily disarmed. I can't believe I have nothing skeptical to say about my "Loving-Kindness Meditation Retreat," but I don't. I went home feeling calm, although no more so than after yoga. But over the next few days, I was spectacularly productive in an effortless way. And whenever I felt myself getting annoyed with someone, instead of adding up all my watertight reasons for feeling that way, I tried forgiving the slow cashier or the churlish friend. This certainly took up less room in my mind. And it made me realize how often my censure of others is rooted in self-recrimination.

The workshop had managed, in its oblique way, to demonstrate how judgment, particularly self-judgment, compounds pain. People in pain blame themselves for not getting better and for complicating the lives of those around them. Therapists who treat them find it tempting to judge them as well. As Dr. Kelly mildly put it, "Chronic pain is very complex. What people need most of all is encouragement and ways to help them feel better. We shouldn't limit ourselves to one kind of medicine."

Dr. Kelly comported himself like a scientist who works around the limits of his science. He also had a way of saying something useful and then erasing his tracks, like the Cheshire cat who evaporates to nothing but a floating smile. And then there was that surprising little laugh. *Hee hee hee!* I have no idea where that giggle comes from.

6

PHANTOM LIMBS

THE ABILITY TO MAKE SOMEONE FEEL AGONY in a limb that isn't there is one of pain's most impressive sleights of hand. And phantom pain is not a rarity or a fluke: Among people who have had a limb amputated, almost 70 percent will end up suffering some form of phantom pain. Nobody knows for sure what causes it. It may take weeks or years to develop—and it can last for a lifetime. Occasionally, over time, the pain may recede, although no one knows why. And although surgeons may snip away at nerves or stumps in an effort to alleviate it, phantom pain remains notoriously difficult to treat.

People report specific kinds of pain—burning, stabbing, or aching. They feel the pressure of a nonexistent ring on a missing finger, or fingernails digging into the palm of a phantom hand. For all its ghostliness, phantom pain is explicit about where it hurts and how it feels—warm or wet, gritty or metallic. The sensation is said to be almost holographic. If ever there was evidence for pain being "all in the head," phantom pains provide it. They

1

also demonstrate that pain is sometimes a complex perceptual illusion involving vision, body image, and sense memory.

Surgeons can cut the nerves that lead from the limb to the spinal cord (a rhizotomy). But cutting nerves is not considered a very effective way to treat phantom pain, which is too intimately connected with the dance of perception itself to be plucked out like a splinter.

The Civil War physician Silas Weir Mitchell came up with the name phantom limb pain. In those days, lopping off limbs was the most efficient way to prevent infection or gangrene. This led to a bumper crop of amputees, who began to report bizarre sensations or excruciating pain in their missing limbs, a phenomenon that Mitchell wrote about in detail. But the first mention of phantom limb pain goes back to the sixteenth century in descriptions by the French surgeon Ambroise Paré. And Lord Nelson also experienced it. In 1797, when he lost an arm in battle and discovered that he still felt the presence of his fingers, Nelson declared that this was proof that the soul really does exist. If his arm could persist when its physical attributes were gone, surely our spirits can survive the demise of the body.

Sometimes phantom limbs have an active life as well. They will "gesture" or try to carry on with their previous lives—absent arms that rise to swing at tennis balls, missing hands that reach for a cup. One man said his phantom hand still reached for the check in restaurants ("Oh, my phantom will pay—trust me"). For equally mysterious reasons, phantom limbs can also be paralyzed or become stuck in awkward positions. Amputees with frozen phantom limbs will automatically make room for them when they walk through doorways and protect them in tight situations.

For years, phantom limbs were treated almost as part of medical folklore—exotic case studies that made for lively reading in medical monographs. But for people who suffer from phantom pain, it is as real as having a broken neck in a halo cast.

As I rummaged through the literature, I was struck by how the successive historical explanations for this weird phenomenon—from the soul to the current concept of neurogenesis, or the brain's ability to grow new cells—also reflect the way we've conceived of pain in general.

Phantom limbs were initially regarded as something that couldn't be touched scientifically—they were the body's equivalent of an alien abduction. In fact, Mitchell was so unsure of his speculations about them that he published his first article on the subject under a pseudonym in a popular magazine instead of a scientific journal.

This also reflected the nineteenth-century attitude that pain wasn't legitimate unless it could be pointed to, probed, and measured; otherwise, it was "hysteria," "neurasthenia," or simply madness.

The next phantom pain theory, which lingers on, is that it arises from inflamed or irritated nerve endings, called neuromas, in the stump. Some doctors have tried to treat phantom pain by surgically removing these neuromas or even by doing an additional amputation. Occasionally this helps, but each new amputation can also breed a new phantom, raising the specter of a hall-of-mirrors effect and an infinite number of phantoms-within-phantoms. Finally, in the middle of last century, the attention shifted to the brain.

In the 1940s and '50s, the great Canadian neurosurgeon Wilder Penfield began to map the brain in an alarmingly straightforward way. Since the brain itself has no pain receptors, he was able to do surgery on it using local anesthetic. Patients remained conscious. While the brain was exposed, he stimulated particular parts of it with an electrode. Then he asked the patients on the operating table what they felt as he poked about.

What they reported was remarkable—a kind of jump-cut movie that involved feelings, images, and vivid memories. Penfield was like a puppeteer, pulling the strings attached to different parts of their lives. One of the things he discovered was a narrow strip that runs down both sides of the brain and contains a representation of different parts of the body. If he stimulated an area at the top of the brain, the patient felt sensations in his genitals. If he moved the electrode down a bit, the patient then reported a tingling in his feet. What Penfield learned was that different parts of the body—the tongue, the lips, the hands, the genitals, and the face in particular—

have a disproportionately large area of representation in the brain. It was an early version of "brain maps," which now number in the hundreds, and it gave rise to that odd little medical-school character known as the Penfield homunculus.

Students encounter this troll-like figure when they first learn about the somatosensory sites in the brain that correspond to parts of the body. Since the hands and the mouth have the most complex nerve endings for touch, warmth, and pain, they have accordingly large areas in the brain map. But the torso doesn't need to discriminate so finely in its sensations, so it has a smaller area of representation. The resulting Mr. Homunculus (looking a bit like some licensed action figure) has gigantic lips, tiny little arms, and big steam-shovel hands.

From the point of view of phantom limb pain, what was revealing is that the map for the foot is right next to the map for the genitals, and the hand area is adjacent to the area representing the face. This may help explain why sensation in a missing thumb can be triggered by light stroking on the lips; according to some scientists, this is a result of the sensory input migrating from one area of the brain to its neighbor.

The problem of phantom limb pain gets right to the heart of our misunderstanding of how pain works. In the past, we assumed that pain originated in the injured body part. Cut it off, or cut the nerves, and the pain will end. Also, any pain that couldn't be located in the body was a trick of the mind, a delusion, and therefore untreatable. But some researchers in the area of phantom pain— John Dostroevsky and Joel Katz at the University of Toronto, Ronald Melzack at McGill University, and neurologist V. S. Ramachandran at the Center for Brain and Cognition at the University of California in San Diego—have carried out studies that illustrate what Melzack has always argued: Pain is in the brain. "You don't need a body to feel a body," Melzack wrote. "The brain itself can generate every quality of experience which is normally triggered by sensory input."

Melzack agrees that the brain has a map of the body, but he argues that the map is innate and genetic. Otherwise, how could one account for phantom pain in people born without a limb, with no possible "body knowledge" of pain in the missing part? Melzack has studied this phenomenon in 125 people, most of them teenagers, who had either lost a limb before the age of six or were born without a limb. About a quarter of the people missing a limb since birth reported feeling, sometimes vividly, the arm or leg that they had lost. "One woman's phantom arm reached out to prevent a cupboard door from slamming shut and to catch a falling egg," Melzack wrote in a 1998 article in *Discover* magazine.

These findings persuaded him that "the body we perceive is in large part built into our brain—it's not entirely learned." He thinks that a network of neurons forms in the embryonic brain to link up the somatosensory thalamus and cortex (regions that enable us to sense the location of our limbs) and the limbic system, which is involved in feelings of pain and pleasure and is the area that helps us learn from our experiences. These connections prepare the brain to respond to body parts that may not even form.

"The brain needs to have information about what is going to happen to it," says Melzack. "The brain is not just born into the world willy-nilly, waiting for anything to come bombarding in from the senses. It anticipates that it will be getting information from a body that has limbs and other organs, that there will be a mother and two breasts and sources of food. And even if we are missing a part of the body, the brain is still able to generate the perception of that part."

(This observation makes you wonder about conditions that involve persistent distortions of body image, such as anorexia nervosa. Is our body image laid down long before we look into a mirror?)

Melzack called this convergence of connections in the brain the neuromatrix, and attributed to it the totally convincing, detailed, baffling sense of pain in a limb that is no longer there. This is one theory. In truth, nobody knows why or how phantom pain arises. But nothing could illustrate the primacy of the brain in our experience of pain more dramatically than this utterly real, utterly "invented" pain.

The neuromatrix argument is compelling, however, because it

takes pain out of the mechanical, tissue-damage, signal-transmission domain and makes emotions an integral part of pain "wiring." It suggests that cultural attitudes toward pain—the meanings we attribute to pain—can play a profound physiological role in how we feel it. On the one hand, the neuromatrix model may look like another cuts-of-meat, reductionist argument; on the other, it offers a metaphor for what geneticists are discovering about the perception of pain as an inheritable, individual expression. (Melzack writes about each person's "neurosignature.") The concept of a neuromatrix suggests that pain is not an invasive, alien force or a learned response but part of the map of who we are. Pain should not surprise us (a point of view the Buddhists have been teaching for some time).

The neurologist V. S. Ramachandran takes a more . . . neurological view of things, as one might expect. In *Phantoms in the Brain,* his entertaining 1998 book, he describes a number of off-the-wall experiments with people who suffer from phantom pain, where he manages to visually trick the brain into revising its mistaken body image. While his experiments don't offer any practical treatment for phantom pain, they do illustrate just how integrated the experience of pain is with other senses, especially seeing and hearing. (Elaine Scarry reports in her book *The Body in Pain* that forcing their victims to look at the instruments of torture is one of the strategies that torturers use to increase the intensity of the pain.)

Ramachandran's book addresses itself first to the old conundrum of how the brain gives rise to the mind. We know the topography of the brain, but how does the activity of 600 billion neurons define "self"? By looking at a number of odd neurological syndromes, he not only comes up with enticing theories about the "how" of perception, but, in the course of his experiments, finds himself able—temporarily at least—to manipulate the pain intensity and posture of phantom limbs. These involve smoke-and-mirror strategies that Ramachandran reports with boyish enthusiasm, like someone demonstrating his prizewinning science-fair project.

Some women, Ramachandran notes, have reported phantom breasts after radical mastectomy, complete with sensation in phantom nipples. Men who have had the misfortune of losing their penis have reported phantom erections. Ramachandran tells a story of a patient who confided to him that ever since his leg had been amputated from below the knee, he was experiencing strange new sensations whenever he had sex. His orgasm had spread, as it were, to his phantom foot—which, as he pointed out, offered more terrain for sensation. He seemed to enjoy his new, enlarged pedal orgasms, but he wanted to know if they were within the realm of normal phantom behavior. (They were.)

Ramachandran did a simple experiment on a man who had lost his arm and hand below the elbow. Using a Q-tip, he stroked various parts of the man's body. When he touched his cheek and other areas on his face, the man felt the sensation both in his face and in his phantom hand. He could travel from baby finger to index, by slowly moving the Q-tip from one facial area to another. Soon Ramachandran had mapped out the whole hand—on the man's face. The only explanation for this weird correspondence between missing hand and sensations in the face, Ramachandran felt, was the fact that the brain maps for the hand and the face were side by side. ("More Descartes thinking," Melzack humphed when I asked him later about Ramachandran's theories.)

When amputation interrupted signals from the hand, Ramachandran believes, sensory fibers belonging to the face began to invade the "empty" hand area and become active there. Neural colonialism, if you like, or squatters' rights. As he writes, "This finding flatly contradicts one of the most widely accepted dogmas in neurology—the fixed nature of connections in the adult human brain." Contrary to what is taught in textbooks, he continues, "new, highly precise and functionally effective pathways can emerge in the adult brain as early as four weeks after injury."

The brain, formerly thought of as fixed, is capable of change and remapping. This idea of neuroplasticity has emerged only in the last twenty years, and it has far-reaching implications for pain patients and for people with nerve damage from strokes or injury. It means not only that there is a possibility of nerve cells regenerating or invading damaged areas—"like ivy growing over a brick wall," as one doctor put it—but that there may be a built-in redundancy to the brain: When one area conks out, another can kick in.

But how does phantom pain arise? That was still a mystery. The brain cells might make new connections. Or maybe the "volume control mechanisms" involving pain go awry as a result of the remapping. Ramachandran likens it to a wa-wa pedal in the brain that creates a jumbled, echo effect that is eventually perceived as pain. The fact is, he writes, despite our progress in locating what happens where in the brain, "we really don't know how the brain translates patterns of nerve activity into conscious experience, be it pain, pleasure or color." In matters of the brain, *where* is less important than *how*.

Ramachandran found that although he couldn't cure phantom pain, he could sometimes "conduct" the missing limbs. A patient with cancer came to see him with a vivid phantom limb that was doing very strange things. It would sometimes go into a clenching spasm, and nothing could get his phantom hand to open. He even felt phantom fingernails digging into his palm, and it was excruciating.

The neurologist did an experiment using a simple device that involved a vertical mirror in a box with two holes in the front. He had the man put his good arm inside the box on the right side of the mirror and "insert" his phantom on the left. Then he asked his volunteer to use the mirror to superimpose the image of his good right arm on the missing limb. This gave the man the visual impression that his left arm had been restored. Then Ramachandran asked him to clench and unclench his good hand. This, of course, resulted in the image of both hands unclenching. As a result of this visual feedback, the man felt his phantom hand opening up. Not only that, but the pain went away. It stayed away until another spasm arrived, which responded again to the mirror-box exercise. The mirror-box not only gave the image of his hand back to the man, but also erased the pain. Alas, the results faded after a while.

Is body image a mere hallucination then? And is this why one-hundred-pound teenage girls can look in the mirror and still say, "I'm so fat"? Since vision accounts for thirty brain maps itself, and even plays a role in pain perception, the idea of the brain as a collection of fixed "modules" begins to look hopelessly old-fashioned. Ramachandran concluded that "pain is an *opinion* on the organism's state of health rather than a mere reflexive response to an injury. . . . There is so much interaction between different brain centers, like those concerned with vision and touch, that even the mere visual appearance of an opening fist can actually feed all the way back into the patient's motor and touch pathways, allowing him to feel the fist opening, thereby killing an illusory pain in a nonexistent hand."

What we are learning about neuroplasticity suggests that the brain is both site-specific, with certain functions organized in certain areas, and dynamic, with the ability to change and reorganize itself. Far-flung areas of the brain are linked up in such "simple" activities as seeing. And, as Ramachandran's mirror-box proves, even vision can affect the pain we feel. Seeing is not just believing— seeing is feeling, too.

7

HARDWIRING, GENE MAPPING, AND BRAIN IMAGING: DESCARTES NEVER DIES

NEUROSCIENCE AND THE FIELD OF GENETICS have generated two seductive metaphors for how we think about ourselves: We now talk about being "hardwired," and ever since the human genome was decoded, we feel "mapped" as well. V. S. Ramachandran's phantom limb experiments and the appealing notion of a homunculus in the brain—the little man with deformed thumbs who "maps" the body's somatosensory representation—can both be used as more fuel for this new reductionism. More and more, we like to think that the brain has fixed areas where certain messy aspects of being human are rooted. In other words, if something complicated like sexual jealousy arises from a tangle of neurons and amino acids in the amygdala, all we have to do is find the master neuron and tie it off like an artery. This slant on things makes me wonder if Descartes is really dead.

The news is full of such explanations. London cabbies, one item reported, must study three years to acquire The Knowledge—the seventeen thousand higgledy-piggledy routes through the labyrinth of the city. Someone recently went to the trouble of measuring the posterior hippocampi (the hippocampus is the area of the brain related to long-term memory storage) of a number of London cabbies and discovered that they had rather bigger ones than other people. According to Steven Pinker in his book *How the Mind Works,* desert mice who have to cache seeds, and therefore remember where they hid them, also have bigger hippocampi than other mice. (This news makes me want to get a silicon implant for my own hippocampus, so that I can find my car in underground parking lots.)

However, nobody bothered to investigate whether only fellows with overdeveloped hippocampi sought out cabdriving in the first place. This experiment struck me as a slightly more sophisticated version of the once-fashionable nineteenth-century "science" of phrenology. Phrenologists claimed that a person's capacity for love, anger, violence, and other aspects of being human could be read through the bumps, dents, and topography of the skull. They used maps or marble busts of the skulls, targeting avarice here and altruism there, labeled in quadrants like a butcher's guide to a side of beef. These were our first crude brain maps.

Of course, it happens to be the case that reasoning tends to take place in the cerebral cortex and that our sense of smell arises from "older" regions of the brain. Certain functions do arise from particular crannies. For instance, neuroscientists have isolated the part of the brain associated with religious epiphanies. Stimulate this area of the limbic system with an electrode (the left temporal lobe, but don't try this at home), and you can induce the feelings associated with spiritual rapture. But the ability to isolate *where* it happens in the brain in no way explains *why* it happens, or the human longing for some sort of faith. To use another example, one part of the brain, quite distinct from the area that controls speech, is involved in cursing and swearing. This may shed some light on the affliction of Tourette's syndrome, but it doesn't explain why the urge to say "fuck off" seems to be such a deep-rooted part of human nature. Being able to prod this zone and elicit a few curses invites a stimulus-response view of human nature that is not so far from Descartes's naked man with his foot in the flame.

Descartes's view of pain still sounds pretty good—a stimulus that begins at the periphery of the body and travels up to a fixed location in the brain that then translates sensory information into the perception of pain. But in this scenario, the body is demoted to a sort of carnal FedEx. Its role is simply to box and deliver.

But what became "science" began as a speculation rooted in the culture and politics of the time. It's no coincidence that our views of the relationship between mind and body often mirror the politics of the period. In the seventeenth century, the body was the humble servant of reason, a benevolent monarch who acted to protect his people ("Remove our foot from the fire, now!"). Today, we prefer more shifting, democratic, cybernetic models for this relationship: The mind "interacts" rather than simply "orders," and the concept of "neuroplasticity" (the brain as Lava lamp) is gaining ground on the "hardwired" genetic metaphor. But the power structure is still very clear, and it's mind *over* matter.

Cartesian dualism dies hard. The first question that people inevitably ask when they learn that I'm writing about pain is: Do you mean physical or mental pain? It's what David Morris calls "The Myth of Two Pains," and you can hear echoes of it in the hardwired metaphor or in a phrase like "it's all chemistry," to explain just about anything. But this is how we read science, not necessarily how science reads us. As the gene researchers themselves are the first to point out, it's one thing to compile a dictionary and another to write a poem. Mapping the human genome just means that we have the dictionary.

The downside of the hardwiring paradigm is what the philosopher Daniel Dennett has called the Specter of Creeping Exculpation—a growing sense that we're not accountable for who we become. This view suggests that we're mapped from birth, or even at the moment our parents' chromosomes collided, and this genetic blueprint determines whether we fail math or play the violin.

More maps and blueprints are emerging from the hot science of brain imaging, where researchers track the electrical activity in different parts of the brain, sometimes even while the person being "imaged" is conscious. They use an MRI machine to surgically probe a patient's brain with an electrode. This produces a kind of aerial view of "hot spots" where the electrical activity is most intense. A few years ago there was some excitement at the University of Toronto, when a research team announced that they had located the "pain cells." This discovery inevitably suggests that pain cells can be switched off, or surgically removed, leading to a "cure" for pain. Brain imaging can provide information that is invaluable in cases of neurological damage, such as strokes, but it can't corner pain; it's just dusting for fingerprints at the scene of the crime.

Pain scientist Patrick Wall liked to poke fun at the brain imagers. He pointed out that this "fixed" pain center was surprisingly nomadic in mice brains, showing up in one place under certain conditions, then lighting up an entirely different area under others. In other words, there really is a pain center—it just keeps moving around.

Although I don't understand the science involved, I tend to agree with Wall. To be human is to be all over the map, and pain is not going to be reduced to one area of the brain, or to a single aspect of existence. Brain imaging is a closer, more sophisticated picture of Descartes's bell-rope; now we can count the strands. But the music of the bell—the experience each of us calls pain—still eludes our understanding.

Many scientists and geneticists reject this reductionism, too. In *How the Mind Works,* Steven Pinker reminds his readers that any dualistic view of nature versus nurture misses the point. "If the mind has a complex innate structure," he writes, "that does NOT mean that learning is unimportant. Framing the issue in such a way that innate structure and learning are pitted against each other, either as alternatives or, almost as bad, as complementary ingredients or interacting forces, is a colossal mistake. . . . Every part of human intelligence involves culture and learning. But learning is not a surrounding gas or force field, and it does not happen by magic. . . . We need ideas that capture the ways a complex device can tune itself to unpredictable aspects of the world and take in the kinds of data it needs to function." Pinker does resort to mechanical metaphors involving data and tuning devices, but my explanation for this is simple: He's a guy. Nevertheless, he can make the brain sound like the ultimate high-end amplifier and still challenge a dualistic view of how the mind works.

I once ran into Sydney Brenner, a world-famous molecular biologist, at a science conference. He is also a bibliophile and a voracious reader who seems to relish the unpredictable plot created by the four stuttering letters of the genetic code, *ACGT*. But when I glibly referred to the genetic code as a narrative, he corrected me. No, he said, the genetic code is not so much a linear story as a representation, "a description of life, just as the laws of a society are a description of how one ought to behave." The science of genetics is still on page one. In his address to the conference, Brenner said, "We're now like the astronomers who first charted the starry heavens." And we all know that Orion's belt doesn't really look like one.

The most creative scientists respect the limits of their science. They don't confuse mind maps with a description of how consciousness works. But the rest of us long for maps and would rather surrender the issue of pain to science and medicine. That way pain can remain a technical topic beyond our grasp, something best left to the experts. But when we forfeit pain to science, we forget that some of the most diligent cartographers of pain are artists, philosophers, and meditators.

The lure of hardwired thinking is simple: It helps absolve us of social responsibility. If people are programmed to become violent rapists, it's much easier to either lock them up or treat them as helpless victims of their genes. If pain is the result of a single misfiring cell, there is no need to address the relationship between chronic pain and childhood sexual abuse, for instance (which has been shown to exist). And the metaphor of mapping feels authoritative, even when we don't know what we're talking about. Christopher

Columbus did an excellent job of putting San Salvador on the map when he first sailed west. The only problem was that he thought it was India.

A belief in innate structure or an understanding of pain mechanisms in the body doesn't have to diminish the role of environment or culture. I drag in Pinker and Brenner here because I don't want to confuse the new dualism with science itself, only certain areas of it. We're too indoctrinated by three centuries of mind-body terminology to give it up quickly or easily.

The technicians in brain imaging and the gene mappers are providing us with vital new information. But it's only data, and only part of the story. What we can't map are the ways in which family, environment, and politics shape who we become. We exist inside a larger membrane than our own skin—the womb of culture and the values we grow up with feed us in certain ways and starve us in others. The impact of culture may not be felt in the same visceral way as a scalded arm, but it leaves its marks. A father's silence, a mother's disappearance, a country's neglect of its artists, and a political environment of revenge are forces as real as a whipping to the person we become. A thought is a physical event.

How we treat each other as a society eventually becomes part of our chemistry. If we're taught to feel fear when we see someone with a different skin color, that response releases an adrenalized, biochemical brew that, sustained over a period of time, turns into hardwiring, too. ("Anyone who has been tortured, remains tortured," wrote Primo Levi of his time in Auschwitz.)

I have been wondering if this modern Cartesian way of thinking is creating a new version of the mind-body split. Now the "mind" is this bio-neuro-geneto-cognitive creature—complex to be sure, but more and more predictable. And the "body" is culture itself, a Cartesian mechanism whose role is to deliver the goods. The environment still has the status of the messenger that tweaks and stimulates and prods the motherboard of the mind. Our relation to the physical environment and our ability to neglect it for so long demonstrate the sense that this larger body that we inhabit is "not us." And as long as we prefer living in our neo-Cartesian world of maps and hardwiring, we will be hiding from what pain could tell us about ourselves.

In his book *Pain: The Science of Suffering,* Patrick Wall puckishly reported that Descartes's tombstone had the inscription "*Bene qui latuit, bene vixit*" ("He who hid well, lived well"). What was he hiding? René must have known—intuited?—more than he was saying.

I SEE AN UPSIDE to the hardwiring metaphor, however. To suggest that something like shyness is genetically hardwired is at least an admission that we aren't meat puppets animated by a more ethereal consciousness. The ghost in the machine doesn't describe us anymore. As poet and songwriter Leonard Cohen put it, "Your body is really, really, really you."

The other helpful term that brain research has thrown up in terms of defining ourselves is *neuroplasticity.* We change. Brains change. We now know that the brain is capable of radical reorganization and even cell regeneration. If a stroke damages one part of the brain, other areas are capable of pinch-hitting for the lost cells. The more mapped we become, the more we also need to acknowledge how exquisitely responsive our blueprints are to the experience of living in the world.

This is taken for granted in other fields. We know how crucial the first three years of child rearing are to the development of intelligence. We know that children thrive only when they receive human warmth and love. In the same way, society either nourishes or stunts. Ideas enter us like nutrients—or toxins—in the water supply.

The "psychoanalytical century" may be over, but it is worth remembering that Freud began as a biologist. He brought a biologist's taxonomic urge to his exploration of the unconscious, and his inquiry into human behavior proceeded along formal rational lines. And now, our preoccupation with the psychological, and with Freudian notions of the subconscious, the unseen, the unmappable, has circled back to a renewed emphasis on biology, neurochemistry, and genetic research. We have become highly trained, sophisticated phrenologists, reading the bumps and dents on the human genome.

Descartes's error was to imagine that the mind was the master of the body, and that messages flew up, but not down or back and forth. The raw meat of reason had yet to be explored. Melzack and Wall's work on pain demonstrated that the reign of pain is mainly in the brain. This shed a whole new light on the phrase "all in your mind." When a doctor used to tell a patient suffering inexplicable pain that it was all in his head, it was a dismissal of his pain as something imagined—and therefore unreal. This suspicion toward chronic pain conditions is still strong among patients, their families, and their doctors.

But for decades now, science has been telling us that pain is in the brain—and that the imagination (for lack of a better word) can amplify or suppress our experience of pain. So pain really is "all in the mind." We got the phrase right, but our understanding of it was muddled.

Pain will never come down to a matter of nerves, chemicals, and tissues. Pain is also made of time and the echo of one's earliest injuries and trauma. As the sufferers of post-traumatic stress syndrome understand all too vividly, abuse and torture can become hardwired, too. The body's memory is detailed, and unforgiving.

Fixed systems no longer make any sense. The fact is, we are hardwired to be endlessly fluid, plastic, and adaptable social creatures. The more we map, the more we dissolve into ceaseless circuits of change. Brain imaging won't fix pain, but it will contribute to the ability of science to target drugs to certain areas of the brain. More detailed genetic monitoring will allow us to tailor medication to the individual, rather than clobber everyone with one-size-fits-all pharmaceuticals. Analgesics will be titrated according to age, gender, and genetic characteristics—as they should be. Our current system of dispensing drugs will come to look as barbaric as trepanning and leeching (but then, leeching is back).

And more and more, science will connect with the traditional experts in the unpredictable, the painful, and the unmappable—

artists. As the gap between mind and body narrows, thanks to science's deeper understanding of the biochemistry of our behavior and the popular swing toward alternative forms of healing, the distance between science and the arts will shrink as well. It's not a matter of either/or. It's and/and from here on in.

Why this whirlwind tour of the way science has mapped and remapped us? Because pain, in its refusal to be reduced to either wiring or "psychosocial factors," keeps us honest in our exploration of identity. Brain imaging and gene mapping capture our imagination now because they give us detailed information; they offer a close reading of the very stuff of life. But we still don't know how to assess the health of the body's second skin, our culture—the world of family, love, art, commerce, and all the bruises and caresses that culminate in who we are. The paradox that science, and the rest of us, now has to accept is that we're both hardwired and endlessly in revision.

8

A BACK STORY

I'M A SLIGHTLY CROOKED PERSON, THANKS to a bit of scoliosis in my back, which is why any kind of pain tends to run, like bilge water, toward one side of my body. Correcting my crookedness has always been on my "to do" list, so when I saw a bulletin-board notice for a "Feldenkrais Back Pain Workshop," I signed up. I didn't have back pain, but I knew that Feldenkrais addressed body alignment. It also turned out to be a roomful of great bad-back stories.

Feldenkrais, like the Alexander Technique, makes you think about how you move or hold your body. Through a series of gentle, precise exercises, it tries to correct damaging postures and habits. Developed in 1957 by a physicist and mechanical engineer, Dr. Moshe Feldenkrais, it's supposed to work not just on the muscles and joints but on the brain and nervous system, too. Good. I felt I could do with a brain gym.

Marion Harris, a long-established Feldenkrais teacher in Toronto, is a rather glamorous older woman, not the typical mascara-free "bodyworker." The session was held in her high and bright studio lined with mirrors, so the crooked can view their crookedness. Most of the women were assorted middle-aged leotard-clad shapes, except for one flexible, fit young woman, Debbie. And it was Debbie, it turns out, who had the most horrible back story of all—four years of schlepping from expert to expert while back pain whittled her life down to zero. But something had obviously worked for her—she was very bendable now. She agreed to meet after class to tell me her story.

Debbie is a former paramedic. She was walking home from her job one winter night when she slipped on a patch of ice on the sidewalk and did a cartoon flip onto her back.

"It was a good fall—it knocked the wind out of me," she said. "Some people saw me go down and rushed over to help."

Debbie is slim and has a pretty, angular face and straight chin-length blond hair. Before her fall, she was "super-athletic," she said, working out six days a week for two hours a day. At thirty-two, she had just finished her training as a paramedic, a job she loved, and was looking forward to her career. Life was ticking along nicely.

"The fall was no big deal. I thought I'd be sore for a few days, and that would be it. I mean, I was in *really* good shape. I laid off working out for a week or so and waited for the pain to go away. My lower back was sore, and my shoulder hurt a little, too."

As she told me this, Debbie's attitude was bemused, as if she still couldn't fathom what this little tumble on the ice had done to her life.

"When the pain didn't get better, I went to a physiotherapist. She pushed me to do all these exercises that hurt me and didn't help at all. I began to worry about my job; you have to lift people and move them around as a paramedic. You need strength.

"Everybody started giving me advice. Some would say, 'All you need is rest.' So I tried doing nothing, and that didn't help. Then I went to that institute," she said, her green eyes turning flinty.

"The famous back place, run by the famous back doctor?" I asked.

"Yes, and if I see him, I am going to kill him. They told me to 'work through the pain.' I knew it didn't feel good, but I forced myself, and what they gave me to do hurt me. They insisted they knew what was wrong with me. They called it 'mechanical back pain' and said I had to push through the pain.

"But I'm not a coward. I know how to work out. I stuck it out for three months and by the end, my pain was the same—excruciating, constant, a seven and a half out of ten."

Debbie seemed to be balanced and credible in every way, but at a certain point in listening to anybody's pain story, doubt creeps in. Instead of focusing on what doctors don't know about backs, you start to wonder what the person is doing wrong. Is this the story of one unlucky fall and its consequences, I thought, or just the latest drama in someone's neurotic relationship to pain? But this is what pain does: It makes people doubt themselves, and it has the same effect on anyone who hears their stories.

Debbie was furious at the medical treatment she had received. All the experts she saw told her they could definitely help, and none did. She spent four years in severe pain.

"I tried a chiropractor. He used that TENS thing on me— transcutaneous electrical nerve stimulation. That made it worse."

What about her GP, I asked. Was anybody guiding you through this maze of therapy?

"Oh, I liked my GP, and she kept referring me to new people. She was sympathetic, but basically she didn't know how to help me."

Didn't you have anyone, I asked.

"I had a boyfriend." Slight eyebrow arch. "I did notice that driving in the car with him really aggravated the pain. We would have these fights in the car all the time, about how he drove." They broke up a few months after the fall, though she thinks "the pain was a separate issue."

I asked about her family. She laughed, sort of.

"Well, my mother basically thought that if I got a *real* boyfriend and had two children, my pain would go away. She thought it was all in my head!" She waved her hand, as if shooing a fly away.

"The doctors I saw couldn't find anything physiological at all, but my pain continued. The only thing that seemed to help was

Advil. I tried various medications, but I hated the side effects, and they didn't really work. From time to time, I would panic. What if this doesn't go away, I thought. How will I work? How will I take care of myself? At that stage, the high point of my day was going to bed and sleeping. When I *could* sleep. The advice I was getting from people began to drive me bananas. . . . Everybody thought they knew what back pain was, but they didn't. Nobody knew what I was going through. I wasn't able to work out or do my job full-time—my life was awful."

She gave the back institute another whirl, doing everything to the letter this time. Nothing changed. She consulted a rheumatologist.

"And you know, all these appointments take a long time, months, to set up. Basically, when you're in this kind of pain, you wait and you wait and you wait, and you hope and you hope and you hope. And each doctor has these set ideas about what is wrong with you.

"I tried a private pain clinic, too. I had to wait six months for that appointment, and then I spent four hours in the waiting room. I'm not exaggerating," she said. "I wrote it down. It was four hours. The doctor gave me an injection of some local anti-inflammatory, and the pain got worse after that. I gave that up, but not before having a big fight with him. Which is not like me. I yelled at him. I even wrote a letter to the College of Physicians and Surgeons. *Then* I went to an oncologist to see if I had bone cancer! Which I didn't. He did tell me that I'd be better in six months, and at least that eased my mind."

People in pain get used to shutting up about it, lest they bore you. So when they get a chance to tell their story, it all comes out, complete and pressurized. There was no self-pity in her report, just incredulity.

"I had CT scans and bone scans. Did acupuncture, took herbs for three months. Got a massage from an osteopath that nearly killed me. By this point I was sure I had some terrible disease. And the scans did show wear and tear on the vertebrae. I was also starting to isolate myself. I didn't want to have fun. I didn't want to go out with people because no one really . . . got it. There was no one supportive in my life at the time.

"At this point, I was obsessed—the pain dominated my entire life. I didn't just want to sit around and talk about it with people, I wanted to get better! I started to think there was something wrong with me emotionally. My mother certainly agreed." She laughed. "I liked my GP, though. I would go to her and cry my eyes out. I had given up the idea of being a paramedic and had to take a more sedentary office job, in telecommunications.

"Despite all this, I had a new boyfriend, and we went on a trip to France. I made appointments with a couple of elite doctors there, who said the usual things and gave me even stronger medication. The Europeans are good for that! By then I wasn't sleeping well. I could *see* the pain in my face, and I was barely able to take care of myself. Most people get around to fixing up their apartment or whatever, but I just didn't. I let things go. I think I was depressed at this point and didn't know it."

A lot of people, I said, would have been depressed a lot faster.

"Then my GP suggested I check out yoga, which I did. It calmed me a bit, but I couldn't maintain it. By April or May of 1998, I hit my low point. I couldn't hide it anymore; a day at work was too much. I went into my boss, who knew nothing about all this, and basically broke down in his office. He was incredibly supportive and told me to take whatever time I needed.

"Finally, as a last resort, I went to see Marion," she said, referring to our Feldenkrais teacher.

"So you clicked with her," I said.

"No, Marion keeps her distance. She's not the touchy-feely type. Her approach is that your body can heal itself, you just need to give it a chance. Plus, I was really hostile at this point! I was mad at all the doctors I'd seen and tired of being disappointed over and over. I didn't want to get too hopeful about anything. But after the first week of classes, something amazing happened. I began to sleep at night. For two whole weeks I could sleep—which was staggering for me.

"The other good thing about taking Feldenkrais was that I started meeting people who understood what I was going through. And Marion was asking me to practice acceptance instead of fighting the pain and hoping to be fixed. That seemed to help.

"I went twice a week to classes and then did fifteen minutes of exercises a day, and by the end of three months, I was pain-free. I had to take a four-hour flight to Calgary, and I was dreading it, but it was fine. I even went hiking in Banff."

A happy ending, for once. There's no way to determine whether Feldenkrais in particular was the key, or if the inner focus it encourages—taking responsibility for getting better—came along at just the right time. Self-directed therapies like Feldenkrais work best when the person in pain is fed up with doctors and ready to throw in the towel. They no longer expect to be cured. That's where Debbie was when she gave Marion a shot.

"I have a measure of control now. If I do the exercises and take care of myself, I can expect to be pain-free. Occasionally I slip up, or if I get really busy at my job, it will flare up. Whenever I experience that old level of pain, even briefly, I cannot *imagine* how I lived with it. But I did."

She looks happy now or, at least, in line for happiness. It's as if every day that doesn't include her old pain already has this rapturous aspect. And she has learned something most people don't know when they are young.

"I was in excruciating pain for years. I lost my job, my security, and my identity. It has changed the way I look at people. Now I know what that kind of pain can do to someone."

9

PAIN AS A BORE

PEOPLE TALK ABOUT THEIR CHRONIC PAIN as if ratting on the other partner in an unhappy, toxic marriage. They fall out with their pain, they have screaming fights with it, they make up again. Or they try to run away with some attractive little analgesic. But pain has their cell-phone number and won't let them escape. Living with chronic pain can be a grinding form of intimacy.

I thought I was over my Munchausen tendencies, but for the past few days I seem to have come down with someone's else pain again. Not mine, surely. My body has been aching everywhere: head, neck, legs, feet, hips. A whole-body migraine. It feels like being trapped across a dinner table from a bore. The coffee is cold. Everyone else has gone home. Pain just drones on and on.

Tonight, Pain is wearing a greenish wool Roger Ebert V-necked sweater under a slightly too small sports jacket. "Have you noticed how incredibly tight your back is?" Pain says to me, gnawing away on a drumstick. "And by the way, I hope the sofa bed is made up, because obviously I'm not going anywhere tonight." Pain then talks about his car, a Ford Taurus, and how he feels about power windows.

"Oh, and the way the tendons up and down your spine audibly pop and crack when you lean over to weed the garden," he says, wiping a smear of grease off his chin. "That's definitely getting worse. I can hear them from yards away." I say nothing and toy with the stem of my wineglass.

"Plus check out that constant, low-grade morning headache—it's like a stain, isn't it, the way it just keeps spreading." I nod bleakly. Pain is dragging a french fry through a blob of mayonnaise in a saucer. "This little minimigraine of yours has been gathering density and weight now for, what, three days? It's worse in the morning, of course, because you refuse to stop drinking red wine with dinner." I empty my glass and glower at him. "In fact, the more I nag you to stop, the more you insist on two glasses instead of one, or three, and then you feel bad in the morning. It's a pain-pain situation."

Pain has polished off the chicken and is now picking his teeth with the shish-kebab skewer.

"So now the muscles down the back of your neck have turned into concrete columns, rigid little flying buttresses of pain. And it's your fault, isn't it, for not tending to my minions of misery right at the beginning. You thought you could ride through it. You forgot! Migraines are like tax auditors—sooner or later, they will track you down and make you pay."

He is right about that.

"Let me guess: This particular headache is one of those faintly nauseating, low-grade ones that never quite peaks, it just simmers along. I could tell by that Pekinese furrow in your brow when you opened the door. My dear, you look so pinched and drained. It really does add years! But what is it you always say? 'Just let time pass.' Although when you're in pain—when you're on my turf—time just drip-drip-drips along, doesn't it?" He gets up and clatters the blinds shut.

As usual, Pain has a point. My headache is not the sort that drives me mercifully back to bed, not the obliteration of a full-blown migraine. No, it is woven into the texture of my day, accompanied by wavelets of nausea and a jittery sense of having been skinned. Too much light, too much noise, too many people.

But the headache must be tended to, like a yapping dog. And you can't blame the dog. It's the owner's fault. My headaches have not been trained properly and now they run roughshod over my day.

Pain flicks cigar ash in my saucer and prattles on.

"Now, this morning, as you left the house, didn't I hear you literally *groaning* when you got into the car? There you were, massaging your hip as you drove—fat lot of good that will do! And the headache, in its third day, is like a tight bathing cap, and that feeling in the shoulders, like violin strings being wound tighter. Which reminds me . . . when you played the violin the other night, what a *dreadful* sound you made. Thin and mean, just like me! I was so proud. To get between you and music—that's progress. And as you well know, the violin never lies. It amplifies whatever state you're in: in this case, blocked, congested, and defeated."

Pain exhales a wreath of pungent smoke and smiles.

"You're locked up like Houdini, babe—and I've got the keys."

Damn. He is quite attractive, when his mouth is shut. As usual I feel obscurely appalled by my relationship with Pain. It brings with it a kind of shame, as if you are cheating on life itself. Tuned in to your own pain, other people irritate you with their blithe openness. The happy are louts. Walled off by your pain, you feel unloving and stingy. Why can't you get over or around this wall? If you just try harder, surely you can rise above it. But after a certain point, like a child having a tantrum, the body in pain can't be cajoled or reasoned with. Then it's not the severity of the pain that requires attention, but the story behind it that demands to be heard.

Pain draws a chalk outline around you, as if to say that any sense of connection with someone, any self-forgetting ecstasy, is a lie. No, what is true (Pain argues) is that you're alone in this body, feeling its borders and contours as a constant, mild, and grievous ache. Pain electrifies the fence between you and the rest of the world.

This sensation isn't one of self-pity, but of cool, irrefutable fact.

The pain feels like a boring bit of death lodged in you like a splinter, and it has to be worked out. Which can only begin to happen when you stop trying to overcome it. Pain demands submission.

"You know, I feel like a single-malt tonight," Pain says, just when I am longing to go upstairs to bed. "Do you mind?"

I go to the liquor cupboard to root around for the single-malt. I haven't had any for years because . . . it gives me a headache! As I'm looking among dusty bottles of holiday rum and sweet liqueurs, I recognize a pattern to the week that has just ended. I had gone from a high to a low. Five days ago I was happy. I had finished a piece of writing that had been bugging me for a year. It was off my desk, and the sense of relief was enormous. I went to a friend's fortieth birthday party, where we drank sangria. I made some music with some other, better musicians. They played the blues, slowly.

The next morning the headache began—part hangover, part the inevitable migrainish down spiral that happens when I stop writing and the deluded nova blast of optimism cools down. I can feel something falling in me like mercury in a thermometer. I lose ground, literally. I begin to feel jittery, weird, and disembodied. Even on a slow night, the TV news makes me weepy.

Whenever this happens, I know some chemical in me is ebbing. Some hoodlum neurotransmitter. All I can do is sit tight and wait it out. It will pass. Chores help, but writing is out of the question. I'm befogged.

Is this depression? I think so, or at least the outskirts of it. It's as if I go from being in a warm, well-lit house to a dark and drafty one. And this is when I start to feel rattled and achy, wrapped in a skein of low-grade pain, not to mention vulnerable to slights and the blunt, obnoxious confidence of the material world. Stores full of shiny things unsettle me, crowds make me think I'm going to topple over, lunch with a friend is a matter of putting things in my mouth and trying to focus on what she says. I mean, I function. In between are glimpses of release, seconds when I think, Yes, I'll make it. I won't die of this immateriality.

What is left is this muscular brown river of dull pain that moves through me, sluggishly, while the rest of the world recedes.

In this dissociative state, the pain alone assures me that I'm here, I can feel—that, in fact, I can't stop feeling.

So Pain isolates me, but keeps me company, too. Everything that found such an intense connection in someone else or something else a few days before coils back in on itself. How sordid it must feel to be hostage to Pain all the time.

All I can do in this state is go through the rosary of the places I hurt: behind my eyes, in my neck, down my aching legs, and in the bottom of my feet, with their rigid arches. It's as if a few days before, I was one of those snow globes, with glittery bits floating up, suspended in a buoyant medium. Now all that has fallen to the bottom of me. It's as if I've literally sunk into my feet and contracted there—a homunculus in a tight curl.

I exaggerate, slightly. It's not the immobility of deep depression. Whenever these biochemical episodes arrive, I can carry on as usual. Make my calls—in a lusterless monotone, if necessary. Work a little, cook dinner, joke with my family. Life goes on. But I know that for a few days there, feeling good, I had the current with me. Then depression came along and it was all upstream again. It's not so out of the ordinary; one in ten go through this.

Back at the dinner table, I pour another big shot for Mr. Big Shot across from me, and one for myself. He is fond of certain phrases like "Be that as it may" and "Hel-lo? I don't *think* so." Now Pain is telling me about an online source for cheap printer ink, and why was I so foolish as to pay full price? It's this bully aspect of him that I dislike the most. But I notice something odd. As soon as I give in and accept that Pain isn't going to leave, I instantly begin to feel better. Less cornered. I take a deep breath. All in good time, I tell myself as he goes on about his dog (a pit bull called Juggs, short for jugular). Pain keeps up his braying monologue, and at last I fall asleep.

10

ALICE

FOR A WHILE, THESE PAIN-AND-DEPRESSION bouts made me wonder if I was developing fibromyalgia (along with shingles). I knew a friend, a most vital woman, who had recently been diagnosed with this modern blight, and she had used the same phrase, a "whole-body migraine," to describe the pain of a fibromyalgia flare-up. I arranged to meet her. In the meantime I waded into the voluminous and contradictory literature on the subject.

Fibromyalgia is one of the best examples of the black-sheep status of many chronic pain conditions: It is invisible; no one knows what causes it; no clear treatment for it exists; it is not life-threatening; and it can derail your life in almost every important way. Some doctors consider it a "wastebasket syndrome"—something they diagnose when every other legitimate condition has been eliminated. Others consider it the second most common rheumatic disorder, after osteoarthritis. While doctors and researchers argue about whether it's a disease, an autoimmune disorder, or the fuzzy constellation of symptoms known as a syndrome, millions of people—mostly women—live with the reality of it.

A whole rainbow of complaints, from digestive disturbances to chemical sensitivities, is associated with fibromyalgia, but the main symptom is muscular pain. It can be stiff, aching, stabbing, or burning, over the whole body. Fatigue and disrupted sleep patterns are an important part of the disorder as well, and some researchers have speculated that whatever it is that undermines sleep may also trigger the syndrome. REM sleep is essential for the production of the hormones that control the release of endorphins, substance P (one of the body's own painkilling substances), and serotonin—all of which relate to mood as well as pain.

Concentration and memory problems are common with fibromyalgia, and more than half of the people who have been diagnosed with the condition have a history of depression. What causes fibromyalgia is still a mystery, but it sometimes develops after an accident, injury, or viral infection. Often, though, it just turns up, usually in women between the ages of twenty and fifty. It's unpopular with doctors, because the symptoms are all over the map, and it can only be managed (with antidepressants and exercise, among other things), not fixed.

In the 1980s and early '90s, fibromyalgia was often lumped in with chronic fatigue syndrome, but these are now thought to be two separate disorders. Allergies, irritable bowel syndrome, insomnia, and sensitivity to noise and light can all be part of the fibromyalgia picture. But a rheumatologist will look for four main symptoms to make a diagnosis: sleep disturbances, fatigue, eighteen designated tender points on the body, and muscle pain.

Well, that counts me out, I thought. I sleep too well. My husband claims that I look young because most people my age have logged more waking hours than I have. But I was slightly disappointed not to have a label, some reassurance that these aches and passing brain fogs were not just a neurotic response to ordinary life. One wants a meaning and a name for one's pain. Other people may see it as a sentence, but arriving at a diagnosis of fibromyalgia almost came as a relief for Alice.

ALICE ARRIVES FOR OUR lunch wearing a bright red coat and a black scarf. She is a writer, a teacher, and the editor of several volumes of journals by the great romantic writer Elizabeth Smart, author of *By Grand Central Station I Sat Down and Wept*. I remembered seeing Alice at a party years ago, dancing in a red dress. She's full of vitality—except when she isn't. Fifty-one, blond, and athletic, she has a fine-featured face that gives her a passing resemblance to Virginia Woolf. There's nothing wan about her, no clue that in the past she had lost years to serious episodes of depression (including two hospitalizations) or that sometimes she must lie low for days on the couch. Bouts of debilitating pain come and go. The week I met her for lunch was a good week.

I remembered running into Alice during a down time. She had just moved to Toronto from the west, where she had acquired a Ph.D., taught English, published poetry, and been involved in a long, rocky relationship with a man. After years of conflict over various potential identities—academic? poet? editor?—she made some choices (or at least made moves that turned into choices). She left the relationship in Vancouver and came east to teach at the University of Toronto. She bought her own house and eventually embarked on a live-in relationship with a new man, which lasted five years before they parted. Now she lives alone and enjoys it. Fibromyalgia has set certain limits for her, but in other ways it has allowed her to stop chastising herself for "not coping," and to enjoy new pleasures—gardening, friends, yoga, solitude, reading, and writing fiction. She teaches only once a week. She doesn't think of herself as a writer any longer, but the private writing continues. A diagnosis for her health helped her rethink her work and reclaim a creative life.

After lunch we went back to her house in east end Toronto to continue our conversation. It's a gabled "worker cottage," a peaceful and feminine spot. The light streamed into the living room from the back garden, and her two cats, clearly spoiled, swished against my legs as Alice went looking for her cigarettes. (She has since quit.)

"Oh, God, I remember now. They're in the fridge."

"Why in the fridge?"

"I just started up again. It helps me cut down to keep them in the fridge."

"Why did you start again?"

"No discipline," she said, although her garden and workroom suggested otherwise. "Plus, I need a few pleasures."

"What are the other ones?"

"A glass of red wine now and then. Reading, listening to music. And my cats. I adore my cats."

Alice was the close friend of a mutual friend, and someone I saw perhaps twice a year. Her friendship with the fierce and unruly Elizabeth Smart, a romantic who paid a big price for her passion, said a great deal about her, I thought. Alice had always struck me as someone with a similar appetite for life who for one reason or another sat apart from the banquet. She could be passionately negative about certain things, registering a visceral horror toward people or books she couldn't abide. But there was an aliveness to her resistance. The edge and appetite are still there (no eerie Paxil implacability), but she seems to have found a measure of calm now. I asked her how she came to be diagnosed with fibromyalgia.

"I STARTED TO FIGURE it out in the middle of a deep depression, when I felt too bad to exercise. I've always been a runner—I started running when I was in my twenties and used to do ten kilometers as a matter of course. For the first time, I stopped running. I just couldn't do it."

"Were you in physical pain, too?"

"Yes! I would get up in the morning stiff, with headaches, and think—Oh, I've been exercising too much. And headaches have always been part of my life, anyway. But in the middle of this terrible depression—I ended up being hospitalized—I realized that I was also having a lot of physical pain. The term I use is 'migraine of the body.' It was like my whole body was on fire."

"Did you tell anybody?"

"No," she said, laughing. "I was too depressed! Then one night I tripped going up the stairs and twisted my ankle so badly that I stayed in bed. It took a lot longer to get better than it should have.

All of me hurt. I eventually went to my doctor, described the pain, and she said, 'Well, you really shouldn't be feeling that much pain at this point.' I realized that since I had stopped exercising, the pain had increased. But at that point I had never heard the word *fibromyalgia*.

"I was in therapy, and my psychiatrist insisted I go see this guy at the university teaching hospital who does a clinic for depressives. I think he saved my life. He didn't care about the pain, he cared about the depression. I had been through about two years of trying various antidepressants, and he wanted to try me on this new high-serotonin one, Effexor. I took it, and after a while, I started to feel better. The depression was lifting. I was thinking, Isn't this marvelous? I was even thinking about doing some work—but this pain kept traveling around, from my back to my neck.

"So I went back to my doctor, and she sent me to a rheumatologist. I think I had seen him for ten minutes, and he said, 'This is classic.' He examined me, went boom, boom, boom, boom, down these points on my body, and everywhere he touched I went, ouch, ouch, ouch. He said, 'It's fibromyalgia, but if you want a backup diagnosis, go see somebody else.' "

I was getting used to these multiple-doctor narratives. The average seems to be five or six visits before people in pain run into someone who knows anything about it.

"I did see another doctor, and he asked me a lot of questions about sleep. Now, anybody who's known me will tell you that I'm the most neurotic person in the world about sleep—basically can't sleep, don't sleep, don't like to sleep—unless I'm depressed. Then I sleep during the day. . . . Anyway, he sent me off to a sleep specialist, who explained the link between sleep disruption and fibromyalgia. Next, I saw Dr. Bombardier here in Toronto, a rheumatologist who is also a fibromyalgia expert. She explained how sleep problems prevent you from going into the stage known as restorative sleep. That's when all the serotonin is produced, and the endorphins, and growth hormones . . . so I finally had this profile and a diagnosis. I was this person with fibromyalgia.

"Suddenly, everything from the past started falling into place. I had always been known as the little-princess-and-the-pea at home—I had to have the best bed and have things dark and quiet. Everything had to be arranged around my 'sleep disabilities.' So I began to ask, 'Well, why *can't* I sleep?'

"And this doctor asked if I had had any kind of trauma in my life. I said, 'Well . . . when I was a teenager there was this . . . sort of abuse.' . . . I mean, you know, in the scheme of things, considering what other women have gone through—" She pulled her hair back off her face, then let it go. "Okay, if you want to put it on a tally sheet of one to ten, it would be about a four. It was nothing—I mean, yes, it affected me, and yes, I had to work to fix it.

"But the more obvious trauma was a car accident I was in when I was sixteen. I lost the hearing in one ear, and I lost two friends, one of them a boyfriend, in the accident. After that I suffered terrible fits of dizziness for about two years. I think that loss—his name was Blake—I think the loss of him affected me quite badly. And I think I repressed it.

"A decade later, when I started to unravel, I realized how much the accident had affected me. What I still have problems with is understanding the connection between all that and the physical pain. I mean, physically, I have this superwoman side—apart from this fibro business and depression, I have been almost overly healthy. I don't get flus and colds or viruses that other people are stricken by.

"So in one respect I was very strong but also overly sensitive to light, sound, and to pain. Irritable bowel syndrome, migraines—the whole fibro profile is totally clear now.

"When I was first diagnosed, I tried it out on a couple of people. One friend said, 'Well, that's all in the mind, you know, you just have to get a grip, find a good therapist, and work it out.' But I'd *done* all that. I *had* worked on it.

"Right now, I'm free of depression"—she knocked on the wooden table beside her—"and back to exercising. I'm stiff and sore when I get up in the morning, but it doesn't really cause me problems. I live with it. But if I overexert myself, put myself through something tense, or stop sleeping, then I'm subject to flare-ups. Before, I could never predict when it would happen. Now, when it happens, it means three days on the couch, unable to move. I can barely walk up the stairs—it's total misery. But I know the flare-ups last three to five days, so I'm okay with it. I get down, but so far I don't get depressed. I can deal with the physical pain."

Which is worse, I asked—fibromyalgia or depression?

"Oh, depression!" she said gaily. "Having experienced both excruciating depression and excruciating physical pain, I'll take the physical pain any day—as long as I know it's going to be over in three to five days. It's finite. With depression, there have been periods when I've lost five years at a time. Five years, before I could have a life again. Five years before I could think, talk, socialize—it's the scariest thing in the world.

"I still see my psychiatrist every other week, and now I find I dream about depression. I dream that I am immobilized by depression—it's so visceral. It's like I'm not really there. Then when I wake up, I'm *so thankful* not to be in it! It's always there—and when I slip, and go down a bit, I think, Oh my God—am I going to stay here? So far, it's just been a few down days. Winters are hard. Everybody has those ups and downs. But when they happen to me, I get panicky. I could get lost in it.

"I now think of depression as pain. It's a kind of living death, a nonfeeling that is its own sort of agony. The problem was, I always knew exactly how *dead* I was, how my mind had shut down. There was still this consciousness of what I was losing. Everybody who is depressed is aware of what they've lost. That's the real hell of it. I remember the last depression I was in—the physical pain, when it was really intense, was almost welcome. I could focus on it. There is almost an exquisite quality to it."

We took a break to talk about the Literary Depressed: Virginia Woolf, Samuel Johnson, Lucy Maud Montgomery, William Styron, and on and on. So many writers. If they're not drunk, they're mad; if they're not mad, they're depressed. Some, like Andrew Solomon, the author of a recent study of depression called *The Noonday Demon*, come to feel a certain gratitude toward their affliction. "I would rather feel the pain of sorrow any day than to lose the capacity to feel at all," writes Solomon. Being exiled from pain—the preferred status in our culture—might, in the end, be more costly than the capacity to live with it.

Alice went into her office to find me a copy of Woolf's first novel, *The Voyage Out,* which has long passages on Woolf's own depression, filtered through the consciousness of her character, Rachel Vincrace. She opened it to a passage, and I read:

" 'She shut her eyes and the pulse in her head beat so strongly that each thump seemed to tread upon a nerve, piercing her forehead with a little stab of pain. . . . [T]he recollection of what she had felt, or of what she had been doing and thinking three days before, had faded entirely. On the other hand, every object in the room, and the bed itself, and her own body with its various limbs and their different sensations were more and more important each day. She was completely cut off, and unable to communicate with the rest of the world, isolated alone with her body.' " The physical sensation, the altered time, the tyranny of pain, the isolation—all there, in one easy paragraph. This is the sort of case study that medical students should be reading, I thought.

"But I think the most painful thing I can remember about being depressed," Alice said, "was waking in the morning and having to face the day. It was like . . . waiting for time to pass, until you could go back to bed again. Now, I hate to go to sleep—it seems like such a waste of time. But I used to crawl up to bed at nine, desperate for unconsciousness."

Fibromyalgia hasn't yet acquired the status of a disease; it's officially known as a syndrome, a cluster of symptoms under one name. Until science determines whether it's an autoimmune disorder, a neurological condition, or something else with a genetic basis (there is evidence that a predilection to fibro is inherited), it will remain slightly suspect. Some critics of the syndrome school think that fibromyalgia and chronic fatigue should not be treated as diagnoses at all. Medical labels, they argue, only attract the whiners and complainers who want some sort of validation for their vague malaise. One doctor believes that fibromyalgia is not a medical condition at all, but a narrative. It's what people use to describe something they can't control in their lives. (The only problem with this view is that our preferred narratives still end up being heavily pathological: She's manic-depressive. He's obsessive-compulsive. They're recovering alcoholics. We're social phobics. Self-diagnosis is not much better.) I asked Alice what she thought about the antisyndrome argument.

"Oh, I loved having a diagnosis," said Alice. "When the first rheumatologist saw me, he said, 'Well, I have good news and bad news. The good news is that it's fibromyalgia, and it's not life-threatening. The bad news is you could be totally disabled by it.' " We both laughed.

"For me, the diagnosis allowed me to accept myself and my limits. I no longer had to see myself as this crazy, neurotic woman. Okay, I'm fifty-one and it's not great that I have this syndrome. It's real, I can't help having it. But I *can* accommodate it and deal with it."

"So what did you do?"

"I started reading about it, and there I was, in the literature. This was me. For a year, I went to a support group. I even went on a three-day fibromyalgia weekend, but I left early. I just couldn't see myself as a middle-aged, disabled woman in a wheelchair, or with a cane. I couldn't identify with them.

"For me, the answer is exercise, although it's very tricky. Too much, and I get a flare-up. But if I go three days without doing some kind of physical exercise, I might get into trouble, too. My regimen now is two days of running about three kilometers, and yoga three times a week.

"The thing about yoga is the stilling of the mind. I have one of these minds that will not settle. For me, it's been a real revelation, learning how to breathe, how to settle down. So I'm religious about yoga. I'm religious about nothing, except yoga! I do it once a week in a group, and here, on my own. I have a tape. I love it. So I think for anybody who has fibro—which has so much to do with sleep and the mind—yoga is probably essential."

"Do you think people are generally in more chronic pain now than in the past?"

"I don't know. Maybe this is just our word for what used to be called rheumatism or neurasthenia. . . ."

"Don't you think it's possible that these chronic pain conditions may come about partly as a result of the long-standing split between mind and body in medicine, and that now our bodies are finding ways, sometimes painful ways, to force a reintegration?"

"That's interesting, because my therapist used to say to me, 'Why do you always refer to your body as *the body,* as if it were a separate part of you?' I wouldn't talk about my feelings, I'd talk about my stomach problems or my headaches. She said, 'It sounds as if you're making your body the enemy.' And that was the first awareness I had of how much I did separate the body"—she laughs at the same reflexive phrase—"and my mind. I had always thought of 'the mind' as being pretty bright—if only it weren't housed in this wretched body!"

"What about the possibility that depression in one generation manifests as chronic pain in the next?" I asked. "Sometimes I wonder if my mother went through a postpartum depression, one that she might not have even taken seriously herself, but it sort of echoed through me and eventually found expression in pain."

"I don't know. If that's the case, then I'm a candidate, because my mother suffered a lot. And when I was thirteen, our family went through a terrible time—my mother lost a baby at nine months and was so depressed she didn't speak for five months. Then he came along—the uncle of a family friend—and took an interest in me."

"The guy who abused you?"

"It wasn't even that . . . somebody was finally paying attention, giving me affection—someone was there for me. My being just opened up to him. The only thing that was traumatic about it was . . . he left. He just disappeared. My first really passionate love!

"I told a friend of mine, who is a therapist, and she said, 'Well that's abuse, all right.' He was thirty-eight, and I was thirteen, after all. But I have trouble with the word *abuse.* He was a real love. Physically, he went beyond what he should have, but it wasn't like he was unprovoked. My friend says I'm just blaming myself, but I know I was needy as hell. He kept saying he liked the way I thought! He kept asking me my opinions, telling me how bright I was. It was the first time anyone had ever said anything like that to me."

"And I bet he thought you were cute."

"He did, he thought I was hot. I remember looking at my body back then and thinking . . . Well, you really are something!"

"I don't know. I think for it to be abuse, it has to come from someone who is supposed to protect you."

"I felt very protected by him."

"Until he left . . ."

"I was brokenhearted, for the first time. This is how abandoned kids must feel. I thought, My heart will never be broken again—and it never has. I have walked out of every relationship I ever had since then."

"Gosh."

"Pretty classic, eh? I spent ten years with a man in a close relationship, but all the time I was testing him. I was bad, bad, bad. Affairs, and rubbing them in his face. And he loved me. I know that now, but I didn't know it then. The sad part is, I loved him, too."

We had segued from body migraines to childhood trauma and a love story without seeming to have changed the subject at all.

"So much pain comes from all those unsorted-out things," she said. "When I finally got my depression under control, I had to deal with losing that relationship. Five years had gone by. Then my body went through a real bereavement, this terrible aching for him.

"Some people talk about pain as a journey toward sight—toward seeing clearly—and I believe that's what happened to me. I see the world much differently than I ever did. I'm not religious, but there is a real dimension of spirituality, of feeling a deep connection with the physical world, that I never felt before. I long to be closer to the physical world now.

"But when I was going through the worst time, I just wanted to shut myself away. I couldn't bear to be around other people. I remember when I was almost at the bottom, I saw my doctor, who put me straight into a cab to the hospital. And I remember feeling such relief. Someone was going to take care of me. I didn't have to fake it for other people."

"So you checked yourself in . . ."

"Toronto Western, psychiatric unit. Know it well. They have two units. You go left, or you go right. Fortunately, I went right—I had outpatient privileges if I wanted them. If you went left, you were in a barred space. Those were people who had no contact with the outside world. Every day we had to have our group discussions. I'd sit there with people who were almost inarticulate. Our favorite thing was to be in the room with the television strobing. Toward the end of my two weeks there, though, I did start to have a kind of friendship with a young guy who didn't make it. He ended up killing himself.

"With depression, it's the loss of energy that saves people. . . . I would lie there in bed most days thinking . . . If I could just get into the bathtub and get a razor—but the thought of getting up and getting into the bath was too much. I just couldn't do it. It's a comfort to fantasize, though." (Andrew Solomon echoes this in *The Noonday Demon,* noting that some antidepressants only give people the wherewithal to launch their suicide plans.)

"Then I got it into my head that my ninety-seven-year-old grandmother was going to die before I saw her again—not such a crazy idea—and even though I was in terrible shape, I checked myself out. I got a friend to drive me to New Brunswick; he was shocked, but he did it. I was so stoned on Ativans—I had what they call an agitated depression—and I was retching, my whole body was shaking," Alice related, like someone saying, "I was a little chilly on the ride." "But, you know, I had to see my grandmother. Oh, it was wild."

"Was your grandmother glad to see you?"

"Yes, but she was worried. Everyone was. I looked terrible, and I'd lost weight. My family knew I'd been in hospital. But when I got there, I relaxed."

"Did seeing her help you?"

"Yes. And she died, three months later. When I came back to Toronto, I was still depressed, but I didn't feel suicidal anymore. I could function—at least, I could sit there at the table, pretending to read a book. That's when my doctor said he wanted to try me on this new antidepressant, Effexor. And six weeks in, I had this epiphany.

"I was in Montreal, Christmas shopping with some friends. I was looking forward to meeting my friend's family and having a glass of wine with them. We had just left Place des Arts and were walking down the street. It was dark, and I looked up into the sky. I saw snow coming down and thought—This is so beautiful! And it shocked me. It shocked me. I hadn't felt that normal happiness for so long."

A LOT OF PEOPLE tackle chronic pain as an either/or situation: either "learn to live with it" and meditate, or go on major medication. But doing it all isn't a bad idea, either. Accepting pain as something you must live with doesn't mean you shouldn't try everything from Pilates to Paxil to get rid of it. Giving in doesn't mean giving up. There's always a turnaround moment with pain—I recognize it from the migraine cycle—when you say, Okay, I'm not going to fight it any longer; pain can have its way with me. And, paradoxically, that's the moment it begins to lighten. But it's not a moment easily arrived at, as Alice's story demonstrates. You can't just skip over the denial-and-resistance stage. This is where a medical diagnosis can be helpful. It tells someone with fibromyalgia, and the people around her, that the pain is real and is not going to be wished or willed away. The sooner the reality of pain is acknowledged (and in our culture it often takes a disease to do the trick), the faster you can focus on improving the rest of your life.

In Alice's case, accepting the fact of fibromyalgia freed her to rediagnose the rest of her life. And now that she no longer thinks of herself as a writer, oddly enough, the writing seems to go along. Pain in some ways cleared that path. Which is not to call it a "blessing in disguise," or to characterize fibromyalgia as something other than the real affliction it is. But being a disciplined, full-time negotiator with pain may also be a sound route to the self-protection and solitude that feeds the writing of a book.

Our dependence on a medical diagnosis may be a symptom in itself—that we have pathologized pain, or that we need to pathologize it before we can deal with it all. But it is better to have pain that has a name, I think, than to suffer something wordless.

11

A SPY IN THE HOUSE OF PAIN

WE GO TO THE DOCTOR TO HAVE OUR PAIN
named. But who names pain for the doctor?
It was time to slip across the border into the
world of pure science, where the idea of pain
—the how and why of it—is under radical
revision.

The Ninth World Congress of the International Association for the Study of Pain
was scheduled to take place in Vienna. The
combination of this particular gathering in
this venue, the city where Freud first inhaled
cocaine, was one I found impossible to resist.
It would be a chance to crawl under the big
top with several thousand of the world's leading pain scientists and researchers. Part of me
was curious to observe the social habits of
pain experts at play, too. What could be more
relaxing (I wrongly assumed) than a cocktail
party of anesthesiologists?

I'm sure Vienna was chosen for its convention facilities rather than its own history of
wounds and woundings, but it seemed to me
that there were unavoidable ironies involved.
In this most civilized of cities, anti-Semitism

114

and extreme right-wing politics have flourished, too. It's a culture that has produced the music of Mozart, the gilded melancholy of Gustav Klimt's painting, and the frank anguish of Egon Schiele's hollow-eyed portraits. Hitler dreamed his dreams here, along with Freud, Trotsky, Brahms, and Wittgenstein (a pain expert himself). Talk about a civic mind-body split.

The World Congress on Pain, an event that takes place every three years in different corners of the globe, is mostly a gathering of pure scientists and researchers rather than clinicians. It is pain at its most theoretical, original, and abstract. Perfect for the city where Freud struggled to create not just a theory but a science, a neobiology, of the unconscious. Perhaps it was the Viennese coffee—strong and very good—but I found that the congress and the city both conspired to produce thoughts on the same imperial scale as the art museums and the virile rooftop statuary. Everything was very big; dinky thoughts were out of the question.

It was possible to die of dehydration, for instance, before getting from one end of the famed Kunsthistorische Museum to the other. I was looking for a particular Brueghel painting, an apotheosis of pain called *The Murder of the Children in Bethlehem*. A postcard of the painting is tacked on my Wall of Pain, which features Frida Kahlo, Betty Goodwin, and this particular eerie portrait of infanticide by Brueghel the Elder. But after backpacking through a dozen art-stuffed salons, I had an attack of museum fatigue and postponed my search.

I stayed in an old-fashioned third-floor pension near the museums. The place had seen better days, but I loved its creaking, crate-sized lift, and the wide staircase where decades of feet had worn shallow curves into the stone. My room was spartan but absolutely vast (of course), with high ceilings, a huge armoire, and a balcony that let in an ocean of light. It was August, and the weather had a military uniformity—clear, sunny, and blue every day. This was not a slipshod town.

Breakfasts were served in the pension's old-world dining room by a shy, mousy waitress. They never varied—a bun, some marmalade, thin, damp sheets of cheese, and an indeterminate cold cut.

But I came to appreciate all that protein, because the days at the congress were long, and the cafeteria was heavy on almond torte. My fellow pensioneers were for the most part genteel professors doing research. It was the perfect spot for an academic gate-crasher like me.

I had a day to kill before the congress got under way, and since Vienna invented the concept of the coffeehouse, I betook myself to one. I ordered a *mélange* in the Café Centrale, a palatial hangout that Freud and Trotsky favored, but it seemed to have devolved into a tourist spot. I made my way across the cobbled Karlsplatz, where I remembered that I am afraid of large squares, and scurried down the closest narrow street. There I took a seat at the equally legendary but still bohemian Café Hawelka. It was a dark and pleasantly shabby cubbyhole, with worn velvet banquettes, inky wooden floors, and waiters in white shirts and black waistcoats who carried small silver trays. The Hawelka served only coffee and two items of food, both cake: the marble and the plum sponge. Each thick-lipped cup of coffee arrived with a silver spoon balanced across the top. A few dollars for a coffee mostly buys time—hours of idle sitting, thinking (a Viennese specialty), reading, or even sleeping. Across the room a blond American traveler was slumped over her backpack, napping, and the girl beside me in cat's-eye glasses was marking up the galleys of her book. I ate my swirly marble cake, drank my rich coffee, and decided that I was going to have to suspend my whipped-cream embargo while in Vienna.

From the city, I commuted across the Danube River to the vast, circular convention center where the congress was being held. The first session I attended was a workshop on philosophy and pain, a "refresher" course intended to broaden scientific horizons. The panel included Ned Block, a hotshot New York philosopher, and Mark Sullivan, a psychiatrist and philosopher from Seattle. The room was full, and for the first time I heard people address all those questions that medicine doesn't touch, questions that explore the relationship of pain to consciousness, memory, and identity.

I was half-lost—philosophers can be as technical in their terms as molecular biologists—but totally exhilarated.

There was a long and spirited discussion of qualia, the things we think we feel we know. Block's example was orgasms. It's possible to describe one in perfect, recognizable detail, but there's something missing that only the *experience* of an orgasm can deliver. Qualia seem to be the leprechauns of the philosophical world: Many swear to their existence, but no one has actually seen one. Pain is rife with qualia. Mark Sullivan got up to speak, and established a different frame of reference. He talked about how we take a "first-person state" ("I hurt") to the doctor, where it is turned into a "third-person state" ("your disease"). He thought it was time to consider looking at pain as a "second-person state" instead—as something closer to a dialogue. "When you know someone is in pain," he pointed out, "your first question isn't 'How do you know that?' but 'Why are you telling me this?' " Sullivan agrees with Wittgenstein, a son of Vienna, who said that pain is not essentially private, but "an invitation to a dialogue."

Pain excites philosophers, because it seems to erase the border between the subjective and the objective. But perhaps the body event we call pain is so synonymous with our emotional experience of it that any distinction becomes irrelevant. Block's cheery bottom line was "I think everything is physical."

Simon Vulfsons, a ponytailed doctor from Israel, argued that hypnotism is one example of a treatment that turns a first-person state—"My hip hurts"—into a third-person, dissociative state: "There is a hip that hurts that appears to be mine." Vulfsons found that hypnotism helped his patients in chronic pain. It's not often that you find yourself in a room where hypnotists and philosophers can agree.

I took copious notes about "the blueness of blue" and other pressing matters, but the minute I left the session, all the sense evaporated out of them, like champagne bubbles. It was so easy to lose your grip on the pure pursuit of pure pain.

When I interviewed Sullivan the next day, he seemed dispirited. Perhaps it was exasperation with my questions, or the sense of irrelevance that a philosopher might feel in a convention heavy on rats-and-mice science. Although the congress was theoretically an ideal blend of hard and soft science, of nurses, dental workers, and psychologists with neurologists, geneticists, and cellular biologists, in practice, the hard sciences prevailed. The focus was more on the mechanisms of pain than on its possible meanings.

At the press conference for the congress, Dr. Allen Basbaum, a neurobiologist from San Francisco, was the most picturesque speaker. "I think of pain as a disease," he said, "but it's invisible. There are memories of injuries that cause a reorganization of the brain. Pain does not work like a telegraph, but like voice mail—it leaves messages. These messages alter the way pain is processed." He even ventured an analogy between pain and beauty. "You can't see where beauty is. One person will look at a Mondrian painting, and the tears will well up, and they'll take out their checkbook and want to buy it. Another person will look at it and go . . . *pffft*. It's the same stimulus, but with two very different reactions. There is an emotional quality to pain."

In scientific circles, this was news.

THAT NIGHT I TAGGED along with a cadre of Israeli doctors who embarked on a pub crawl in the "Bermuda Triangle" nightclub quarter of Vienna. A pretty young physiotherapist from South Africa was part of the group. When she overheard me talking to someone else about the importance of uncovering the meaning or story that underlies someone's pain, she sidled over to me and took my arm. "I'm so glad to hear you say that," she said, "that's what I found in my work. A word, a certain kind of touch will bring the tears, and people in pain need to let those emotions come to the surface. It's not so much what you do, as the quality of the contact." She said she was doing more and more "laying on of hands" as part of her therapeutic work. But we spoke almost furtively, as we walked through the streets behind her physician friends. Therapeutic touch doesn't yet have a seat at the high table of science.

Over the next few days, I attended as many workshops as I could squeeze in. I had high hopes for "Sex, Gender and Pain," but it was largely about methodology in gathering statistics, and its findings were inconclusive. Women report more pain than men, but the question of whether they *feel* more pain than men is still up for debate. Another crowd-pleaser was the workshop on the use of cannabinoids for pain, which told us what most people already know: Marijuana can be a good pain reliever for certain conditions, but there are legal hurdles. (The use of marijuana for medical purposes, including pain relief, has now been legalized in Canada.) I went along to the migraine workshop, where the speaker used his laser pointer to run through a chart of the newest triptans. I was surprised to find that I already knew everything he was talking about, so I left.

What did strike me was the aesthetics of the science world. Each day for five days people buzzed about from workshop to workshop in a triple-tiered hive of halls, all of them offering a performance of sorts. Experts needled one another and traded in-jokes. Most workshops were conducted as panels made up of three or so international experts, who would address the topic at hand: possibly "The Role of Neighboring Intact Dorsal Root Ganglion Neurons in a Rat Neuropathic Pain Model." The congress abstracts alone were as thick as dictionaries. Most of the speakers wielded a laser pointer, directing its jittery red light to diagrams or charts on the screen. Cartoons were popular, too. The congress was dedicated to Patrick Wall, who happened not to have much hair. But in one cartoon Wall was shown with his "hair gene" altered to create a pompadour look. And the highest praise for a scientific study was the fashion word *elegant*. An elegant study, I gathered, arrived at its conclusion cleanly and inevitably, like a diver entering the water with no perceptible splash. This contrasted oppressively with my own task of writing about pain from every possible angle. In my case, a great deal of splashing was involved.

It seemed I was the only "cultural journalist" on board, a role that was so detached that I might as well have been a scientist myself. The convention brought together a number of different disciplines, and each cabal traveled mostly among their own: gene people with gene people, cancer folk with cancer folk, and so on. The science reporters filed their stories daily from the press center, where I tapped away, too—a spy in the house of pain.

But the workshop on back pain was more down to earth. As well it should be. Low-back pain is the leading cause of workplace disability, affecting 60 to 80 percent of the working population, and a staggering 93 percent of low-back cases are idiopathic—without any identified cause. It costs the economy billions of dollars a year in lost work, and we spend billions more on therapies and curious devices to cure it. What was striking about the session was that all the experts agreed that they didn't have a clue how to fix back pain.

The room was packed to overflowing, and the moderator, London pain expert Dr. Chris Wells, began the session with a quote from Chekhov: "Where many remedies exist, you can be sure there is no cure." The panel participants included Nikolai Bogduk, an Australian doctor with a booming voice, a somewhat Elizabethan vocabulary, and a reputation as a respected high-tech back-pain expert with no time for touchy-feely therapies; Gordon Waddell, a Glasgow orthopedic surgeon "by profession if not by nature" and the author of *The Back Pain Revolution;* and Chris Mains, an English psychologist and pain specialist.

Dr. Wells introduced the Glaswegian Waddell by suggesting that the English view a Scot "like a case of hemorrhoids. Those that come down are all right so long as they go back up. It's the ones that come down and stay down that cause the problems." (Only an Englishman and a doctor could get away with this sortie.) Then they laid out the premise for the debate: You're on a desert island with severe back pain, you do not know what you know now, and you want some advice to help you cope with the pain. A hot-air balloon is being sent to help you. There is only so much room in the hot-air balloon, and a whole spectrum of back experts to choose from. So who would you allow on board?

Although Bogduk has a reputation for having all the answers and being a bit of a "needle jockey" who travels everywhere with his little vial of painkilling bivucaine, his presentation in Vienna surprised his colleagues. Instead of talking up the latest surgical intervention, he spoke about addressing the patients' fears and anxieties, and "getting inside their heads." He emphasized that what was most important was to first eliminate "red-flag conditions" that might be (but probably weren't) causing the back pain, and then to reassure the patient that the back would most probably get better and not worse. He still believed in judicious painkilling, but what was more important in treating back pain, he had found, was communication and reassurance. Preventing acute pain from turning into chronic pain was often a matter of "treating the patient nice and convincing him that there is nothing so horribly wrong."

The psychologist Mains, not surprisingly, said that chronic pain arose from our beliefs and attitudes toward pain. "The problem of pain is psychological," he summed up, "and chronic incapacity is psychologically mediated. . . . It doesn't mean you're crazy, it means you're a human being. In order for you to overcome what has been a dreadful physical problem, you understand that it's necessary to regain control over the impact it has on your life." His hypothetical treatment involved a patient who gradually educated himself about pain, attended a pain-management clinic, and got on with his life. "When you break down back pain, a lot of the time you will find that you can cope with it."

But the surgeon Waddell was the most outspoken. "I'm an orthopedic surgeon, so I can give you a bigger, better screw than Nik Bogduk can," he began, in true surgeon style, to laughter. Waddell, whose book is one of the bibles of back pain, is a defector from his own profession. He told the story of a friend who calls his orthopedic surgeon a white rhino, "because he's thick-skinned, difficult to find, and likes to charge a lot."

"Surgery is not the answer for back pain, and it doesn't work," he went on, "so I'm now going to jump out of this hot-air balloon and leave the other two hot-air experts to battle it out. But the trouble is, it's very easy for back specialists to set themselves up as experts. Beware of amateur experts who step out with their own specialty. Beware of high-tech experts who blind you with science or pseudoscience. And beware most of all of the bullshit artist who can sell the idea to you and convince you that their treatment is better than everyone else's—odds are, they're wrong. So throw out the experts and fill up the balloon with malt whiskey, which will probably do your back more good than the experts."

When the professionals in the audience jumped into the discussion, a physiotherapist reminded the doctors that there was "no laying on of hands" at the congress, or mention of the role of exercise and manual manipulation. He pointed out the importance of working with posture and exercises to help prevent future injuries. So the physiotherapist was voted on board. But "dry needling" (a euphemism for what amounts to doctorly acupuncture) was nixed. The congress does not have much truck with popular but unproven alternative therapies. Even something as mainstream as physiotherapy was pretty marginal here.

But what was surprising was how the high-tech experts were willing to admit failure in their treatment of back pain. Most ordinary back pain will resolve itself in two or three months. But when backs get better, anything and everything can be credited as the magic wand. These doctors, who had long experience with people in pain in addition to their traditional training and schooling, had discovered that nothing happens without communication, treatment based on evidence of outcome, and what used to be called a good bedside manner.

"Be aware," Bogduk addressed the congress, "that simple intervention—the time spent with a patient—is a very powerful ingredient of the patient-doctor contract. The evidence is against the traditions such as surgery being true—the evidence says it doesn't work." This new focus on the relationship between doctor and patient, as opposed to the drive to cure an isolated symptom, was a radical change of tune for the doctors. And this was one of several workshops that touted "evidence-based medicine," an approach that judges different treatments based on how well they work. Hasn't anyone thought to look at outcomes as a logical way to figure out what really works? Not until recently. That tells you how far out of the picture the patient has been.

Down in the cafeteria, debating once again whether to eat another sausage or a slice of cake, I ran into Dr. Basbaum, who had dared to include an analogy to art in his press conference address. Basbaum, a Canadian who is now director of anatomy at UCLA, is a large, ruddy man with a sharp wit. He is a leader in the hot science of studying transgenic mice in order to locate the proteins involved in the transmission of pain. As a student, he worked with both Ronald Melzack and Patrick Wall; the subject of his graduate thesis was "mice and cats who could be conditioned not to kill." But he never published it, he added. Why not, I asked. "The Vietnam war was on, and it didn't seem to be the right time." Basbaum is a former director of the congress, and pain has occupied his whole career. His wife happens to be a leading expert on cystic fibrosis, he added, "and so when people see us coming, they say, 'Oh, here comes Pain and Mucus.' "

At the top rung of science, I was beginning to notice, you will find researchers who have a surplus of intellectual mischief and warmth in them. Melzack and Wall have these qualities, I would discover, and so do the gene guys, Jeff Mogil and Basbaum. I asked Basbaum what it was like to study under Melzack and Wall.

"Wall is really a scientist, he has never let go of research, and he is a sweet guy. But if he disagrees with you, he'll needle you. He finds the brain-imaging people a little too narrow in their focus, and he lets them know it. Melzack is right off the scale in terms of niceness, and he would never say anything bad about anyone."

I shuttled back to my pension that night and went to a restaurant full of carousing university students. They ordered steins of beer and plate-sized schnitzels—the gargantuan theme again—and I followed suit, while making notes.

Vienna Pain Diary

DAY ONE: *Headache (jet lag), sore shoulder (heavy bag—too many abstracts), stiff neck (sleeping upright on plane). Notice that jet lag seems to disarm my own "endogenous painkillers." What role hormones? Cf. Melatonin as anti-jet-lag remedy. Did not bring melatonin. Right shin has neuritis. Right hip aches. Wrong shoes! Last-minute veto on sneakers as too "Canadian." Why only stilettos and platform mules? What was I thinking?*

DAY TWO: *Front door of pension massive and very heavy, like a vault. Almost crushed when trying to quickly get in before it slammed shut. Viennese diet of coffee, almond torte, sausage, and cheese not exactly high-fiber. Amazed that Viennese not all massive.*

DAY THREE: *Decide once again that I am crooked and misaligned. Stiffness all down right side. Must try to carry bags on left side instead.*

DAY FOUR: *Fillings of teeth flaking off. Grinding, no doubt (technical term: bruxism). Sore right forearm from taking notes longhand. Laptop shoulders—hotel desks are never the right height for typing. Blister on left ankle, raw, unsightly. Catastrophizing somewhat over that—good entry for staph infection? Flesh-eating disease? Luckily, many, many doctors readily available in town.*

THERE IS A DEFINING moment in *The Graduate,* when Dustin Hoffman's character is cornered by a stockbrokerish guy at a cocktail party. He wants to give Hoffman some life advice. "One word," the man says. "Plastics."

It's hot-tip, commodities language, and I heard an echo of it on another night out on the town at the congress. I was sitting with a table of pain doctors who, I was learning, are no strangers to pleasure. We were occupying some picnic tables close to the Danube River; I could feel a slight chill coming off the water. Beside me was a British pain specialist slightly in his cups. To make conversation, I asked him what the new star was in the firmament of pain treatment. He leaned over.

"Botox," he slurred. "It's huge."

This was well before *The New Yorker* magazine featured the fashionable wrinkle-eraser in a cartoon. (A husband carries his wife under his arm like a stiff cardboard cutout; the caption reads "I think you should probably lay off the Botox for now.")

"It's a biological toxin," he continued dreamily. "It paralyzes the muscles so they can't go into spasm."

Botox is the trade name for a botulinum toxin type A that is produced from the bacterium *Clostridium botulinum.* The product was first developed in 1989 for use in several neurological disorders affecting the eyes. Then doctors discovered that Botox had the alluring side effect of paralyzing the facial muscles that contribute to lines and furrows. Botox has since taken off as an alternative to cosmetic surgery. When it's injected into the muscle, it blocks the release of a neurotransmitter called acetylcholine, which causes muscle contraction. Botox temporarily mummifies the muscles it targets. It does erase lines, although it might be impossible to frown or lift your brow. One injection lasts six to twelve months.

Now doctors are using Botox to treat migraine, back problems, and the sort of chronic pain related to muscular tension or spasm (myofascial pain).

The pain approach is to zap a little Botox into the traumatized, contracted muscles and then follow up with diligent physiotherapy. If you can get over the idea of doctors charging money to inject people in pain with toxic bacteria, it sounds reasonable, maybe even better than living on painkillers.

The congress, like any professional convention, was also a bazaar of commercial products: sleek new opioids, drug delivery systems, electrostimulating machines, and all the other gizmos that might offer relief from pain. The stuff was kept downstairs. On the last day of the conference, I took the escalator down into this hopeful Hades of pain products, where I ran into Mr. Botox again, beside the Botox booth. Commuting back and forth between how we see pain and how we sell it turned out to be illuminating.

The first thing I saw was a long line of people waiting for free T-shirts stamped with their own handprint, from the makers of Tramal, a synthetic opioid. Their slogan is "Tramal—as individual as pain is diverse." I wove through a souk of pills, potions, and devices from the Bristol-Myerses, Parke-Davises, ASTA Medicas, and Allergans of the world. (The IASP gratefully acknowledges up front "educational grant support" from sixteen pharmaceutical companies.)

I could feel a headache coming on from the buzzing lights and information overkill so I strolled over to the Zomig booth, hoping for a handout of triptans. No free samples. There was an array of TENS (transcutaneous electrical nerve stimulation) devices, little boxes with electrode patches that deliver a mild electric current, and there were neurostimulation systems that deliver drugs straight to the spinal cord, like the one that Lori Biduke, Dr. Mailis's patient, had had implanted in her abdomen.

Much of the new technology of pain treatment is quite mechanical and involves more efficient ways of getting the same drugs into a narrower target area. Despite the promise of the previous congress to take pain studies "beyond morphine," the bazaar was overwhelmingly devoted to pills and machines. There were few signs of the alternative world of massage, shiatsu, biofeedback devices, magnetic therapy, herbs, hypnotism, cognitive approaches, or even the widely accepted elder of the nonmedical world, acupuncture.

Actually, acupuncture was there in theory, but not in name. In the doctor world, acupuncture is sometimes reconfigured as "dry needling" or "electrostimulation," to get around the lingering bias against its Chinese origins. One company sold something called an "AS Super 4 needle stimulator," which simply adds a current of electricity to needles inserted into the traditional acupuncture points, along with the reassuring contours of a stereo amplifier. If you can attach a little appliance with multiple dials to an ancient therapy, North Americans tend to have more faith in it.

The favored advertising image was a body part—hand, arm, or face—attached by wires to a mysterious box with control dials. Just you and your pain machine.

Here was the familiar Cartesian dichotomy at work. Upstairs, at the congress workshops, it was pure science. Upstairs, you could lose yourself in "elegant" studies of the molecular, genetic, or neurochemical behavior of pain. Upstairs, the body of the noisome pain patient had been successfully amputated.

Downstairs was where they kept the corpse. Here was an old-fashioned, mechanistic world of pills and powders, needles and unguents, all designed for the dull, thick world of physical pain. The pain bazaar was not about working with pain in the world, but about modifying or blocking "pain impulses," either with drugs or counterstimulation. The more integrative approaches to pain, which might combine physiotherapy with hypnotism and a morphine patch, too, were mostly missing. This is partly because most alternative pain treatment is a process rather than a product.

Powerful pharmaceutical companies are still the engines that drive gatherings like this one. The narrowing gap between research and profit has affected even the most august medical journals, the *Journal of the American Medical Association* and the *New England Journal of Medicine*. The editors recently announced that they would no longer publish articles based on research funded by pharmaceutical companies, because they had become alarmed that these studies were not unbiased. Sometimes there is more science than meets the eye in the alternative therapies and less than we want to believe in "controlled studies."

The basement was also reserved for a charming scientific tradition—the poster sessions. Here, in an area that resembles a bustling high-school science fair, researchers are able to post their individual papers, often on hand-lettered pieces of bristol board that address topics like "Rat Tail Withdrawal Tests." This is where students get their first exposure and where the most marginal, original work can be found. The rows and rows of homemade posters create a scientific shantytown, where, at certain hours of the day, the authors stand by their posters, ready to discuss or argue their work with the crowd.

When I wandered into the poster hall late on the second day, only a few of the presenters still stood wearily by their work. Most of it was incomprehensible to me, but not being hooked into the detail let me register the bigger themes. Each corridor was reserved for different areas of study: gene expression, inflammation, analgesics, neuropathic pain, myofascial pain, "illness behavior," opioid therapies. It was as stunning a spectrum as the biggest, brightest supermarket where you can buy everything from car mats to star fruit in one visit. All of pain was here, atomized into the tiniest of fragments:

"Effects of Midazolam in the Spinal Nerve Ligation
   Model of Neuropathic Pain in Rats"
"Pain Coping Strategies in an Iranian Population of
   Chronic Pain Sufferers"

"Heterogeneity in the Electrophysiological Properties of
Tetrodotoxin-Resistant (TTX-R) C-Fibers of the
Frog Sciatic Nerve"

"Non-verbal Expressions That Nurses Use to Determine
Pain in Individuals with Severe or Profound
Cognitive Impairment"

"Gabapentin Potentiates NMDA Responses in Gabergic
Dorsal Horn Neurons"

"Migraine in Tunisia"

"Pain in Painting Art" (from Norway, Edvard Munch's
home)

How odd it was to wander these corridors thick with data and
realize at the same time how little we know about easing pain. It
wasn't a futile feeling—people were already benefiting from the
work reflected on these hopeful squares of bristol board and Magic
Marker. But it wasn't a hopeful feeling, either.

What would a person in pain think, wandering through these
halls? He might conclude that pain was the provenance of scientists,
and that science could be as exclusive as a golf club. He would sur-
mise that his favorite physiotherapist or masseuse would not feel terribly valued here, and that the role of diet in pain treatment was not
nearly as sexy as gene research. He would surely recognize that the
pure science of pain is his first hope for some relief, next month or
next year. But as someone moving slowly down the aisles, as a figure
who represents both the human side and the unfixable nature of
pain, he might feel out of place.

ON MY LAST DAY in Vienna I did some gawking around St. Stephen's
cathedral in the Graben, the city's main gathering place. Sometime
after buying a tourist torte at Demel's, the former confectioner to the
emperor, my wallet was pickpocketed out of my backpack. My
flight home was early the next morning and I had no money left.
Upon hearing my story, two strangers at the congress immediately
forked over $150. This was my double-blind study on empathy
among pain scientists, and I found the results reassuring. Then I

hustled back to the congress, where Ronald Melzack and Patrick Wall were signing copies of the fourth edition of their textbook on pain. Yes, even the pain world has celebrity signings.

Melzack was pacing around the booth. He looked a bit like Marshall McLuhan, with more hooded eyes. I chatted with him and asked him what the focus of the congress would be in ten years. "Oh, the brain," he said, waving a hand. "Pain is in the brain." He introduced me to his protégé Jeff Mogil, a psychologist and gene researcher, and said, "But this is where the action is—genetics." It was crowded and noisy in the hall and I didn't feel equipped to interview Melzack in depth, so I stepped out of the fray.

Over by the wall, I noticed Patrick Wall sitting with his tea by the *Lancet* booth. An old buddy with a hearing aid sat beside him. Tall and lanky, Wall was the very picture of a Shavian intellectual, or perhaps a Chekhovian actor playing the philosopher-doctor. He drew on a cigarette, relighting it whenever it went out, and balanced a cup and saucer of tea on his leg, tipping his ash into the saucer. He was in his seventies and had prostate cancer. He looked a bit papery and frail, but when I introduced myself, his face crinkled up genially. I asked him to sign my copy of his book *Pain: The Science of Suffering* and complimented him on its subversive nature. "Well, that was the idea, to wake people up," he said. I asked him why there weren't more workshops on the social and political issues around pain.

"Because the old are all in pain," he said, with a slight brow lift that acknowledged his own membership in this club, "and when they don't feel like going out anymore and voting, they have no voice." I made a joke that the next congress might be overthrown by an insurrection of lab rats, and he laughed at that. I was, in fact, waiting for someone to point out the obvious and unpleasant irony of the congress, that is, inflicting pain on animals in order to study how to erase it in humans, but it never happened.

When the gate-control theory of pain developed by Wall and Melzack was first published in 1965, it was roundly attacked for flawed physiology. Critics now agree that a few details were off, but the general concept was sound. Wall wasn't admitted to the Royal

College of Physicians and Surgeons until he was sixty-four. When I encountered him, he still had the air of a gentleman renegade. In the summer of 2001, at the age of seventy-six, Pat Wall died.

BY THE END OF my week in Vienna, I had a pocketful of generalizations about the scientific study of pain. Science can quite successfully cocoon you from suffering, and the gap between knowledge and application was exasperating. Scientists doing research into pain get to tinker in their labs with specially bred mice, far away from the frustrations of treating pain patients in clinics. Even in the space of a week, I found myself almost seduced by the Elysian Fields of pain studies. It is so *elegant,* unlike the crude reality of pain. The best pioneers in pain studies—the John Bonicas and Cecily Saunderses and other pain revolutionaries—never lost sight of the patient in their research. Once the patient slips out the picture, "pure" science risks pursuing nothing more than pleasing arabesques of reason and conjecture.

Given the congress's multidisciplinary philosophy, I was surprised by the absence of alternative pain approaches—the whole spectrum of cranial-sacral massage, healing-touch therapy, and other hands-on skills that are a lifeline to many people with chronic pain. Alternative therapies are hard to evaluate, but that's no reason not to explore them. The other omission was a deeper consideration of the cultural dimension of pain. Well, the congress *was* about science, not art. But writers and artists have articulated pain in ways that science is only catching up to now.

I had just enough time left to stalk Brueghel again before I left Vienna. I hustled into town to the Kunsthistorische Museum, paid my hundred schillings, and in my foolish footwear mounted the stairs, oppressed on all sides by marble, gilt, and swagged drapery. There is no such thing as "casual Friday" in the Kunsthistorische. I made my way from one claustral salon to another, pausing at the Caravaggios, until I was rewarded.

In salon ten were the paintings of Brueghel the Elder in all their surface calm and swarming, happy-nasty humanity. Skies that looked like a recipe for a tornado. Lapidary landscapes with small figures tucked into them. I took in *The Tower of Babel,* which seemed to have some relevance to my week at the congress, with its cold-faced king striding in among his groveling stone masons. Then I turned to the surprisingly small canvas entitled *The Murder of the Children in Bethlehem.* From a distance the painting looks almost festive, like a village celebration on a snowy day. The figures could be skaters on a pond, except that they are soldiers killing people. Up close, you see that they are not dancing but bending backward in disbelief and despair as their children are killed. Men in uniforms rip infants out of mothers' arms. The spectacle is beautiful until you inspect the details of it. The composition is as serene as a constellation of stars.

"About suffering they were never wrong, the old masters," wrote the poet W. H. Auden on the subject of a Brueghel painting. He was right. It was only a picture, but I needed to see pain put back in some context, even such a horrific one as this. I wanted to be reminded of the ability of the artist to look and not turn away. Then I staggered out. We're really not meant to see that much art at once; it's like downing ten eggnogs in a row. The ideal gallery would show only four paintings, one for each vast wall. As I made my way out of the gallery, onto the football field of the grounds, I stuck my hand through the pruned borders of the topiary, right into the dense tangle of branches.

Perhaps pure science, I thought, practices a kind of intellectual topiary—nature translated into the mind's cool geometry. In its own way, the congress had been a gallery, too, as Basbaum's link between pain and painting had suggested. The evening air in the gardens felt good. I had been inside too much. Navigating by several naked rooftop sculptures that I now recognized, I found my way back to the pension, where my passport and plane ticket home were safe inside my enormous armoire.

12

BROKEN BONES

THE PAIN CONGRESS WAS OVER. ON THE flight back home, I opened my copy of Patrick Wall's *Pain: The Science of Suffering*. Although I was exhausted, I couldn't stop reading. Despite his long years in the field, and a deep engagement in the anatomical and intellectual questions raised by pain, Wall never lost sight of life outside the lab, especially the plight of the elderly and the poor who put up with pain.

The message of his book is simple but radical: Pain is unique to each person who suffers it. Science can't cut pain out of the body and must learn to look beyond symptoms and "pain centers" to the bigger picture: the person in pain and his world. Like a piece of art, pain presents us with a wordless picture. Wall's advice was not to look at the brushwork under a microscope—or, at least, not to look at pain in only this way. He was, after all, a physiologist, a detail man himself. We also have to stand back and take it all in—shape, color, line, form, and social context. Pain asks scientists to respond more like artists. Wall was someone who understood just how far a stretch this can be for science.

We'll never find a single rigid system for pain in the body, Wall claims, because the interplay of mind and body with history, politics, and economics will always enter into our experience of pain.

The only shortcomings I could detect were Wall's lack of curiosity about the alternative spectrum (the section on massage consists of one word: "delightful") and a certain understandable haste, given his health, in the writing. When the book first appeared in England, the *Guardian* was lavish in its praise. But the prestigious science journal *Nature* was dismissive. Too much mushy talk about social issues, not enough hard data.

As I read along, I became more aware of the people around me in the plane. My seatmate was exceptionally fat, which was no surprise. Only obese people sit beside me on intercontinental flights. Right away, he oozed my way and staked out "our" armrest. He was also strangely inert. He read a Dutch textbook, then put his head back, closed his eyes, and for six hours, neither moved nor got up to use the washroom. Perhaps he was catheterized. His stillness became almost as unnerving to me as restlessness. It was like sitting beside something with thick insulation, like a ceramic kiln.

As everyone else drooped and nodded in the gloom of the plane, I took out my yellow highlighter and proceeded to underline every other sentence in Wall's book. By the time the blinds went up and breakfast was served, the pages were as yellow as dandelions. Three aisles over, a baby wailed that worst of all possible wails—the gasping, escalating shriek that says "I need comfort, and so far experience has taught me I won't be getting any." I could see the back of the mother's head; she was as inert as my seatmate.

Passengers eye babies on planes like tiny lepers. I sympathize with parents who have to cope with not only a restless baby but also the pressure of not disturbing everyone else. But the escalating hysteria of a baby who has already learned that his mother may not respond is one of the most intolerable, heart-wrenching sounds in the world. Whenever I hear the wails of a baby who is being willfully ignored in public, I feel as if I'm witnessing a stabbing on the street. This is the primal pain: a baby crying for a mother who is tantalizingly there, but not there. Early suffering sets our thermostat for how we respond to later insults and injuries. For some, affliction becomes a kind of default setting. Neglect opens up channels for pain that may never close. In this way, pain trains us. All sorts of cultural conditions—child-rearing customs that teach us to ignore a crying baby—may end up contributing to chronic pain conditions later in life. Or at least, that's my theory.

I think Wall might have agreed. In essence, his book says don't just analyze the pitch of the cry—pick up the baby. Whether or not we can draw a map of pain in the brain or trace its electrical storms in the body, the first thing we need to do is to overcome our desire to deny it.

Finally, a flight attendant went over, took the baby in her arms, and the crying stopped. I never did find out what was up with the mother.

I thought back over my week at the congress. On the one hand, I was rather seduced by the world of pure research. Pain takes the mind to new places. For academics and philosophers, the subject is sort of like a hooker standing in the doorway of consciousness, saying, "Hey, sailor, looking for a good time?" Pain is consciousness in extremis. I had also been expecting a gathering of the careworn and the furrow-browed. *Au contraire.* There was a giddy postdoctoral zing in the air and plenty of humor in the lectures. Pain could be a fun world, if you weren't actually feeling it.

I got home on the weekend to find that my sixteen-year-old son was sick and required soup making, which I was happy to perform. On Monday morning, still cobwebby with jet lag, I sat down to transcribe my tapes. The phone rang.

It was my ninety-one-year-old father. I keep forgetting he's ninety-one. He and my eighty-nine-year-old mother still live in the house where I spent my teens. He drives; she cooks; they manage very well. My sister Jori and brother Bruce live not too far away and, unlike us, they know how to install handrails and bathtub grips. My parents have also been so brilliantly self-sufficient for so much of their official old age that I eventually stopped waiting for that dire call—which, of course, is always when the phone chooses to ring.

"Oh! You're there," my father said, having braced himself for our answering machine. "Marni, uh, Olive had a little fall last night."

Here it comes, I thought. He cleared his throat.

"I was just changing the bulb in the porch light, I was on the little stepladder, and she insisted on helping me . . . she was going to hand me up the wing nuts, and she went to step up onto the porch—it's a big step—and I guess the toe of her shoe must have caught the edge of the step. She fell onto the cement with her full weight and her arm under her. It broke her shoulder and her wrist, too. She's down in Brant hospital right now."

Okay. Rewind. Erase.

"She just about passed out because of the pain, but I got her sitting in that lawn chair we keep on the porch. We had a heck of a time getting her inside, but somehow the two of us managed. Then, of course, she wouldn't hear of going to the hospital, but Jori came over at midnight and thought we better get things checked out. So we called an ambulance. The paramedics came pretty quickly, and they were quite good, I must say. And now we're waiting to see what the orthopedic surgeon says."

Poor dad. He operates like a guy at least ten years younger—but still, that makes him eighty-one. The two of them run a tight ship—in my household, the porch light would have stayed burned out for six months. This sort of mundane chore has nearly done them in before. A year ago, my mother was standing on a chair, trying to reach a tray on top of the fridge, when she caught the edge of the fridge door, fell, and broke her wrist—the same wrist she'd apparently broken again. At eighty-nine, you can't afford to be falling off chairs and porches. My mother is smarter than twenty CEOs laid end to end, but recently she has become dependent on a body with bones that can break like breadsticks.

I made some mental adjustments. A long stretch of caretaking might be ahead of us. But my heart didn't sink—I was relieved that it was only a broken-bone call. However, the irony was unavoidable. I had come home from the theory of pain to the fact of it.

The next day I drove out to Burlington, with its hissing summer lawns and well-tended gardens. I expected to find my mother in bed, but I walked in to see her dressed and reclining on the den couch. She looked quite festive, in fact—her left arm was in a navy blue sling and there was a neon pink cast on her wrist. Her skin was pale, but her spirits were suspiciously jaunty. I attributed this to codeine and her relief at being out of the hospital and back home.

"That's a nice top," she said to me. "I bet you wear that all the time." I was a little unnerved at these social graces but happy to see her in good spirits.

I made some lunch for my father. The two of us sat down across from each other at the kitchen table. "Scrambling eggs is an art," he said. "They're great when they're done perfectly like this, and awful when they're not." My father has always been gracious, but at ninety-one he makes a point of expressing his appreciation to his family. It's a refreshing quality.

Then he made his usual meticulous shopping list—juice, garbage bags, and "bendy straws" so my mother could manage drinks. I offered to go for him, but he wanted to get out and do something useful. He carefully extracted the car from the garage and drove off, while I sat down to hear my mother's story.

"You know, no matter how awful it is, you always learn a lot from these experiences," she said. She has been in the emergency room two or three times before, with heart attacks and weird reactions to her various heart and cholesterol medications. She always treats these ER episodes as a kind of Nepalese trek to perilous but fascinating new terrain. It's an adventure—especially when you survive it.

Because our current provincial government is evil and barbaric, there were no beds when my mother arrived at the hospital. She lay in a hallway all night, waiting for the orthopedic surgeon to come round. She was told not to eat or drink because they might operate, so for twenty-four hours she didn't have anything to drink. "I was so thirsty, I kept dreaming of orange juice." The surgeon was overworked, as most doctors and all nurses are under the current system. When he finally saw her, he took X rays, checked her age, decided not to operate, and sent her home.

The cries of the man in the next cubicle during the night stayed with her. "He seemed so fit and jolly when he came in," she said, "a big man, joking away. But in the middle of the night I heard these awful shrieks. I kept wondering what was wrong with him to make him scream like that." The next day she asked the nurse what the man was in for, and he told her it was kidney stones. "So, that was the sound of kidney stones," my mother noted.

I asked her what her own pain had felt like. Shoulder pain is supposed to be bad. "Oh," she said breezily, "it was pretty agonizing, until they gave me a needle. But when it wore off, I kept throwing up from the pain. I felt sorry for the little male nurse taking care of me, but I guess he's seen it all before. He was good. And he finally got them to give me something more for the pain."

Along with my sister, my brother and sister-in-law, who have both worked in hospital environments, were there to run interference. My mother was sent home with a sling that nobody knew how to get on or off and a prescription for painkillers that somebody had to fill. Luckily there were three family members in a flying wedge to help her navigate the transition.

For almost two hours she told her story, full of concern for the overworked nurses and other patients with no one there to help them. "You even have to bring your own Kleenexes," said my father, marveling. My son, who had come along with me, joked that this was our new medieval version of universal health care—a cart that comes around to your door with somebody ringing a bell and yelling, "Bring out your dead!" My mother was already coming up with solutions as she took a swig of water from the plastic sport bottle she kept handy.

"I don't know why they don't give every patient their own

water bottle, so they don't have to ring for a nurse just to get a drink," she said.

ONE THEORY WALL WRITES about is that pain is a "plan for potential action." It helps us avoid things that might kill us, for starters. In the acute stage, it automatically makes our hand flinch away from a flame. Our reaction is unthinking. This is the "fast" pain, moving up to the brain and back without mediation from other cognitive areas. Then another "slow" kind of pain sets in, accompanied by inflammation, which urges us to withdraw and keep still, so the body can devote its energies to healing.

AT THE MOMENT, MY mother was overriding pain's agenda. She sat up, leafing through the paper with her good hand. That first day, I was struck by the expressiveness of her right hand. She is normally left-handed, but now her other one kicked in with a riveting, mobile sort of intelligence. It was as if her will and spirit were now flowing down and out of those cocked fingers, hanging on hard to life. A newborn has the same powerful grasp—it can support its own weight with the grip of its hands. They turned on a British sitcom with Judi Dench that they like to watch. "She's heavier than she used to be," my mother noted. They both treat watching television almost as a sport, going at it with interactive verve. My dad remains a boundless marveler, and my mother has sensible but unorthodox opinions on how the world should sort itself out. Cynicism is something they have yet to arrive at.

At five o'clock, we sat around with our sherries, as usual. It was weird. My mother was now semicrippled, and life was going on as if nothing had happened. "There's still some pie in the freezer," she told me as I went in to assess the pantry situation. Later on we watched the news. It was all about damage and dying, of course— plane crashes, fresh murders, bombs in malls, small children being strangled by ordinary curtain cords. Mayhem all around. One could step up to change the porch light and fall down in a heap.

The important thing was that my mother could still dress,

however painfully, and make her way into the bathroom by herself. That was the Maginot Line between invalidism and independence.

The next afternoon, my parents napped, falling into that deep, slightly frightening abyss of sleep that the elderly practice. I slipped out for a walk down to the lakeshore. There was a cool breeze, very faint, like a fresh thought, coming off the water. I looked at the Riviera Motel, with daily specials of $44, and balconies that look over the water toward the smudge pots of Buffalo, and thought, I could move in there, and nip in and out to check on them. The prospect seemed quite bohemian: living in a motel room in my own hometown. I lay down on the cement breakwater for a long time. Two retired folks walked by me, then looped back. When I sat up, they seemed relieved. "We thought you were dead," they said gaily. People in Burlington normally don't lie down on the breakwater.

When I got home, my father was looking pale but still game. That first day at home, when Mother was riding on her codeine and we had our little drinks safely in their coasters, I saw my father in his chair briefly tip his head back and close his eyes. He could afford to relax now, just for an instant. Then the old vigilance surged back and he opened his eyes again.

In the middle of the second night, when they both woke up, I heard them murmuring and talking in the bedroom next to mine. It sounded so convivial, so loving. Their roles are no longer aimed in two divergent directions—toward kids and house or work in the world. All their work is for each other now.

The next day, my father had a doctor's appointment. When he left, he leaned across the wide bed to kiss my mother on the mouth.

"That must have been sweet," she said tartly, having earlier announced that her mouth tasted like a sewer.

"It *was* sweet," he said.

The next morning, reality hit home. My mother was pale, exhausted, and nauseous, either from the pain or the codeine or both. Just sitting upright left her clammy with sweat. She didn't ask for her glasses. Her one good hand didn't reach for the cantaloupe I had cut up for her. I longed for her to show her usual spirit. In the aged, spirit comes and goes, just the way it does in infants, like the sun going behind a cloud, then coming out again.

My father was worried. He hovered, fussed, and swept the kitchen floor. He hates things to break down. He decided he really needed a permanent marker to label the blue recycling box, and he went out to buy one. When he got back, the battery in the smoke detector chose this moment to run down and emit imperative chirps. I drove instantly to the No Frills store to buy a new battery. My father and I installed it together, to avoid any further ladder-climbing incidents. The whole apparatus dropped out of the ceiling. This entailed fixing it with duct tape, which he allowed me to do. When the detector was finally working and shoved back into the ceiling, he sat down in his chair in the den. I brought him tea.

Meanwhile, we had to organize home care. Until I showed up, my brother and sister-in-law had been the front-line workers, and my sister came by every day. But they had jobs, too. My mother's doctor came by—a house call!—examined her gently, then phoned to arrange for nursing care. A woman phoned to say that someone would be around in the afternoon to assess my mother's "situation and needs." Situation and needs! The bureaucracy of the language was music to our ears. There was a system, a worn, depleted, under-funded, and perhaps dying system, but on this particular day it came through for my mother.

A woman radiating competence arrived at the door shortly. In a twinkling, the home-care lady was up in my mother's bedroom, her strange purse slumped on the floor, her rather dog-eared note-books splayed on the bed. Her name was Anne; she wore glasses and had thick straight white hair. A pen with a coiled cord was attached to her shirt. She was efficient, with just the right touch of humor. She showed us how to pivot my mother out of bed with an arm behind her neck and one under her knee. We all gazed at the psychedelic bruise on my mother's right leg from being hauled into the house after her fall.

Anne showed us how to fold a pillow behind my mother's back so it wouldn't spring out again. She advised my mother to take the pain medication every four hours, not to tough it out, and to expect constipation: "Whatever you're doing for regularity, double it." She wasn't too nursey, which was important—any sort of cooing would have appalled my mother. Everything Anne said was practical and ingenious.

My mother was helped into a more vertical position, but I could see she wanted to lie down again and rest. I could feel her energy wax and wane, like a current of air in the trees. It's as if I had a kind of seismograph inside me that registered her tremors. My body ached, too, everywhere: transdermal pain.

Anne left us with the documents that would inform the incoming nurses of the situation. There would be a Debbie, or perhaps a Julia, who would come every day, for half an hour. This seemed to put the world right for a few hours. My father positively beamed, because he is an engineer, and this was a system, and the system was working smoothly. When we finally sat down to our belated lunch, my father said, "You know, this has really been a good house—every window you look out of, you see trees. It's like living in a park."

My mother looked a little unhappy at the prospect of strangers in her house, but she didn't resist. There were new things to learn, and these were the people who would teach her.

13

CITIZENS OF FOUR A.M.

Pain—expands the Time—
Ages coil within
The minute Circumference
Of a single Brain—

Pain contracts—the Time—
Occupied with Shot
Gamuts of Eternities
Are as they were not—

EMILY DICKINSON

EMILY DICKINSON, WHO SUFFERED FROM headaches and loneliness, wrote often about pain, but in a crisp meter that expunged any self-pity or languor. She was a scientist of her own suffering. And there were compensations, she noted:

After great pain, a formal feeling comes—
The Nerves sit ceremonious, like Tombs—

This might be the first endorphin poem, a portrait of the exalted calm that can arrive in the lee of a migraine.

Poetry is consoling in part because its meter marks time. This is why we still need poets—not just because they locate words for heartache and other kinds of wounds, but for the way they put terrible events back inside the flow and order of time. Poetry uncovers a pulse, a pattern, in the ungovernable. It can temporarily repatriate our lost ones—loves that end, friends who die, a picture from childhood. Poetry allows us a little bit of dominion in the matter of time.

Pain also changes the way time works. My mother's wait on the gurney in the halls of the emergency ward, the minutes between pressing the hospital buzzer and the arrival of the nurse, the bottomless last quarter of the fourth hour before the next morphine injection . . . nothing chops time up into such fine and cruel increments as pain that won't end. Like an especially bureaucratic form of LSD, pain insists we tour the hidden contours of time—Blake's world in a grain of sand, hellishly inverted. We scour each inhospitable moment, looking for a door out, a better view. So much time! Nothing fills it up, makes it as palpable and visible as a dye squirted into the veins, the way pain does.

Manufacturing its own minutes, pain cuts you off from the distant galaxies of Before Pain and After Pain. As Emily Dickinson wrote:

> Pain—has an Element of Blank—
> It cannot recollect
> When it begun—or if there were
> A time when it was not—
>
> It has no Future—but itself—
> Its Infinite realm contain
> Its Past—enlightened to perceive
> New Periods—of Pain.

Pain-time progresses as slowly as a story told by the most excruciating bore at a family reunion of people you are not related to. Inside pain, in the hospital, you feel doomed to witness the machinery of everything—the way the traffic noise down in the street swells to a blur during rush hour, the rattly trundling of the lunch trays down the hall. Pain becomes a bad-tempered Picasso, breaking time down into Cubist elements, then reassembling it in brutal and disarming ways in order to make you say . . . Ah, yes, I see how time works now.

Night is something else. Even in a hospital room, the light will change in the course of a day, but the hours after dark are one solid color, identical to pain. The first night on a hospital ward, in fresh pain, is a rotten banquet of time. Beside you in another bed is someone else, perhaps wandering through another landscape of pain—or worse, asleep. Sighing. Mumbling. The sound of the nurses down at their station, their island of bright light and banter—nothing could seem farther away. Darkness becomes a cave in which pain swells, until the night feels engorged with it, like a tick full of blood. The world outside the circumference of this pain goes blank and becomes unimaginable. And whoever you normally are in your life—the person who buys navy blue pajamas, or tells a joke in a certain way—has fled. Instead, you have turned into an easily shamed servant, frantic to please your humorless master, pain. He's a bully in a too-tight collar. You are obsequious and apologetic as you pray to neglected gods and promise total reform if only the bully will take his foot off your neck.

In pain, you become grateful for the smallest things. A nurse adjusts a pillow under your shoulders. You want to marry the nurse. There are no ordinary attendants when you're in pain, only angels or sadists.

Then, as soon as the agony passes, time snaps back into its old elastic ways, fitting you with more forgiveness. A whole morning can drift by, a branch carried on a current. But if the pain comes back, its random power to strike makes you feel temporary as a sand castle. One minute you're on the beach, an impressive, crenellated edifice with moats and turrets. Then a wave of pain breaks over you, and everything is first blurred and then demolished. Nothing is left in your spot but a great, liquid muscle of pain.

Chronic suffering creates its own chronic sense of time—a thick, stoical knowledge of how long a day takes to be digested, and of the secret folds and creases of time that a sleepless night conceals.

Each portion of the twenty-four hours has its own touchy mood as well. The hours before midnight are sometimes hopeful; the darkness seems fresh, and almost like sleep. Even the minutes between one and two A.M. have their mild drama, the sense of a solitary tryst with the self. And in the middle of the night, the need to be brave for the sake of others is mercifully suspended. Everyone else is asleep. Bodies are at rest.

But the time just before dawn requires serious negotiation. These are scary, bottomless hours. It's as if every night at four A.M. you have to sign a new contract, with many little riders, agreeing to wake up the next day. And this is when the prospect of going under becomes seductive. Struggle seems bogus, the work of a bad actor. At four A.M. fear and the imagination take over, interpreting every new symptom as hemorrhagic stroke and heart attack. Tumors are nocturnal. Like a dog with a bone, pain runs away with you.

Then there is the loneliness. No one else is up at these hours, and if they are, they don't want to be. Partners brew tea, droop, and chain-yawn. Even books seemed closed and shuttered for the night. Late-night radio channels voices from the other side—a kind of wacky Australia of exiles from the daylight world. Only wolves, ghosts, new mothers, jazz DJs, and people in pain inhabit this corner of the night.

At four A.M., you have no choice but to lie there and accept the weight of time. Lie submerged in it like a boulder in a cold stream, half in the water, half breaching the air. You are bestride two elements now, like an artist in dialogue with the self. Pain has split you into subject and object, where, like Emily Dickinson, you can observe yourself decked out in the coffin of the moment.

14

AN ARCHAEOLOGY OF PAIN

He had never realized before that underneath every action, underneath
the life of every day, pain lies, quiescent, but ready to devour.

VIRGINIA WOOLF, *The Voyage Out*

SUMMER. I WAS WALKING UP THE INDISTINCT
path from the dock to our rented cabin in the
Laurentian Mountains of Quebec. There was
no proper path, just a daily decision on the
part of the three of us to take this or that route
down through the long grass and wildflowers
—Indian paintbrush, small buttercups tipped
up on their angular stems, and blank-faced
daisies growing not just along the path but in
it. Each day we would make our way down
this slope toward the lake and a dock that had
been slightly buckled by the winter ice in this
cold part of Canada. The dock seemed about
to execute a wooden twirl. We got used to
lying on it at a slight tilt, as if lounging inside
a satellite dish. No straight lines, no flat surfaces: nature.

It had rained almost every day since we arrived, so the path now had muddy parts and crossed a line of unsteady rocks at the foot of the dock. These rocks required a certain amount of last-minute decision making and agile hopping. In fact, at each stage, the path was 100 percent choice and revision—this way or that? The buttercups could be avoided, but the grass at some point had to be trod upon. The users of the path—my husband, our teenage son, and me—had agreed with our feet to take the most logical route. Canoe hauling, with its more lumbering gait, had revised it, too. The path was always in progress for the month we spent defining it day after day.

Paths are great liberators of the mind. Paying full attention to where you step frees up your train of thought. Each time I picked my way up or down the slope, I found myself changing my mind about something. The thought of a *planned* path, a straight line from cabin to lake, seemed distinctly unappealing. This got me thinking about pathways in general—which, as it turns out, are central to the way we understand pain.

What is the path that pain takes in the body? Since Descartes, scientists have stayed very attached to the idea that pain can be linked to one neural pathway, a single pain cell, or one Grand Central pain depot in the brain, even though these magical centers and cells continue to elude them.

The allure of this theory is easy to understand. If pain travels through us like some hidden version of a garden hose, then surely we can figure out how to tie it off or root it out. A hopeful view.

Science, in other words, is superstitious, and prefers to prove what it wants to believe. I've already compared pain to the invisible but beguiling Sasquatch, but a better comparison might be the Lost Continent of Pain, or the mythical city of Atlantis. Convincing "scientific" evidence can always be marshaled to prove that Atlantis really did exist, off the coast of Greece or Florida or Greenland. In the same way, evidence for pain centers can always be found in the thalamus, the hypothalamus, the midbrain, or other regions of the brain. Science tends to lay down a straight paved road before exploring where the existing paths might lead.

In crude terms, the pain-pathway concept seems logical. When I cut my hand slicing a bagel, something obviously happens at the end of my arm that ends up as a very intimate event in my consciousness—pain. A body-event transforms itself into a spasm of the self. How?

There are two schools of thought about "pain pathways": one is the paved-road sort, the other more like the patterned chaos of an English roundabout. First, we went with the telegraph-line theory. The knife cuts your index finger. This unpleasant sensation, the so-called nociceptive impulse, travels from the nerve endings of cut skin up the cables of a dedicated pain pathway, into the spinal cord, up the "pain and temperature tract" to the brain, probably the cortical region, which—here's the tricky part that no one could explain—then interprets these signals as pain. In other words, *pain in, pain out.* This is the concept that dominated science from the days of Descartes until the gate-control theory of pain was published in 1965. Melzack and Wall hypothesized that pain was a two-way highway, with signals going up to the brain and other chemical messages descending to modify the pain input. The whole picture of pain began to evolve from the idea of simple transmission to the notion of a dynamic interaction. As with most things modern, the idea of a "center" didn't hold.

Scientists began to look at things differently. "Nothing can properly be called 'pain,' " William Livingston and his team of pain investigators concluded, "unless it can be consciously perceived as such." "Pain is in the brain" is how Melzack puts it. There is no fixed pain pathway that we can magically yank out of the body, like a varicose vein—there are only various transactions between peripheral signals, the central nervous system, different regions of the brain, and our individual response to the world. "Pain is never just a matter of anatomy and physiology," David Morris writes in *The Culture of Pain,* "it happens at the point where bodies, minds and culture meet." Elsewhere he reminds us that "our pain, now officially emptied of meaning and merely buzzing mindlessly along the nerves, is the product of its own specific modern history."

In the past fifty years, we have moved toward what could be

called the postmodern picture of pain—shifting, interactive, fluid, and relativistic. (As Martin Amis pronounced in his dentally dominated, pain-sodden memoir, *Experience,* "Shaw was wrong: suffering IS relative.") Using new imaging techniques, neuroscience is now able to track in detail the electrical activity that pain elicits in the brain. What do they find? Basically, that pain moves around. No central pain station has emerged—instead, we should talk about pain storms, or pain patterns, or even pain prints (the brain's version of fingerprints).

The fixed-path theory arose from the mechanistic view that "we" live inside our bodies like a suit of armor. "We," greasy little mind stains that we are, simply don the various technical bits that help us walk around and have sex. The idea that pain is a mutable, context-dependent, subjective event keeps it more unmappable, and suspect. If the more dynamic theory is correct, then pain becomes part of each person's neurological signature. Accepting the subjective nature of pain challenges the experts, since each person then becomes the only possible expert in his or her own private pain.

In the fixed-path school of pain, there was assumed to be a simple stimulus-reflex arc. The worse the damage, the greater the pain. But as many have learned to their sorrow, chronic pain doesn't necessarily work like this. A minor injury can heal, yet months later mysteriously trigger intense, persistent pain. And people who sustain dramatic wounds—even a leg shredded by a land mine—may feel no pain at all at the time of the injury. Pain has no logic.

What happens in the cases of chronic pain related to nerve damage is that an injury can hypersensitize the central nervous system, until it may register pain when there's no detectable injury or cause. This is the mystery and misery of "central pain" (related to the central nervous system, and not to be confused with a pain center), and one of the more dramatic ways that pain can be seen to alter the architecture of the nervous system and the brain.

It now seems as if pain carves a path through us in the same way that water creates a route down the side of a mountain. It flows where it must. Chronic pain is the result of flooding on that pathway, until it erodes a deeper channel, or creates new ones. And those channels are where even a trickle of water will flow next time. This is why it is so important to treat acute pain early, before it digs in and begins to reroute the flow. After six months or so, pain becomes set in its ways.

The longer and deeper pain flows, the more it lays down a sensitized trail for future pain. And this can become the conduit for other kinds of pain—divorce angst will head straight for that channel, until body pain and life pain become indistinguishable. This is why some people get a toothache when a friend dies, or others succumb to back episodes when stress hits. We all develop our own pain pathways.

Lumbago, sciatica, headache, a touchy, tender knee—take your choice. Pain provides a language for wordless events like loss. Sometimes I think that pain is just the body thinking out loud.

WHEN I ARRIVED AT the cabin for our holiday, I brought with me an ear infection that had been simmering away in the background. And the day before I left the city I had had a mammogram for a suspicious cyst in my breast. It was probably nothing, but I was going to have to wait for the results. All these aches and possible pains ran into one another and became one dark thing. I spent the first night of my vacation (as usual) lying awake calculating how far it was to the nearest hospital as my mind raced with unpleasant possibilities. An imminent stroke, I assumed. Funny how pain changes its locus as you get older. The panic attacks and heart leaps of my twenties had been replaced by more smoldering alarms.

In my thirties, for a long stretch, I had endometriosis. This is a rather modern kind of pain caused by estrogen-fed "wandering uterine tissue," and it was less common in the days when women had one child after another. Patches of endometrium for some reason grow outside the womb, in other parts of the pelvis, and then continue to respond to hormonal waxings and wanings. The stray tissue grows plush with blood just like the womb lining, doltishly preparing each month for some fertilized egg to drift by, even though it's in the wrong neighborhood entirely. Sometimes endometriosis is symptom-free, but in millions of women it causes monthly cycles of dragging, debilitating pain.

A digression on hysteria is called for here, because pelvic pain has often been misdiagnosed in women as *hysteria,* from *hystera,* the Greek word for womb. Hysteria was linked, especially by Freud, with suppressed, overstimulated, or otherwise unruly female sexuality. This way of thinking still feeds the notion of psychosomatic pain, and the notion of hysteria has cast suspicion over female reproductive pain to this day. "Hysteria," writes David Morris, "both ancient and modern, provides important evidence that pain is constructed as much by social conditions as by the structure of the nervous system. It allows us to understand how women and men may face illness in cultural contexts so different as to create what can only be called male pain and female pain."

Plato took a strikingly different view of things. He believed that the womb was a separate creature entirely, a *small animal* that lived inside women. He was quite serious about this. When this little creature wandered around, it caused trouble, as you might imagine. So Plato believed in a "wandering uterus," too, except in this case, he was referring to the womb itself. As is often the case with the early philosophers, these colorful theories would eventually bear some resemblance to scientific fact. Endometriosis does in fact behave like a small runaway animal in the pelvis.

In the nineteenth century, the neurologist Silas Weir Mitchell specialized in treating hysterical women, who had previously been shipped off to asylums. Mitchell didn't believe in asylums. Instead, for nervous afflictions in women he prescribed his famous "rest cure"—isolation, a high-fat diet, and absolutely no more than two hours a day of intellectual stimulation (the Häagen-Dazs-and-sitcom cure). He saw women as morally superior, oversensitive creatures who really shouldn't think too hard—or God knows what might happen. The womb might pick up and move to Paris.

Anyway, endometriosis represents a kind of estrogen poisoning, in the sense that it feeds on estrogen and is linked to years of uninterrupted menstrual cycles. Women no longer go through the sequence of pregnancies and miscarriages that was their lot in the past. But biologically speaking, the female body still equips itself for reproduction month after month. Laparoscopic microsurgery can improve or even eliminate endometriosis, but the other thing that will always (temporarily) cure it is pregnancy—an insidious biological argument for remaining barefoot and knocked up.

It's true that pregnancy cured it in me. But long before I got pregnant, I began to characterize the pain of endometriosis as a blatant, somatic pining for children. Not as a subconscious Freudian trope. I didn't just *imagine* that my body ached for children—it really did. The condition itself—the monthly swelling of the body, the dreadfully named "chocolate cysts" and "blueberry cysts" that cobweb the pelvis and can grow to invade the bladder or colon—is real, and colorfully visible on videotape.

At the time, I had met my future husband, but he wasn't ready to have children yet. So my body clamored away like this for several years. I developed odd ways of dealing with it, apart from hot-water bottles and many Tylenols. Part of my analgesic strategy was just to be with my husband. His proximity somehow cut the pain. It was like having a homing device implanted in my body.

The texture of this disease, and the pain it causes, I decided, is the same texture as thwarted longing. It feels like desire that has gone off.

Eventually I talked my future husband—to his eternal gratitude—into having a child. The hormone shift of pregnancy banished the endometriosis. Minor bouts came back when I went on very low doses of estrogen during menopause. But the pain was no longer linked with baby lust, and so it caused much less suffering.

Coming up the path to the cabin, remembering the undercurrent of longing during those years, I thought about how pain becomes imbued with . . . what is missing in your life. Pain keeps uncovering the past, making us vulnerable to old wounds. As I walked through the grass, with my attention focused on skirting the dew, the question floated up again: Why did I choose to write about this subject? I could, after all, be writing the history of the tango, or something more fun. And why do minor episodes of ordinary pain arrive with such urgent undercurrents of meaning, like indistinct forms under ice?

As if signaled by the waving daisies, thoughts of my family arrived. Stories of a great-great-grandfather who was murdered in a doorway, in Scotland, on his way to deliver the company payroll to the bank. Stabbed with a knife, family legend has it. His widow and five children then emigrated to Canada—that random murder was what brought my ancestors to this country. I thought about my mother's early life on a Saskatchewan farm before the Depression. My father as young boy, losing his dad. These were just the things I knew. A time and place where nobody talked about whatever pain they were in.

I decided that writing could be a path taken toward past pain. Not even my own. Pain with the sense, as Saul Bellow put it in his latest novel, *Ravelstein,* of "having come from 'elsewhere.'" In this expansive novel about his great, contentious friend Allan Bloom, Bellow refers regularly to Plato, and the fall from completeness that leaves us yearning for our missing half. "In Platonic theory all you know is recollected from an earlier existence elsewhere." In my case, this circling back to pain didn't feel platonic, but it did feel ancestral. Old pain.

Can pain echo down through generations?

Science now accepts that untreated pain in the body can wear new grooves in the nervous system, altering and amplifying the neural pathways. Could pain that was ignored or silenced in one generation surface as chronic pain—or at least an unusual attunement to pain—in the next?

Pain might be more than an erasable memory or something to "overcome." It might be a permanent memory, embedded in our cells and genes, changing the way future generations respond to the world. A big, Vienna-sized thought that overtook me on my grassy path.

This even makes some evolutionary sense. If one society permits a great crime to flourish in its midst—the Holocaust, for instance, as an example of the greatest crime, but terrorism could be cited, too—then the ability of the species to "pass on pain" could

presumably lead to a greater investment on the part of later generations in preventing similar crimes. Empathy isn't an idea. We learn
empathy *through actively feeling the pain of others*. So a nervous system especially primed for pain may actually be a form of history. A
"flair for pain" may be inherited, just as shyness is partly genetic. If
war attunes us to the pain of others, it may help us survive.

This is why, I decided, it is not just a "health issue" to address
the matter of silenced pain, and why the study of pain is not about
documenting whiners. To be fully human, we need access to a
deeper dimension of pain as well as joy. And to truly be able to
imagine pain, we must "think with pain," as the writer Viktor
Frankl has put it.

Frankl, the author of *Man's Search for Meaning* (a book that
sold millions of copies when it came out in 1964), was a psychologist
who survived Auschwitz. He wrote about his time in the camp, and
how people went about salvaging meaning, even grace, from their
experiences as prisoners. It revised his understanding of human
nature. Frankl observed that even in the hopelessness of Auschwitz,
the most important form of independence could still survive—the
spiritual freedom of individuals to create meaning out of their experience. "Fundamentally, therefore, any man can, even under such
circumstances, decide what shall become of him—mentally and spir-
itually. . . . Dostoevski said once, 'There is only one thing that I
dread: not to be worthy of my sufferings.' " Despite the humiliations
heaped upon them, Frankl saw that people could remake their
world, in ways that were invisible and inviolable, simply by looking
for meaning in their actions.

In a certain light, the fact of the Holocaust and the existence of
terrorism in the world seem to argue against both meaning and God.
(Our first response to pain is always "Why me?" It seems illogical.)
But pain is also an opportunity to make meaning. This definition was
offered to me by a friend, a therapist who has spent months immobilized by back pain. At first this sounds a little Pollyanna—"When
someone gives you lemons, make lemonade"—but the process of
working through pain has nothing to do with perky stoicism. The
meaning of pain is transformative.

Frankl was forced to confront an extremity of pain that most people never encounter. "Suffering had become a task on which we did not want to turn our backs," he wrote. "We had realized its hidden opportunities for achievement, the opportunities which caused the poet Rilke to write '*Wie viel ist aufzuleiden!*' 'How much suffering there is to get through!' Rilke spoke of 'getting through suffering' as others would talk of 'getting through work.' There was plenty of suffering for us to get through. Therefore, it was necessary to face up to the full amount of suffering, trying to keep moments of weakness and furtive tears to a minimum. But there was no need to be ashamed of tears, for tears bore witness that a man had the greatest of courage, the courage to suffer."

Like someone who steps inside the negative of a photograph, Frankl survived an experience in which darkness and pain, rather than light, determined the contours. He underwent a reversal of normal values. Normally, we turn our faces away from death and suffering. After all, it's painful to witness pain, and only human to turn away. But Frankl discovered that confrontation with physical hardship and spiritual pain—his own and others'—on a daily basis didn't result in a proportionate amount of suffering. "Suffering completely fills the human soul and conscious mind, no matter whether the suffering is great or little." For him, the aftershocks of imprisonment that followed his eventual liberation from Auschwitz were much worse. Inside the camp, committed to survival, engaged with his fellow prisoners, there were strengths to be found and even peace deep within pain. *It was being on the periphery of pain that hurt the most.*

The periphery, the margins of pain, is where our past attitudes toward the subject have landed us. When medicine zeroed in on symptoms and disease and began to leave individuals and the environment out of the picture, we shut the lid on pain. It began to shed its religious or pagan contexts and exist in a cultural vacuum.

My own gloomy hunches regarding our denial of pain were confirmed when I read the book I have been liberally quoting from: David Morris's synthesis of science, history, art, and literature, *The Culture of Pain*. He argues that our modern era, in its pharmaceutical trance of self-induced anesthesia, has helped create the wave of chronic pain that is upon us.

When the best we can do is throw painkillers at it, we have already set up the conditions for low-grade, elusive, deep-seated forms of pain. Maybe we're now paying the price for the road that pain-phobic medicine has taken for the past several hundred years. If that's the case, we should be as vigilant about the contents of our culture as we are about our drinking water. Culture is a nutrient, too.

The thing is, pain will out. The more we run from pain, the more it will seek new paths. I think this goes for history that diminishes pain as well. If we try to mute or numb the legacy of pain in certain stories, such as the slow self-destruction of aboriginal people, the eruption of phantom pains should come as no surprise. The level of suicide and self-destruction among natives is a form of phantom pain, the result of cultural amputation. The pain emerges when a community has been severed not only from its past but from an acknowledgment of the damage inflicted.

"History is what hurts," Robert Jameson has said. Pain and the visceral memory of pain always work against the lie of revisionist constructions. History that hurts but never surfaces becomes a liminal ache instead, using the body to keep the truth alive.

Pain often poses itself as a question that requires an answer. As the poet Anne Carson wrote, "One of the principle qualities of pain is that it demands an explanation."

AND DOWN AT THE bottom of this archaeological dig of pain, of course, is our fear of and unease with death. Part of pain's urgency is to sound the alarm and remind us that we're mortal. However, despite the slow advance of the palliative care movement, we still prefer to keep death, and its roommate pain, sequestered away.

So we ache in the dark, afraid of what our shadow pains mean. Are we dying? The question arises so quickly and so alarmingly because we have so few alternative meanings for pain. Instead, we try to cultivate a physical and moral numbness as a shield against pain. Pain becomes a ringing phone we never answer. Until we become more frank with death, more accepting of it in the room, we will probably go on letting ordinary injuries metastasize into chronic suffering. Pain is a splinter that has to work its way out. It's when we try to ignore that small, early wound that the radius of pain swells.

LATE ONE NIGHT IN the cabin, I heard a faint, erratic thumping somewhere outside, like a door banging, but there was no wind. Just thick, wild silence. On the edge of sleep, I would hear another restless thump again, a slightly hollow sound. Since there were no other houses nearby, it was hard to diagnose this noise. Then I remembered that we hadn't brought the canoe up on the shore, and the bow, lifted about by waves, was knocking against the dock where it was tethered. I got up, found a flashlight, and made my way down to the dock, glancing up at the stars on the way. Such a profusion of stars. The edge of the dock had already been nibbled away by the metal prow of the canoe. I hauled it up on shore and overturned it, against the direction of the wind.

Coming up the path to the cabin in the dark, my mind open and aimless, strange thoughts popped into my head—that the body with its ordinary pains is also a forked branch that can point to a hidden, underground stream of historical pain. That pain tunes us in to the past.

15

LOSS

I'm going out of my mind
With a pain that stops and starts—
Like a corkscrew to my heart,
Ever since we've been apart.

BOB DYLAN, "You're a Big Girl Now"

THE PATH PAIN TAKES IN US IS ALSO carved out by love. A broken heart hurts. It's physical—a pressure in the chest, the heavy sensation of being entombed in the body. The end of love is a deep, diffuse, crazy-making pain, like a toothache. We go on seeking out and testing the edges of this pain the way the tongue seeks out the jagged tooth or the appalling empty socket.

The first lost love is the template. Evicted from the sunny rooms that love once furnished, the sensation of heartache can feel like a shelter at first, or a trip to the rehab clinic, where withdrawal from love is as intense as love itself. Absence gets turned into presence. But eventually you have to leave that room, too. It's hard to realize how much the presence of love buffers and encloses you until you have to step outside its bulletproof shield.

Living inside love, on the other hand, everything works so smoothly: The world fits, every light turns green in time, the body seems the perfect vessel for joy. The components of life dovetail like a handmade join in a wooden box. Nothing feels broken.

At the same time that love offers shelter, it also improves the view. Even ugly or forlorn places—a ravine full of urban junk, a deserted asphalt schoolyard—seem welcoming. Anywhere is fine. I once kissed someone I was in love with in the middle of a minor blizzard, at night, outside, on a stone bench in a park. I couldn't have felt warmer or more at home. Wherever we found ourselves, under the influence of love, felt hospitable, like a well-lit room. The lucky get to live inside the body that way, too. Even terrible, objective pain can be borne, or at least borne with less anguish, by someone confident in love.

Children can behave with what looks like extraordinary courage when faced with physical ordeals. They endure operations in an offhand, chipper way and bounce back. They lack self-pity and don't cling to a history of pain. Children are right there inside the horrible moments and then, poof, they move beyond them to the next moment. It's not that they feel less pain, although that was the assumption medicine worked from until only recently. Children and babies clearly feel as much—if not more—physiological pain than adults. But when they are too small to use words to express how they feel, the lack of language, combined with the invisibility of pain, can mislead people into imagining they feel less pain. Medicine now uses "facial analogue scales"—a pain scale using a range of facial expressions, from happy through noncommittal to howling tears—so that children can communicate their distress to the people caring for them.

But despite their capacity for experiencing and expressing pain, children sometimes appear as adept as yogis at "not suffering." Well-loved children tend not to doubt themselves. They still *are* their bodies. When they're in pain, they may scream, or cry, or withdraw inside themselves. But when it passes, the sun comes out again. Unless the pain keeps coming back, children don't languish or act wounded. Pain doesn't seem to shake their sense of identity in the same way it attacks the adult sense of self.

This is no digression from the subject of lost love, by the way. Just as cared-for children can confront pain without the fear and anxiety that transform it into more intense suffering, love allows adults to face it with some of the same innocence. When you fall deeply in love, it resituates you back inside the endless, sunny day of the adored child. You cut a swath. Your bodies together throw a tall, gleeful shadow up to the moon, down into the earth. Falling in love, you recover that early, irrepressible sense of power and invulnerability. When you lie on the grass, like children you can once again sense the curve of the earth, the wheel of the universe.

For children, a tent made out of dusty blankets held up with chairs and dust mops is a fine place—the finest place. In the same way, love can redefine a less-than-perfect hideaway and make even pain habitable. We gratefully take refuge inside adult love in the same way we once lived unselfconsciously inside childhood—when we were naturally brave.

Although love and a safe childhood can't shield anyone from injuries or illness, to an almost miraculous degree both can inoculate us against unnecessary suffering. The placebo response is a powerful painkiller, and it is a conditioned one; in other words, the placebo response will not work unless we have *already* experienced relief from pain and have learned to expect that same relief, under similar circumstances. In the same way, safe and loved children have been given a set of hopeful expectations: When something hurts, they are confident that they'll survive and that help will come. In the least sentimental sense, love is the best medicine.

Being loved can help us distinguish between mere pain and bottomless, free-fall suffering. This is why people in chronic pain who live alone are not just at the mercy of a body that hurts. Over time, their pain becomes inseparable from a larger sense of being unconsoled and (much worse) being inconsolable. Their pain becomes a voicing of their isolation—cruel proof that no one can ever really know what another person feels. Pain, in short, becomes suffering.

I can remember being in my early twenties, standing around at some literary event where two older men were talking about a friend who was gravely ill. "But what would you know about pain," one of the men said, in a well-meant but awkward attempt to include me. I felt mildly insulted, of course, but was surprised by my reaction. Even then, in my lucky life, I knew I was no stranger to pain. For some reason, I already felt like a veteran, although nothing to speak of had wounded me.

The Buddhists believe that pain in this life may be a debt to a former one—that stubborn pain is visceral, ancient history. Geneticists believe that a talent for pain can be inherited and is nothing but a matter of peptides. Whatever the origin, I've always hated it when people leave me, either for the weekend or forever, and the sense of being abandoned always plays out in me as physical pain.

In the trade, they call this "somatization." When highly "rational" people don't own up to anger or sadness, the emotions can go underground and surface as pain. Physical symptoms give someone a logical reason to feel bad. In my case, I can always tell myself that "I" am doing okay—it's just my body that has a little problem. Women in particular can have a problem with this, when they feel their emotions are too outsized or inappropriate for their world. The most obvious example is when unexpressed anger in women turns inward and is transformed into depression. But sometimes the feelings come up to the surface in more melodramatic manifestations, like the creature that drives up out of the bodies of its victims in the movie *Alien*.

Loss and brave children are on my mind because I'm alone in the house. My husband has flown off on business to another continent for several weeks. Normally this is the sort of break we both look forward to after living together for twenty-four years. And for the first few days after he has left, I'm temporarily thrilled to live the single-mother life, renting movies he wouldn't deign to watch and leaving dishes in the sink. I feel pretty darn euphoric, in fact.

Then a sense of wrongness sets in, and a soap-opera feeling of desertion comes over me. It's maddening and illogical. He travels often, calls regularly, and it's not unusual for me to take off on my own for a week or two. But when he's the one to walk out the door, however benignly, the needle on my Desertion Meter goes up into the red and the whole pathology kicks in.

The pain starts in the shoulder, moves up the jaw and face, then spreads down the right side of my body. A horrible thought occurs to me whenever this happens: Maybe long-standing couples develop an architectural stability that requires both of them to stay put. Remove one weight-bearing support, and the whole structure gets shaky. That's how it feels, in fact—teetery, off-balance.

Alas, my husband doesn't share my separation symptoms. He feels fine, except he has trouble sleeping alone. It's a trade-off; he needs me to get through the night, and I need him to get through the day. The friction between people under the same roof, which can be so rankling, also gives us borders and makes us feel solid. Separating opens a small but real wound that leaves us more uncovered, more vulnerable to pain.

I took the usual steps to un-somatize. Made an appointment for a massage. Met with some friends. For an evening, I gave up trying to be madly productive with my solitude and just sat around feeling bereft. I thought back to the other times when people have checked out of my life, and I've been "fine," too. Then I would be felled by something physical—dizzying bouts of sinusitis, heart mayhem, or that mysterious muscular voodoo all down one side.

Love really is a drug. Love has major side effects; it lets you fly across the rooftops, like Chagall's wavy-necked couple. Then when it disappears, something as profound as withdrawal from a narcotic happens. No more flying. Gravity reclaims you. The weight of life descends again, and the shoulders droop, the spine droops, the mouth droops. The lighting in the room turns harsh, unmasking flaws in the room you had forgotten about. Things suddenly cry out to be fixed and mended. You feel the creakings of time in your body.

I've learned to recognize this as a cycle that is unavoidable, but transient. By the time my husband has been gone for a week, I have adjusted to my single status and realigned myself. And when he comes back, I know there's going to be that rocky reentry phase for both of us. Like a satellite reentering the earth's atmosphere—a period of intense friction, followed by alarming heat and near-meltdown and then, restabilization. Calm.

Rehearsing loss is the price of sleeping in the same bed with someone for a long time. Even in its most married version, the business of separating can still make me feel the raw, unhealed edges of every other lost love.

16

RAIN ON THE ROOF

Our wounds are far less unique than our cures.

JIM HARRISON, *Just Before Dark*

WHEN PEOPLE IN PAIN TALK ABOUT WHAT they do for themselves to feel better, they begin by rattling off a list of medications or therapies. But sooner or later they will mention, apologetically, the odd unmedical thing that helps. A certain rocking chair. A purring cat asleep on their chest. And more than once, I was told that the sound of rain on the roof was a particular comfort. Obviously, this didn't come from a scientist. I heard the rain-on-the-roof remedy first from Jim Harrison, the American novelist, poet, and screenwriter, who has negotiated his way through a whole smorgasbord of pain in his customary unorthodox fashion.

As a writer, Harrison is an agile shapeshifter who can crawl inside a broad spectrum of characters that includes wolves, bears, dogs, Native Americans, and women. Although best known as a novelist, Harrison also wrote the movie *Wolf* and the screenplay based on his novel *Legends of the Fall*. His novella *Dalva* inhabits a profoundly female imagination with the utmost grace. Nothing seems beyond his ken, and certainly not pain. When I met him after a reading, I asked him about a column he once wrote in *Esquire,* which described the aftermath of a sinus operation. He said that the pain of having his sinuses reamed out was roughly on a par with his sojourns as a screenwriter in Hollywood.

And yet Harrison is a guy's guy, an ursine fellow of girth and appetite who likes to hunt, eat, and cook with Hemingway brio. In person, he is charming and shy, an effect intensified by the fact that you can't tell whether he's looking at you or someone else over your shoulder, because his eyes don't match. He agreed to be pestered on the subject of pain by fax, when he got back home to Minneapolis (although he added that he thought book tours, "which in general are a shit monsoon," should be in the pain index, too).

"The earliest pain I can remember," he wrote back, "and perhaps most severe, happened when I was seven years old. I was playing doctor with an unkind little girl, and she jammed a broken bottle in my left eye and blinded it. I don't suppose pain medication was as effective at that time, and after a month in the hospital there were several more months of acute discomfort that I didn't know quite how to express. The only thing that seemed to help was rain on the roof of our cabin. Over 50 years later, rain on the roof of my cabin in the Upper Peninsula is still the most soothing remedy for mental pain. After that came a facial fracture in football, the tearing of back muscles and a fall off a cliff. This latter experience involved several years of pain. I suppose I should add sinus and gout. Oddly enough, gout is relatively simple to deal with despite the severity of the pain because you can distance yourself from it, which you can't do with the head and the back."

I asked him how pain changes the way we look at the world.

"Pain makes us more conscious of our mortality," he wrote, "but then we should be. In Zen, you try to die a little bit every morning so it won't come as a big surprise. Acute pain is too over-whelming to associate with it, although you are a lot better off if you stop short of writhing around."

How would he describe his relationship to pain?

"My relationship to pain," he answered, "is that of a suppli-cant in the face of a small, implacable god."

Harrison has a strong bond with his dogs and other creatures. I asked him if he thought that animals feel pain in the same way we do. Does great pain require higher consciousness—whatever that is?

"We have every reason to feel that animals feel pain as we do, though there is evidence that they don't have the immense psycho-logical apparatus that we develop. Once, when our eldest daughter had surgery at age 3, I noted that she was better at ignoring the dis-comfort. Trout fishermen of the catch-and-release variety ignore the fact that fish obviously are in pain, which causes the struggle that we find so entertaining. It is a mandarin approach to fishing. There is no virtue in not eating the fish other than to possibly further the species population. As I have said before, I like to think of reality as an accretion of the perceptions of all creatures.

"But our culture is in denial about pain because it distances itself from all 'otherness.' We suffocate the core of life in an effluvia of lint and detritus. We are daily absorbed in taking a psychic heroin in the form of what the media offers."

Isn't there any purification involved in the experience of pain? Does a hangover, for instance, have its spiritual payoff? "The trouble with the plus side of hangovers is that it's rather rare," he cautioned. "Maybe one out of ten can be instructive in clarifying, perhaps in the manner of a shock treatment.

"The worst aspect of pain is its utterly unforgiving nature. The best is that, properly viewed, it can correct your capacity to dilly-dally through life as if you were a Nerf toy," he concluded. "As Rilke said, 'Only in praising is my heart still mine, so violently have I known the world.' "

AFTER HEARING FROM HARRISON, I began to ponder the rain-on-the-roof phenomenon, and whether it might not have some scientific basis in the gate-control theory of pain. Maybe rain on the roof is an especially effective version of "white noise," a competing aural stimulus. It reminded me of an ad for something called the "Fussbuster" for fussy babies. This is a CD with recordings of variations on white noise—a tumbling clothes dryer, a humming vacuum cleaner, drops of water in a bathtub, the sound of a dishwasher. Nine minutes for each cut. I thought back to the days when my son was a baby with one ear infection after another; I used to calm him by setting his basket on the warm, churning dryer. In addition to offering the interruption of a new stimulus, white noise may also reproduce the muffled sounds of our first environment in the womb. Perhaps our "normal" neurological set point is not silence and stillness, but the rock and roll of our mothers walking, turning, eating, sighing. Perhaps rain on the roof "rocks" us, too, reminding us of the guaranteed analgesia of life in the womb.

I was standing in line in the bank the other day (an endangered activity) behind a young mother with a baby in an infant seat. Whenever she set it on the floor, the seat rocked. It seemed to be equipped with some windup motor. It was a cold February day, and the baby was tucked under many blankets, working away at a pacifier in her mouth. The line was taking forever. Then the baby fell asleep, the pacifier fell out, the motor wound down. Right away, the baby woke up, cried, and the mother set the seat in motion again. How strange and alarming it must feel, after the amniotic Jacuzzi of the womb, to be placed on a flat, still mattress of a crib in an unrocking world: like a sailor losing his balance on solid land. Rocking returns a baby to that safe, gyroscopic, prenatal dance.

Autistic children also rock back and forth on their own, to soothe themselves. Motion and stimulation reassure. The worried parent in the hospital waiting room paces up and down. The teenage boy in the library jiggles his knee, vibrating his foot against the ground. Children swing. We are constantly massaging our nervous system in these small, repetitive, and sometimes unconscious ways. Rocking, tapping, and jiggling may all be versions of the rain-on-the-roof effect.

Rock-a-bye-baby on the tree top. When the wind blows, the cradle will rock. When the bough breaks, the cradle will fall, and down will come baby, cradle and all. In other words, when the rocking stops— watch out.

ALTHOUGH WE ASSUME THAT silence and stillness is what is most calming, we seem to need certain patterns of stimuli that help us engage with our environment. This is the case with light and vision, as well as sound and motion.

I was at a friend's cabin on one end of a fair-sized lake, aware of how grateful my eyes were for the refreshment of this long focal point, across an expanse of silver water. It was a sunny day, with just enough wind to ruffle the lake. Light danced on the surface, a constant, shifting, diamond glitter. Why does soft light on moving water soothe us? Surely there's something more involved in the plea- sure of a view like this than mere beauty. It's not just that such views tend to be associated with vacations, or more time to relax. The dance of light seems to hook the eye, like the pixels of a TV screen, creating a sense of connectedness. The mind busies itself processing this constant but unpredictable pattern of visual events. Nature engages us physiologically, in ways that the simpler contours of an artificial environment cannot.

Perhaps a "good view" like this has a neurological impact, act- ing as a kind of visual massage. The depth of field and the play of light both soothe and stimulate the eye, like a pacifier in the mouth.

In other words, beauty feeds more than the soul. It promotes good health. The presence of art may even strengthen our immunity. No wonder prisons reserve a bare cell in isolation for the ultimate punishment. It is the opposite of rocking, or of rain on the roof. To be deprived of visual or aural nourishment is to be trapped in an environment that amplifies pain and misery.

When pain threatens to isolate us, the sound of rain on the roof puts us back inside the larger body of the natural world.

17

GOOD PAIN (AND GOD'S PAIN)

I'VE BEEN GOING TO THE SAME MASSAGE therapist, off and on, for years. She knows my dents and knots very well. I once came out of a session to discover that my car had been towed away. I didn't care. That's how good she is.

But lately she's been living in the country, making infrequent trips into town, and you must book her weeks, months, in advance. So when nine A.M. on Monday, the long-designated time for my massage rolled around, I had completely forgotten about the appointment. And I thought I didn't need it, either. Monday morning is when I expect to tense up, not relax. But it was too late to cancel so I rushed there anyway. I would consider it preventive—muscle flossing.

Her room has a big shelf of books, which I find reassuring, and she usually doesn't play oceanic tapes called *Bliss* or *Solitude*. Quite often, we chat. She's trained in everything under the sun from cranial-sacral to deep-tissue and uses it all. Although she has volunteered at an orphanage in India and worked on sustainable-resource farms, we may only talk about haircuts. When I arrived, I told her this was a waste of her time. I'm tip-top, I said, and slid under the cool sheets on the massage table. But the minute she started in on my neck and shoulders, it felt like she was squeezing pure muscular misery out of me like toothpaste. Everywhere she went was unexpectedly tender and tense, and yet it felt good to know that. It's odd: A massage is actually mild, reconfigured pain—good pain.

She used her fingers to draw out the tight columns of muscles in my neck and worked methodically from one area to another, like someone ironing a shirt: first the yoke, then the collar, then the sleeves. It brought my Monday-morning thoughts, which had been flying off like crows toward the horizon of work and chores, back down into my arms and legs again.

"Want any music?"

"No, this is fine."

Lying on the table, eyes closed, I replayed the events of the past weekend, which, until I had climbed up onto the table, I would have called relaxing and noneventful.

My husband was still off at the Cannes Film Festival, one of the world capitals of pleasure. The fact that he was swigging rosé in the south of France while I sat in a coffee shop underlining scholarly texts on self-mutilation was not lost on me. I had made plans to go to a movie with a friend, but at the last minute she pleaded fatigue. I went off to the video store instead and glimpsed her driving by in a car, carefully made up, on a middle-aged date. I hate being dumped for a guy.

On Sunday, my son and I drove to Burlington to spend the day with my parents. My mother had pretty well recovered from her broken shoulder, and it was a good, unharried visit, just the four of us tending to some chores around the house. The May weather was sunny, clear, and rinsed. My father sent my son up a ladder to fix a leak in the old metal eaves trough. This involved getting up on the roof and wielding a caulking gun, the sort of thing we don't often do at home. At one point, both my hale but rickety father and my alarmed-looking son were up on top of the patio roof, a wooden grid that bowed ominously under their weight. I ordered my father down. He obeyed and disappeared into the garage. Then he came out, erected a small aluminum stepladder, and climbed to the top of that. From there he instructed my son in the niceties of caulking the eaves trough.

This sort of work was child's play to my father, who is an engineer, but my son had never been on top of a house before. He soon got the hang of the job, however, and my father was good-natured about this switch of roles—the lad of the family moving farther up the ladder.

Meanwhile, my mother gave me two small dishes of seeds, one of nasturtiums, the other morning glories, and oversaw the planting of them. She doesn't like to kneel too much. Her shadow fell on me as I dug tiny holes, pressed the wet seeds into the soil, watered the depression, and covered it up with dirt. We both wore sun hats.

"I want them to go up the drainpipe and the rose trellis," my mother said. I could hear my son's slightly urgent questions—both ends, or just one?—from his perch on the ladder. After an hour or so of this, we all retired indoors, for glasses of cold water and beers. As usual, I went to the upstairs bathroom, where they have an excellent set of mirrors for looking at the back of your hair. I thought I needed a haircut.

Then, with a certain gothic banter, my mother took me on an Inheritance Tour of the house, as she asked me what I wanted. I wanted the things she had painted, or the bowls she had made when she did pottery, and my father's old pastel drawings. I wanted the antique sideboard. We gazed at her "good dishes" with the lily-of-the-valley pattern and discussed whether I liked them or not. They planned to sell the house "in a year or two," my mother said, "depending."

On the way back to Toronto, in the car, Casey and I listened to a tape, *Bird by Bird,* by Anne Lamott. It documents with neurotic accuracy the comical despair of the writing life, and it made us laugh a lot. My son is becoming a good writer. But one night, after having to write an essay on Elizabeth Smart for school, he looked at me over dinner and declared that he never wanted to make writing his problem. This was aimed at me.

The whole weekend, in fact, seemed to teeter on the cusp of things being passed along, or not. Things shifting. Absent mate, aging parents, fledging writer-son. There was nothing overt, nothing that demanded to be grieved or even remarked upon—and that was the trouble. I had spent the past two days shooing away assorted ordinary painful thoughts but they had settled in me, anyway.

The forearms are a surprising secret reservoir of pain, especially if you type a lot. Wendy worked her way down both arms, into my strangely aching palms. Ball of hand. Fingertips. The images on the inside of my eyelids changed, from the usual fuzzy-TV static to a luminous, fluid, dancing blue. I always interpret this to mean that my brain waves have gone alpha (if not omega).

"Your left side is much more rigid than your right. For what it's worth," she added, "and I never know how much of this to believe, they say that pain on the right side is about the future, and pain on the left is about unresolved things from the past."

Over the weekend, I had entertained a very unscientific view of pain by reading *The End of the Affair*, by Graham Greene. "Stop wallowing in medicine and open Graham Greene," a friend had advised me. "The English understand pain." I thought about the story as the massage progressed.

The End of the Affair is a novel in which secular love overlaps with spiritual anguish (as is usual in Greene's fiction). Right from the epigraph, he questions the purpose of pain: "Man has places in his heart which do not yet exist, and into them enters suffering in order that they may have existence." In other words, pain imagines us. This seemed true. Even the pleasurable pain of a massage seems to create new space inside the body.

The novel begins as an exquisitely exact rendering of a tragic love affair. The narrator is a writer, Maurice, who is so smitten with a woman, Sara Miles, that he fears the end of love—and so he works at destroying the relationship instead. It eventually becomes a novel about a jealous love triangle in which the Other Man is God.

The story unfolds during World War II. Sara is married to a good, dull man whom Maurice befriends. During a tryst, the lovers are caught in a shelling, and Maurice is knocked unconscious. Sara fears that he's dead and makes a pact with a God she has never believed in. If God will only spare his life, she promises she will "be good" and deliver a more peaceful life to Maurice, by leaving him. Well, of course, Maurice survives, but Sara keeps her vow. She begins seeing a priest. Maurice is shattered and assumes there is someone else. He follows her, and assumes the worst. Only later does he learn about her unsuccessful struggle to replace human love with faith in God. And then, of course . . . it's too late!

The novel describes love not as a presence but as a potential absence—the theme, it struck me, of my weekend, if not my entire life. The architecture of love oftens turns out to be about how to surround this burning question of empty space.

Maurice eventually hires a private detective, who uncovers Sara's diaries. He reads a page in them where Sara describes a dream. She is happy, because she is climbing a stairway to meet Maurice, but at the top she is met instead by a "voice that booms like a fog-horn."

"Then I woke up," she wrote. "I'm not at peace any more. I just want him like I used to in the old days. I want to be eating sandwiches with him. I want to be drinking with him in a bar. I'm tired and I don't want any more pain. I want Maurice. I want ordinary corrupt human love. Dear God, you know I want to want Your Pain, but I don't want it now. Take it away for a while and give it me another time."

Our body is God's pain—at least, that is Greene's anguished, slightly melodramatic reading. The very tissue of faith and "ordinary corrupt human love" is the pain of longing and the ache of desire.

Lying on the narrow table with the muted hiss of morning traffic coming up from the street, I was able to sort through the neglected bruises of the weekend. The orderly progression of her hands from one tender area to another made room in my body for all that I had been trying to resist.

Pain is what sets you apart, in good and bad ways. It tells us that we have collided with something—that we exist, if only because we ache. Good pain is like having a lover's quarrel with the world. It is proof of our carnal connection to existence. Pain reminds us that even long after children have grown and affairs have ended, we remember love with our body.

WHEN THE MASSAGE WAS over, I went home, ready to tense up and work. Instead, I began to bundle the newspapers for recycling and came across an article in the *New York Times Magazine* about thirteenth-century female saints and martyrs—early cheerleaders for God's pain. It linked up those rebels and visionaries to the modern mortification of girls who fall prey to eating disorders and self-mutilating impulses.

In the Middle Ages, girls didn't get to be anorexic supermodels or TV sitcom stars. They had an even narrower band of choices: They could live a thoroughly anonymous life in which extremes were not expected (or allowed), or they could choose a radical expansion of awareness that manifested itself as spiritual visions, stigmata, or acts of self-laceration. Extreme behavior. Extreme sensations. Punk piety.

Choosing pain—as I will describe in the chapters that follow—can be one way of groping for control over one's life. This is what the author of the magazine article also saw in the unsmiling faces of too-thin models and the triumph of the anorexic over desire: It may feel safer to flirt with death on your own terms than to risk sexual surrender, or to be defined by someone else.

I looked at the up-rolled eyes of these female saints and thought about a more recent martyr, Ally McBeal. The modern woman, semiempowered (or at least wearing the outfit), and still burning, still in pain. That was the "new" thing about *Ally McBeal,* when it first came on the scene—she was a lawyer, a girl with a bit of weight in the world, who still admitted to retro pinings. She missed her boyfriend. It wasn't her nice job that made her so contemporary—it was her game sadness and her starved self. She even had visions, too, if only of dancing babies and her ex.

Germaine Greer puzzled over this state of affairs in her unabashedly cranky book *The Whole Woman*. She wondered why women in the executive suites aren't pursuing real power—the power to shift the world's priorities. Why, she asks, do so many women still get sidetracked into overwrought territorial games with the boys at work, or languish in self-destructive relationships? Is a certain amount of pain the price women now accept for having moved into the corridors of power?

Studies of pain and gender, as I had learned, are no help at all. They're totally inconclusive when it comes to figuring out which gender feels more pain—but one thing is clear. More women than men *report* pain. They are more willing to express it (although gushing stigmata may be overdoing it). The chronic pain patient is most likely to be a woman, most likely older than thirty-five. On the other hand, men in pain demand more morphine than women.

Greene's heroine, Sara, chose spiritual pain instead of human love. A negotiable agony. Do women tend to "get involved" with pain, like a no-account boyfriend, rather than taking on a more viable partner—or even the world? Perhaps we starve ourselves or do things to our bodies in order to remain always a little afflicted, a bit disadvantaged. That way, the question of being totally in charge doesn't have to be an issue yet. If we can engineer our own suffering, rather than being passive to it, pain can even represent a degree of progress. Anorexia, while not chosen, can be a self-punishing form of power. The self-flagellation of the thirteenth-century saints must have felt like good pain, too.

I finished bundling the papers. One of the illustrations for the article was of the famous sculpture by Bernini, the writhing, rapturous *Ecstasy of St. Teresa*. When society stopped burning witches at the stake, some women decided to go on burning, anyway.

18

CUTTERS

SOME PEOPLE, WOMEN ESPECIALLY, DON'T wait for stigmata to strike—they like to make their own blood flow. They use razors, broken glass, or whatever's handy. They want to draw blood and leave marks, but not die.

A good way to keep strangers at a distance in a café, I have found, is to read a book like *A Bright Red Scream: Self-mutilation and the Language of Pain,* with yellow highlighter in hand. Nobody will bother you at all. Marilee Strong's book, with an introduction by the expert in the field, Armando Favazza, is a well-researched study of "cutting," a phenomenon the *New York Times Magazine* declared "the body disorder of the decade" in 1997.

Often misunderstood as a suicide attempt, the act of cutting can be a gesture in the other direction—a survival strategy. Self-injuring, as the textbooks and proliferating websites like to call it, makes psychic pain visible. There is something consoling about a scar, after all—it's a sign of healing. I remembered being a kid at summer camp, and the peculiar solace of counting my mosquito bites. If I scratched just a bit too much, they bled, and the itchy bumps turned into even more satisfying scabs.

Along with eating disorders, cutting offers women a measure of control, however desperate, over their own bodies. In a powerless situation like prison, cutting is a little bit of autonomy. Women can become the author of their suffering. And in some ways, cutters are only more literal examples of a pain-inflicting impulse found in many other corners of the culture.

Piercing is a more conventional form of self-mutilation. It's become a useful rite of passage for teenagers in part because it delivers an unequivocal message to parents: "My body belongs to me now, not you."

But some happy piercers have discovered that the act itself, the punch of the piercing gun through the flesh, delivers an intense rush, and that mysterious peace at the center of pain. Or they become enamored of the daily washing and cleansing of the newly pierced area afterward, which offers a soothing ritual of self-care. Piercings require a lot of babying. For some kids this sort of tender attention to the body might be something new.

Wound pleasure is not confined to the young or the hip. For lots of middle-aged women, cosmetic surgery has become a form of socially acceptable cutting. Some get hooked on the surgery itself, just as kids get off on piercings. There is nothing quite so intimate as having a doctor get under the skin of your face. Although I haven't had cosmetic surgery, the one time I did go under the knife lingers in my mind as a primal and even disturbingly sexy experience.

I had a small benign cyst on my right jaw that my doctor suggested I have removed. Off I went to the referred cosmetic surgeon, who happened to be one of the more well-known gents in his profession. He was handsome and reassuring. It was a routine operation and I breezed in unprepared for the attention he gave me. In the OR, I was given a local and remained conscious as he took a scalpel to my skin and then gently mucked about in the gristle of my face. We chatted. I found to my horror that I was actually . . . *flirting* as he ever so carefully, ever so tenderly, stitched up the side of my face. By the time I tottered off the operating table, we had bonded. My blood brother. And it wasn't because he made me look better; I think it was because he was looking at me and talking to me while he was literally inside me. Erotically, this has always been a hard combination to beat.

For weeks afterward, I had a strange urge. I wanted to go under the knife again. It was such an intimate place to rest.

So I get it, sort of. But being incised by a handsome doctor is a far cry from women in prison who hide razor blades in their mouths.

The other misperception about cutting, I read in Strong's book, is that it is a form of sexual masochism. Cutters don't necessarily even feel pain, and pain doesn't seem to be the point. Instead, the act of drawing blood delivers an endorphin rush and a sense of peace. The women who do it say that cutting grounds them or provides an outlet for a level of rage or anxiety that becomes intolerable. On the other hand, if they feel numb and disembodied, the sight of blood proves to them that they're alive and can feel.

In other words, cutting is not so much about inflicting more suffering as it is about connecting with a reservoir of pain that already exists. Cutting manifests hidden pain; it's a form of wounding that heals. However, some cutters then become compulsive about the act and start to accumulate scar tissue like war medals. The compulsion eventually overrides the original gesture of taking back control. Prisons are full of women, their arms covered in nubbly, leathery scar tissue, who have become addicted to cutting.

I can't help thinking that someone who inscribes her body like this is also writing. She's just chosen the harshest medium possible for telling her story. Cutting, of course, is also melodramatic, and a great way to get attention. We think pain is private and should stay that way. But cutting is pain that won't shut up.

JUST AS CUTTING IS more about a release of anxiety than a rush of masochistic pleasure, some sexual masochists have argued that pain itself is not the point of their erotic rituals. The writer and critic Kenneth Tynan teased out this distinction in a passage on spanking (which he famously enjoyed) in one of his journals: "The apprehension, the preparation, the threat, the exposure, the humiliation—

these are thrilling, and so is the warmth afterwards, and the sight of the marks; but the impact of cane on bottom is no fun at all. (There used to be an ointment on sale that deadened the skin: it was a boon to masochists.) Thus [Wilhelm] Reich is right when he declares that masochism is not—as Freud claimed—a form of death wish in that it seeks not pleasure but pain. The pain is not part of the pleasure of masochism: it is the unpleasant price that must be paid for the pleasure that precedes and follows it."

Pleasurable pain is such a vast and—as we shall see—thorny topic that I am going to leave it in the capable hands of the experts. Despite my wallow in pain for the past four years, I felt the kingdom of S&M was too populous and already well documented to try to penetrate it here. Besides, there's no surprise (or sting) left in the news that, for some people, pain is a turn-on.

In the past few decades, the S&M culture has moved from the cultural fringes into the mainstream. Piercings or tattoos are no longer just for pirates and road dogs. For women, stilettos and bondage-inspired gear have taken over where the floppy bow-tied corporate suit left off. In cartoon culture, the bullet-breasted, cat-suited dominatrix has long been a fixture. And for a surprising number of straight people, going to a leash-and-dog-collar S&M party is just another night out. What used to be considered deviant and fetishistic is now just fashion-forward. Like the volume dial in the movie *This Is Spinal Tap,* everything in pop culture now "goes up to 11 . . . because it's one louder." I could even cite the recent sentimental return of heavy metal music as evidence of the mainstreaming of S&M (or BDS&M, not to exclude bondage and discipline).

The science of S&M is not complicated: Just beyond the pain threshold, and usually stopping short of tissue damage, is the yummy cascade of endorphins. Pain's payoff. What the spankee is spanked for. At least, that's the story on the surface of the skin. The frisson of submission and domination is another sort of conditioned pleasure that has more to do with exercising or surrendering control. But I leave the niceties of all that to the Marquis de Sade and other tireless archivists of pain's erotic footnotes. My own meager experiments in this direction have only led to feelings of being trapped in a bad play.

All that needs to be said is that the option to add caramel squiggles to vanilla sex is now widely accepted.

In fact, you could even say that S&M has been domesticated. That's what struck me when I discovered a website maintained by "The Society for Human Sexuality," which offers horticultural advice—a "Torture Garden" designed by "Chuck G."—for growing irritating, thorny plants, perfect for flogging. I liked the way the site combined the grandmotherly tone of a gardening column with the Ikea-like efficiency that creative tops and subs bring to the tools of their trade:

> STINGING NETTLES: *These lovelies are usually found in disturbed areas in mild or cool climates where there is plenty of moisture or shade. They have the most potent venom when the plants are small. The effects are an immediate and very nice burn, which is not especially intense and wears off after a couple hours, with generally no lasting effects. The term venom is pretty accurate as the plants have small hypodermic-like needles along the stems and under the ribs of the leaves. . . . Fresh plants, applied to any tender areas of the body, should result in some nice reactions in the sub. The venom of nettles can be neutralized by a small plant that grows near it in very wet soil called false or wild impatiens. This plant has thin small leaves and succulent stems and yellowish flowers with brown spots that are bilaterally symmetrical, like small orchids or snap dragons. If I were going to cultivate these nettles in a garden setting, I would confine their roots in a large bottomless planter, or with a thick plastic or tin collar around them sunk at least 1 foot deep and angled slightly outward. Cut them down before they go to seed, unless you are an EXTREME masochist and like painful weeding.*

> CACTUS AND SUCCULENTS: *Most of us are familiar with cactus, and if you like pain as much as yours truly, have experimented with them somewhat. I tested nearly every species for the sharpness and skin-piercing abilities of the spines and found that some have barbed traits also, making them hang on once in place*

in the skin. Some cactus have spines that are decidedly hooked and devilish-looking. One thing to realize about cacti is that they generally do not grow back spines that have been harvested; thus, if you have a nice specimen, it would be best to savor each spine you remove and use in a special way.

More urban sadists may prefer the Violet Wand. This is a spark-generating gadget with a high-frequency circuit, similar to a Tesla coil, that builds up a static charge in a gas-filled glass tube. "If you hold the tube near your sub's body," the instructions say, "each time the charge builds up enough to jump the gap, a spark jumps from the tube to your sub's skin. Unlike shuffling across the rug, though, the Wand can spark many times a second. You can adjust the intensity and rate of sparks depending on your purpose. The nature of the body's response to this type of charge is such that you can use the wand anywhere on the body except for the eyes."

The amateur science of inflicting pain turns out to be every bit as creative as the science of treating it.

19

BOB FLANAGAN, SUPERMASOCHIST

SOME CHOOSE PAIN; SOME ARE CHOSEN BY it. In the case of Robert Flanagan, he lived both sides of the coin. Flanagan was an American writer, performance artist, longtime survivor of cystic fibrosis, and a tirelessly inventive sexual masochist. By making pain a source of pleasure, he gained some control over the suffering he had no say in.

Flanagan was the subject of an unforgettable 1997 documentary that Roger Ebert called "one of the most agonizing films I've ever seen." Co-produced by Flanagan's wife, Sheree Ross, *Sick: The Life and Death of Bob Flanagan, Supermasochist,* also has many tender moments, but the most infamous one involves a scene in which Flanagan nails the head of his penis to a board. Whenever I'm talking to a man about pain and his eyes glaze over (as happens with men on this topic) I can always snap him awake by referring to this little Everest of agony.

Flanagan's personality and wit manage to dominate (as it were) the more shocking elements of the film. The extremes of his life somehow have the cumulative effect of normalizing pain, almost domesticating it. The S&M lifestyle is one based on rituals, conventions, devices, and accessories to the point where it sometimes seems like a direct inversion of suburbia. The movie is also a moving account of Flanagan's relationship to Sheree Rose, his fifteen-year life-and-art partner. Most of all, it's an unflinching, perhaps pro-flinching, portrait of someone who chose "to fight sickness with sickness" and to talk back to pain in its own language.

Flanagan, who died in January 1996, at the age of forty-two, was the world's oldest survivor of cystic fibrosis, a genetic disorder that affects the lungs and pancreas. Most people with CF die before they reach adulthood. It's a dreadful disease, causing an oversecretion of thick mucus that clogs the lungs, making breathing difficult and inviting perpetual bacterial infections. The oxygen depletion caused by the congestion leads to excruciating headaches and fatigue, not to mention the sensation of drowning in one's own bodily fluids.

Flanagan grew up in an Irish Catholic family, spending his childhood either in constant pain or in the hospital, being poked and needled, and in bondage to an oxygen tank. Not surprisingly, he eventually made it his aesthetic mission to explore sexual pleasure through pain. He was a poet, one of the founders of the Los Angeles poetry workshop Beyond Baroque, and he used his own body in mordantly funny S&M performances. For seventeen years, he was also a counselor at a camp for children with cystic fibrosis, where he entertained them with songs like "It's Fun Being Dead" and "Forever Lung," a rearranged Bob Dylan tune. Flanagan found an inspiring dominatrix in Sheree Rose, a West Coast artist with red hair, big breasts, and an M.A. in psychology. On screen, their relationship is so warm/bitchy/ordinary that before long, the novel images of trussed-up genitals, mouth gags, and sessions of mild, consensual torture seem no stranger than the gym-going, dog-grooming, and BBQ rituals of any couple. Sheree Rose and Flanagan just had a different take on the phrase "in sickness and in health."

Flanagan was a brutally honest reporter from both sides of suffering—the obnoxiousness of his disease, as well as the pleasure he got from having pain consciously inflicted. He was an amusing tour guide through pain's red-light district. In exhibits like "Visiting Hours," which toured to major galleries in New York and Boston, Flanagan would lie on a gurney of nails or suspend himself naked from hooks in the ceiling. He also published five books of poetry and appeared in a number of music videos including "Happiness in Slavery" for the group Nine Inch Nails. The video had the distinction of being banned on MTV.

In the last year of his life, however, he was mostly tortured by his diminishing interest in painful sex. ("Just now she wanted to drip hot wax on me, but I said no to that too.") He kept track of this and other aspects of illness is his *Pain Journal,* a funny, fascinating, whiny, banal, human account of what a drag it is to live in pain. He was dying, and he knew it. Originally a website, the journal was published as a paperback, with an afterword from Sheree Rose, in 2000. It tells no lies. Although *The Pain Journal* is not elegant literature, it is as valuable a charting of pain as anything medicine might offer.

"Thought I'd write tonight," Flanagan reported in March 1995, "but found myself mulling over why it is I don't like pain anymore. I have this performance thing to do and I'm shying away from doing or having SM stuff done to me because pain and the thought of pain mostly just irritates and annoys me rather than turns me on. But I miss my masochistic self. I hate this person I've become. And what about my reputation?"

Early in the same month he wrote:

My irritability and depression is amok. I feel like crying all the time. My computer keeps crashing, which is exactly how I feel. I've been off antidepressants since Christmas. Time to go back? I guess. Will it help? Is all this oxygen related? I've got it up to 3 liters. Too much? Not enough? Who knows. The TV is on but I can't hear it because I've got ear plugs in my ears to block out Sheree's snoring. I want to run upstairs and fiddle with the computer to get it working again so at least something's back on track, but it's too late (4 am). I was asleep but I woke up an hour ago with an awful stomach ache and the usual heart ache. Don't know what to do with myself. Took a couple of anti-anxiety pills, Oxazepams, but they only make me sleepy, so now I'm sleepy and anxious. I guess I'm really into the pills now. The age old quest for happy pills. But there ain't none. My body throbs with unhappiness. It's like a big weight, a giant distraction all the time. So I'm always annoyed by it, antagonized from the minute I wake up, till the time I finally go to sleep—doesn't leave room for much of anything else.

Three months later, he writes:

Tonight's notes, before I slip off into my pharmaceutical soup: more aches and pains from the aches and pains department. No Demerol. Some Vicodin. The names of these drugs are capitalized as if they were gods. St. Vicodin. Lord Demerol. Our Lady of Cephtazidime. Let's not forget the great and powerful Zoloft, son of Prosac [sic].

And by October, he is in the hospital, still pounding on the laptop:

Waiting for the nurse to come on who pushes the Demerol, rather than the one who slowly infuses it with the pump. Fuck the pump. Gimmie the push. So what, a 30 second brain rush, is that gonna kill me? With the pump, by the time it's infused I'm wanting it again. Ah, fuck it. Why don't I just start shooting heroin like the rest of the junkies? Because I'm still a good boy. A sick boy, but a good boy. And the worst I'll do is, while the nurse is out of the room I'll take the Damitall out of the pump and give it a little push. Weeeeee! Like jumping into a nice warm pool. Make no mistake, it's a tiny push, and a tiny pool. It's no fucking diving board and I'm certainly not jumping off the roof or anything. But I'll give myself a couple of pushes here and there, and take a leap now and then, the pain doctor be damned. Weeeeee!

Sick: The Life and Death of Bob Flanagan, Supermasochist is not easy to watch—just as it is not easy to sit by the bed of someone who is suffering. But it's liberating to hear the voice of a person who so completely "outs" suffering and sickness: Flanagan is not stoical, he does not rise above it all, and he never worries about boring people with the details of his illness. He keeps himself transparent. His angry courage is palpable, and his intelligence is as unstopped as his pain and pleasure. Even at his most wasted and pale, coughing and skinny-chested, Flanagan remains a funny, charismatic human being.

The hardest scenes to watch are near the end, when Flanagan, mortally ill in his hospital bed, nearly expires on film. There is also an uncomfortable interlude when Sheree Rose begs Flanagan to have sex with her, to "submit" like the good old days. But he's just too tuckered out for the whips and plugs and ceiling hooks. It's like a domestic spat about who's going to take out the garbage, erotically speaking. Despite the S&M paraphernalia, Sheree Rose and Flanagan resemble any family trying to work through a terrible disease.

Flanagan's honesty uncovers something moving about the mercurial nature of pain—how it can slip so easily from one category of experience into another. From a bit of death to a sign of life. In the "Bobumentary," as they referred to it, Flanagan reads his manifesto, a document that explains why pain turns him on. It's also a checklist of the shadowy presence of pain in our culture.

Why

BECAUSE it feels good; because it gives me an erection; because it makes me come; because I'm sick; because there was so much sickness; because I say FUCK THE SICKNESS; because I like the attention; because I was alone a lot; because I was different; because kids beat me up on the way to school; because I was humiliated by nuns; because of Christ and the crucifixion; because of Porky Pig in bondage, force-fed by some sinister creep in a black cape; because of stories of children hung by their wrists, burned on the stove, scalded in tubs; because of "Mutiny on the Bounty"; because of cowboys and indians; because of my cousin Cliff; because of the forts we built and the things we did inside them; because of my genes; because of my parents; because of doctors and nurses; because they tied me to the crib so I wouldn't hurt myself; because I had time to think; because I had time to hold my penis; because I had awful stomach aches and holding my penis made it feel better; because I'm a Catholic; because I still love Lent, and I still love my penis, and inspite of it all I have no guilt; because my parents said BE WHAT YOU WANT TO BE, and this is what I want to be; because I'm nothing but a big baby and I want to stay that way, and I want a mommy forever, even a mean one, especially a mean one; because of all the fairy tale witches and the wicked step mother, and the step sisters, and how sexy Cinderella was, smudged with soot, doomed to a life of servitude; because of Hansel, locked in a witch's cage until he was fat enough to eat; because of "O" and how desperately I wanted to be her; because of my dreams; because of the game we played; because I have an active imagination; because my mother bought me tinker toys; because hardware stores give me hardons; because of hammers, nails, clothespins, wood, padlocks, pullies, eyebolts, thumbtacks, staple-guns, sewing needles, wooden spoons, fishing tackle, chains, metal rulers, rubber tubing, spatulas, rope, twine, C-clamps, S-hooks, razor blades, scissors, tweezers, knives, push pins, two-by-fours, ping-pong tables, alligator clips, duct tape, broom sticks, bar-b-que skewers, bungie cords, saw horses, soldering irons; because of tool sheds; because of garages . . .

Because I was born into a world of suffering; because surrender is sweet; because I'm attracted to it; because I'm addicted to it; because endorphins in the brain are like a natural kind of heroin; because I learned to take my medicine . . .

Because it is an act of courage; because it does take guts; because I'm proud of it; because I can't climb mountains; because I'm terrible at sports; because NO PAIN, NO GAIN; BECAUSE SPARE THE ROD AND SPOIL THE CHILD; BECAUSE YOU ALWAYS HURT THE ONE YOU LOVE.

BOB FLANAGAN.

The poems of Emily Dickinson, the performances and writings of Robert Flanagan, the flat, dry voice of William Burroughs in his book *Junkie*—these artists all give pain a voice. Because they report from the margins, where pain is quarantined, their writing should be read and taught alongside the medical history of pain. And oddly enough, both Flanagan and the history of pain science took me to the same surprising place—Los Angeles.

20

PURSUING PAIN IN L.A.

L.A. IS AN ANALGESIC SORT OF PLACE, A chronic paradise. My desire to tour the UCLA History of Pain Project in L.A. was therefore an occasion for some hilarity among my friends. I would not be eating at La Chinoise, or hoping to catch a glimpse of Russell Crowe buying organic vegetables at the Farmers Market. I probably wouldn't be buying a $6,000 handbag on Rodeo Drive. Instead, I would be up on the ninth floor of the Louise M. Darling Biomedical Library, locked inside the deliciously humid Special Collections room, reading case studies on Civil War gunshot wounds, and happy as a clam.

L.A. was uncharacteristically cool and threatening rain when I landed. I rented a candy-red Mazda as the sun set . . . and set, and set. Dusk in L.A. is a long, drawn-out, blood-red event that seems to involve valet-parking the sun just beneath the horizon. I decided to take La Cienega all the way into town rather than face the freeways. My "merge" problems were acting up.

A friend had recommended I take advantage of special "renovation rates" at a West Hollywood hotel undergoing a face-lift. "We want to make it clear," they had cautioned me on the phone, "that this is major, major renovation." West Coast talk, I thought—major this, major that. But the warnings were not exaggerated. I stepped into a small, temporary lobby behind which was a plywood wall, beyond which was: rubble. Even the marble check-in counter had a major, major crack in it, as if the Big One had already happened.

Nevertheless, the staff behaved as if they were welcoming me to the Hong Kong Four Seasons. I was told to watch my step as I followed a labyrinth of dankly carpeted plywood corridors through what looked like a small plundered village, to a hall where the painters had just passed through. I opened the still-tacky door to my room.

Inside, everything was perfect. The walls were freshly rolled in blender-cocktail shades of mango and avocado. The phone had a dial tone. I pulled up the blinds and looked down into a drained and fetid-looking pool. Then I opened the door and stepped back into the hall, where I had an excellent view through the ruins of the old lobby of the traffic whizzing by on Sunset Boulevard. Everyone carried on as if they were still surrounded by walls.

Meanwhile, it had begun to rain, steadily and hard. The hotel was next door to the House of Blues, and just down the road from the Viper Room, where River Phoenix had partied and dropped dead. A nice little bracket of pain, I thought. And somewhere up in the hills was Our Lady of the Migraine, Joan Didion. In books like *Slouching Towards Bethlehem* and *The White Album,* Didion's neurasthenic prose registered the hidden tremors of California life like a seismograph, and seemed to be the direct result of living in an environment designed to eradicate pain. There was something fishy about America's anodyne culture in the 1960s and '70s, and Didion felt it.

I like L.A. It reminds me of a vinyl record with an A side and a B side. A is a polished, urban production with a techno beat, and B is surprisingly wild and natural. In five minutes, I could drive from the river of cars outside my rubble-hotel up into narrow canyon roads, overgrown with dark, heavy foliage, and the lurid blossoms of spring in the desert. To my starved Canadian senses, cocooned in winter, it was like entering a rain forest. I liked the jittery feel of a place as temporary as a movie set, where even the canyons are nothing but great gouges in what's left of the Sierra Madre mountains as they peter out to the sea. Flash fires, mud slides, and earthquakes are all daily possibilities here. And yet people toodle around the city as if nothing could possibly go wrong. It's like a Road Runner cartoon of the human condition—the coyote has stepped off the cliff and is pedaling madly over thin air, but he hasn't looked down yet. No wonder the secret history of pain is stored here, under lock and key.

The next morning, I drove through fat-palmed, comatose Beverly Hills to the UCLA campus, a little kingdom of peace and vaguely Georgian buildings beside Westwood Village, which itself resembles an architect's model. Up on the ninth floor of the biomedical library, I was met by the archivist for the History of Pain Project, Russell Johnson. He wore a sharpened pencil over one ear and seemed delighted to have a visitor.

Johnson explained the scope of the collection, which is devoted to the history of pain research and therapy since World War II. The archives are named after John C. Liebeskind, a UCLA professor of psychology and a leader in pain research who launched the project in 1993, and worked on it until his death from cancer in 1998. The two current codirectors, librarian Kathleen Donahue and medical historian Marcia Meldrum, continue to add to the collection of books and personal papers, along with historical documents related to organizations like the International Association for the Study of Pain and the American Pain Society. But the most remarkable materials are the thirty-nine oral interviews conducted with pain pioneers like John Bonica, Willem Noordenbos, Kathleen Foley, Cecily Saunders, William Fordyce, Ronald Melzack, Patrick Wall, Ada Rogers, and others.

Although there is not much to look at—no bronze statues of the dorsal horn or circumcision dioramas—a vibrant chorus of voices is gathered here: researchers willing to talk across disciplines and borders about a subject that mutually fascinates them. It reveals a field of science in its earliest and most imaginative form.

Johnson took me on a tour that proceeded at a stately, archival pace. He produced a key and ushered me into the rare books room, where books were locked yet again behind a glass and wooden grill-work. A display case held some correspondence between Melzack and Wall about the development of the gate-control theory. There was also a human skull, for good measure. On one wall a thick vault door led to a tiny back room where the oldest texts are kept, along with something that looked like a box of chocolates but turned out to be an antique case of glass eyes.

"What impresses me is that someone actually painted on the little bloodshot lines," Johnson remarked. Then he showed me an antique scarifier, a small metal device that cuts the skin in a neat design, like a bar code in a supermarket. There were samples of early pain potions, ads, and boxes of Lydia's Liver pills. The shelf of contemporary books on pain was short, for the simple reason that not many exist. We left the vault and went across to the reading room, where I would be spending my time.

What is so rare as a rare books room in spring? The weather inside, designed to protect fragile documents, is benign and un-changing. There were certain rules, a protocol to observe. I was to leave my purse in the library office and divest myself of pens. Johnson produced another key. Inside the reading room, a woman was at work, studying the incidence of tuberculosis in southern California. We exchanged scholarly smiles. On the walls were oil portraits and prints. The desks had green bankers' lamps and wedges of foam rubber to support the spines of aged books. I would order up my documents from the stacks and be locked in and out of the room—a system I wished I had at home. The nearest refrigerator here was nine floors away. Clearly, I would not be eating egg salad sandwiches in the reading room. Wallpapered tin cans held sprays of sharpened pencils. Oh, how happy I was. I presented Johnson with a list of names and said I was especially eager to look at Silas Weir Mitchell's books. "Which ones?" he asked after a tactful pause. The archives have 125 publications by this protean American physician, poet, and novelist. Johnson returned with a stack of Mitchell's writings, and I began to read.

SILAS WEIR MITCHELL (1829–1914) is considered the father of modern neurology and was the first to publish detailed studies of nerve damage. He was a productive and skilled fiction writer, too—in fact, he might never have become a surgeon if he hadn't submitted some poetry to a Boston publisher at the age of twenty. The editor, Oliver Wendell Holmes, rejected the poems and told him to concentrate on his medical career instead.

But he did both, and had the last word. At the height of his fame, in the 1870s, Mitchell was as celebrated for his novels and poetry as he was for his medical work. And on October 16, 1896, Mitchell gave a speech at Boston's Massachusetts General Hospital to commemorate the fiftieth anniversary of the invention of anesthesia. For the occasion he composed and read his own scenery-chewing poem "The Birth and Death of Pain."

> *What awful will decreed its silent strife!*
> *Till through vast ages rose on hill and plain*
> *Life's saddest voice, the birth-right wail of pain.*
> *The keener sense, and ever growing mind,*
> *Served but to add a torment twice refined,*
> *As life, more tender, as it grew more sweet,*
> *The cruel links of sorrow found complete . . .*
>
> *What will implacable, beyond our ken*
> *Set this stern fiat for the tribes of men!*
>
> *Whatever triumphs still shall hold the mind,*
> *Whatever gift shall yet enrich mankind,*
> *Ah! here no hour shall strike through all the years,*
> *No hour as sweet as when hope, doubt, and fears,*
> *'Mid deepening stillness, watched one eager brain,*
> *With godlike will, decree the Death of Pain.*

When Johnson returned with a copy of *Gunshot Wounds and Other Injuries of Nerves*, a collection of case studies based on his treatment of soldiers injured in the Civil War, I opened it and studied a portrait of the author. Mitchell had a long, horse-handsome face, with a wide brow and large, slightly doleful eyes, all of which gave him a remarkable resemblance to the actor Donald Sutherland. He appeared very much the doctor-patriarch he was. Born in Philadelphia, trained as a surgeon at Jefferson Medical College, he studied in Paris and then entered his father's family practice, publishing his first articles on odd physiological topics like cataracts in frogs and the production of venom in the rattlesnake.

When the Civil War broke out, he became an acting assistant surgeon in the Union Army and ended up in charge of Turner's Lane Hospital in Philadelphia. There, along with George Morehouse and William Keen, he wrote detailed reports on the treatment of 120 soldiers wounded in the Battle of Gettysburg in 1863. Mitchell was the first to recognize and document the puzzle of neuropathic pain (which he called causalgia).

I began to read Mitchell's case studies, which at times became as vivid and detailed as Audubon paintings.

"Hiram Weston, 42, a colonel, wounded in the Wilderness, in 1864. He was moving at a double quick, and was shot in the left arm. He felt violent pain throughout the limb. . . . [T]he pain which then began, has never left him. After fifty days, the pain has consisted all along of darting pangs from below or under the elbow, down into the hand. . . . [I]n the hand the pain is burning and tingling, or, as he phrases it 'prinkling.' It is intense and is increasing. It is worse in daytime and in hot weather, and when the hand hangs down. Noise and excitement increase it. . . . [T]he back of the hand is eczematous and mottled in tint. . . . [T]he joints are exquisitely tender, and very stiff and swollen. The patient has kept the hand wet ever since he was hurt. . . ."

Mitchell concluded that this pain was in a class of its own.

"We have here set apart for distinct consideration that kind of pain which we have before spoken of as burning pain. It is a form of suffering as yet undescribed, and so frequent and terrible as to demand from us the fullest description . . . men who describe a pain as burning or as 'mustard red hot' . . . or as a 'red-hot file rasping the skin.'

"The seat of burning pain is very various, but it never attacks the trunk, rarely the arm or thigh, and not often the forearm or leg. Its favourite site is the foot or hand. . . . [I]ts intensity varies from the most trivial burning to a state of torture, which can hardly be credited, but which reacts on the whole economy, until the general health is seriously affected. The part itself is not alone subject to an intense burning sensation, but becomes exquisitely hyperaesthetic, so that a touch or a tap of the finger increases the pain. Exposure to the air is avoided by the patient with a care which seems absurd, and most of the bad cases keep the hand constantly wet. . . . Two of these sufferers carried a bottle of water and a sponge, and never permitted the part to become dry for a moment."

Mitchell observed in his soldiers how pain eventually distorted the personality.

"The temper changes and grows irritable, the face becomes anxious, and has a look of weariness and suffering. The sleep is restless . . . the rattling of a newspaper, a breath of air . . . give rise to increase of pain. At last the patient grows hysterical, if we may use the only term which covers the facts. He walks carefully, carries the limb tenderly with the sound hand, is tremulous, nervous, and has all kinds of expedients for lessening his pain."

This was the sort of invisible, high-pitched suffering that could easily have been dismissed as an invention—and still can be today. But Mitchell put together his physiological knowledge of nerve damage with his attention to the personality and occupations of his patients. He tended to see the big picture, if not always the whole picture—as his opinions on hysterical women (a dime a dozen in the nineteenth century, to judge by the literature) bear out.

In 1904, Mitchell published a fascinating book called *Doctor and Patient*. It begins with a number of sensible observations: "There are very few instances of chronic ailments, however slight," he wrote, "which should not be met by advice as to modes of living, in the full breadth of this term; and only by a competent union of such, with reasonable use of drugs, can all be done most speedily that should be done." This rather wholesome view was part of Mitchell's conviction that "the physician cannot be a mere intellectual machine."

He took the perspective that pain was only as bad as you perceived it to be—a modern perspective, in a sense, but one that could also be moralistic and punishing. It was a "buck up" sort of approach; in his view, moaning and whining only begot more pain. There is truth to this, but Mitchell also believed that women were much more likely to be neurotic whiners and difficult patients. Their inability to stand pain was just one of their feminine defects, and he had much to say on the subject.

"My simple practical thesis is that pain comes to all soon or late," he wrote, "that the indirect consequences are most to be feared, and that endurance in the adult, rational endurance, must be won by a gradual education, which can hardly begin too early. But of what use are these stern lessonings [sic] in the bearing of what none can quite escape? Do they enable us to diminish pain or to feel it less? Indirectly, yes. One woman cries out for instant easement if in pain or distress, unschooled to endure. She claims immediate relief. Another, more resolute, submits with patience, does not give way, as we put it, tries to distract her attention, knowing that even as distinct suffering as toothache *may be less felt in the presence of something which interests the mind and secures the attention* [italics mine].

"Nothing, indeed, is more instructive than to watch how women bear pain—the tremendous calamity it is to one, the far slighter thing in life it is to another. I speak now of transient torments. When we come to consider those years of torture which cruel nature holds in store for some, no one blames the sight of the moral wreck it is apt to make of the sufferer." Here Mitchell is alluding to women who developed an opium habit, who seemed quite numerous in his practice. "On the other hand, there is nothing I ever see in my profession so splendid as the way in which a few, a rare few, triumph over pain." The doctor puts aside his customary fears regarding female patients to describe an exception to the rule.

"I recall well one woman who for years, under my eyes, was the subject of what, with due sense of the force of the word, I call torture. At times she shut herself up in her room, and, as she said, 'wrestled with it.' This happened every day or two for an hour or more. The rest of the time she was out, or busy with her duties, but always in some pain. . . . At her dinnertable, in chat with friends, or over a book, no one who did not know her well could have dreamed that she was in such pain as consigns lower natures to disability. Her safeguard from utter wreck"—again, Mitchell's code phrase for a morphine habit—"was a clear and resolute faith, a profound and unfailing interest in men and things and books, which gave strange vigor to her whole range of intellectual activities. But above all she possessed that happiest of gifts, the keen, undying sense of the humorous, the absurd, the witty. . . . [S]he once said to me, in the midst of a storm of acute suffering, that pain seemed to her a strange sort of joke. . . . [A]ll opiates she disliked and could rarely be induced to take them. 'If my mind gets weaker, I shall go to pieces. . . .'

"To endure without excess of emotion saves her from consequent nervousness, and from that feebleness of mind and body which craves at all cost instant relief. It is the spoiled child, untaught to endure, who becomes the self-pampered woman. There are those, indeed, who suffer and grow strong; there are those who suffer and grow weak. This mystery of pain is still for me the saddest of earth's disabilities."

The "instant relief" was, of course, the nineteenth-century pharmacopoeia of opiates. "If [the physician] be weak, or too tender, or too prone to escape trouble by the easy help of some pain-lulling agent, she is soon on the evil path of the opium, chloral, or chloroform habit."

Addicts were simply lily-livered and weak, in Mitchell's view. "Is it not rather due to the softening influence of luxury, and the fact that we are all being constantly trained to feel that it is both easy and our right to escape pain, however brief?" He thought there was something immoral about pain-shirking and he wasn't alone among Victorian doctors, some of whom were dead set against the use of ether to ease the pain of childbirth. Pain was part of God's plan for us. Mitchell had a mistrust of analgesia, while acknowledging its power. "When people are first given opium, it is apt to be the friend of the night and the foe of the morrow. Repeated often enough, it loses power to constipate and distress. It still soothes pain. It still gives sleep. At last it seems to be in a measure a tonic for those who take it. But after a while it does some other things less agreeable. The mind and memory suffer, but far more surely the moral nature is altered. The woman becomes indifferent, her affections dull, her sense of duty hopelessly weakened. Watchful, cunning, suspicious, deceitful—a thief, if need be, to get the valued opiate—she stops at nothing. It would seem as if it were a drug which directly affected the conscience." (Here he at least gets the chemical tyranny of addiction correct.) "At last, before this one craving, all ties in life are slight and bind her not. Insensible to shame and dead to affection, she is happy if the alcohol habit be not added to her disorder, for if she cannot get the one drug she longs for, the other will serve her at need." And now Mitchell warms to his subject—the destructive power of a fallen woman.

"I know of a woman who took for years ninety grains a day, and ruined a weak husband, a man of small means, by the costliness of her habit." For Mitchell, opium had a particularly devastating effect on females, causing "the general failure of all that is womanly." The problem with woman was that "when she seizes the apple, she drops the rose." It is seizing knowledge that leads to the loss of femininity, which lays the woman bare to all manner of bad things. For Mitchell, it was in the nature of womanhood both to suffer more pain (which is actually the case) and to suffer it badly. Culture or social roles didn't really enter into it. "Nor do I think any educational changes in generations of women will ever set her, as to certain mental or moral qualifications, as an equal beside the man."

In the midst of these rants, I encountered—briefly—the exasperated voice of one of the women under his care.

"'It is easy for you to sit by in your strength and see me suffer,' said a woman once to me," he reports. "She was on the verge of the morphia habit, and I was trying to break it off abruptly."

One wonders why Mitchell had a special interest in hysteria, given his opinion of female patients. "The selfishness of nervous women sometimes exceeds belief in its capacity to claim pity and constancy of expressed sympathy," he declares, adding that the ones with questions are the worst. "The terrible patients are nervous women with long memories, who question much where answers are difficult, and who put together one's answers from time to time and torment themselves and the physician with the apparent inconsistencies they detect."

Perhaps he had one particular woman in mind. One of Mitchell's most famous patients was Charlotte Perkins Gilman, author of the short story "The Yellow Wall-Paper." When she came to him complaining of nerves and insomnia, Mitchell gave his usual prescription—isolation, bed rest, a high-fat diet, and a very minimum of intellectual stimulation. So Gilman was confined to the attic of her house, where her care was overseen by her well-meaning but conventional doctor-husband. Mitchell ordered her not to touch a paintbrush or a notebook. (His "rest cure" was a kind of caricature of the social roles imposed on women of a certain class then.)

Not surprisingly, this interlude only intensified Gilman's madness. In "The Yellow Wall-Paper" she describes how the woman confined to her attic room wore grooves in the floor, pacing back and forth. She hallucinated a crouching woman behind the red bars of the wallpaper. In the end, Gilman ignored Mitchell's orders and went back to writing.

I did stumble upon another unorthodox prescription that was a little less punitive than the rest cure. Mitchell once "prescribed" a camping trip for one woman who was "almost helplessly nervous."

"I said to her, 'If you were a man I think I could cure you.' I then told her how in that case I would ask a man to live. . . . Pitch a tent by the lonely waters of a Western lake in May." She lived there until August and this macho version of the rest cure worked. "In a word, she led a man's life until the snow fell in the fall and she came back to report, a thoroughly well woman."

With regard to women, Mitchell was very much a man of his time (and women being treated for pain are sometimes met with a muted modern version of this attitude). But in other respects he was farsighted and original. In 1871, he published a little book called *Wear and Tear,* which called attention to the "inability of Americans to play." He felt we lived life at too fast a clip and had forgotten how to relax. Perhaps someone will reissue this.

The other publication that caught my eye was a study called *The Relations of Pain to Weather*. As a sinus sufferer, I already had theories about this. Mitchell studied fifty cases of amputees with stump pain and found that "less than half felt unusual sensations upon the coming of an east wind, or during it." The book includes storm maps, barometric charts, and the statement that neuralgia— everything that aches and is related to nerves—was apt to prevail when the northern lights were intense. Mitchell never tackled anything lightly. He concluded that people suffer more pain in the fall, when the atmospheric pressure drops, and that a falling barometer followed by rain "as a rule insures an onset of pain." Mitchell even drew diagrams of the "neuralgic margins of a storm," which he found to be exactly 150 miles before the rain.

It's part of the weather forecast now to include windchill factors and UV scales. Someday we may also have a "pain front" in the weather report. They can call it the Mitchell Factor.

DOWN BELOW THE LIBRARY was the UCLA hospital cafeteria. I took to having seventy-nine-cent breakfast tacos there every morning, among the weary clamor of students and interns in green scrubs. Then at lunchtime, after a morning of reading up on stump pain, I would carry my tray across the street to the six-acre botanical gardens that flank the medical library. I liked the giant white palms and the fact that all the trees were labeled: more archival calm.

But Sunday arrived, and the library was closed. I tried to track down Sheree Rose, Bob Flanagan's widow. Apart from uncovering some gallery shows she had been involved in I had no luck. I spoke with the director of the Flanagan documentary, who was tied up in a new production. There was an S&M society in town, the one that Rose and Flanagan had begun in San Francisco, but I couldn't see sitting around there with notebook and pencil in hand. So I drove up into the hills to visit the daughter of friends, who had had her first child, becoming an overnight expert in another modern kind of pain—a cesarean delivery where everything that could go wrong, did. The baby was fine, but Zoe, the mother, went through hell.

Zoe and her husband, Garth, live in a small house above one of the winding roads that climb out of Los Angeles into the Hollywood Hills. It had been a wet spring; there were wildflowers in bloom everywhere and birds-of-paradise springing out of the ditches. Zoe kept a sloping garden that clung to the hillside and grew in steps, like a rice paddy. Down below, I could hear the BMWs ripping by at high speeds, like hornets.

I walked into the kitchen and saw Zoe in a wolfish hunch over a bowl of cereal—the baby, Max, only one week old, was miraculously asleep, so she was eating as fast as possible before he woke up again. She looked like a tired Russian peasant just back from the fields. I sat down at the table and without any prompting at all the story of her son's birth poured out.

"My water broke, so I went to the hospital, but nothing happened. They were worried about my water, so they said, 'Why don't we put you on Pitocin and get things going,' and that sounded pretty good to me, frankly. I could just *smell* the relief of having him out and not feeling huge anymore. I mean, you're supposed to be big when you're pregnant, but I was, like, *huge,* and so tired of feeling that way. So they gave me Pitocin, and I went into labor and had contractions every two minutes for twenty-four hours, and he wouldn't come out," said Zoe, still wanly amazed. "I kept pushing and pushing and thought, *I'll never be able to do this.* I was screaming bloody murder, too. I've never felt pain like that."

Ordinary labor is right up there on the pain scale, and Pitocin can make the contractions even more intense and unmanageable. This is when, in domino fashion, one little intervention can trigger a cascade of them.

Zoe took her hair band off—the band that keeps her brown hair out of the baby's face when she breast-feeds—and then pulled it on again. Upstairs, Max slept on, miraculously. Zoe's father, Zalman, had flown into town to help out for a while. He was staring into the fridge deciding what to buy and make for dinner.

"And I had all these objects inside me—a catheter, the leads to the fetal monitor, plus there were millions of people in the room—when all of a sudden, the baby's heart rate dropped, and things began happening really, really fast. They wheeled me down the hall and into the OR, and started getting me ready for a C-section." The good thing about monitors is that they can save the lives of babies in fetal distress. The bad thing about monitors is that temporary dips in heart rate, as can happen when the baby passes through the birth canal, and are normal, register as major seismic events on the computer screen.

With the early L.A. light streaming in, Zoe's skin was paper pale. Any minute now the baby would certainly wake.

"The only problem is, the anesthesia didn't quite work—I could *feel* them cutting into me! I could feel them tugging at the baby to get him out. It was a pounding, burning feeling, like my belly was boiling over with lava. And I was still screaming. In fact, I traumatized the anesthesiologist so much that when he went out to speak to my relatives afterward, he actually cried. It was sort of a horror show all round." Zoe is normally unflappable, someone who knows how to calm horses, so this seemed to go beyond the usual why-didn't-anyone-tell-me? labor story.

"But the worst part was afterward, when they took the baby away. They took him up to intensive care, and I didn't get to see him or hold him for ten hours—there wasn't anything wrong with him, it was just that I couldn't get anybody to bring him down. That was awful—to go through all that, and then no baby! I was so afraid something had happened to him, and they weren't telling me. Finally I got in a wheelchair and demanded that they take me upstairs. He was screaming when I came in, but as soon as I held him, he stopped."

A tiny wail just then from upstairs. Max. His father brought him downstairs. Zoe, walking as if there was still a good chance that some organ might fall out of her body, moved gingerly into the living room in order to arrange herself on the Breast-feeding Shrine, a big armchair with multiple cushions and a footstool. This was my chance to hold Max for a minute and look at him. A long-limbed boy, wide-browed and surprisingly strong. He was already lifting his head and trying to look around. Every muscle in him felt alert and alive as he pressed his feet down into my lap. He didn't seem phased at all by his rocky ride into the world.

What little blood was left in Zoe's face drained out of it as Max clamped his jaws on her breast. Breast-feeding can hurt, too. And in the postpartum dip of hormones, each ache sinks in more deeply, rousing a nervous system recently held hostage to hours of labor pain. The few first days after childbirth pass in an uproar of new sensations. But Zoe was, if not cheery, at least stoical, and I watched her face shed every trace of pain when she gazed at Max, watching the expressions, wild and disorganized as clouds, that moved across his face. The runaway birth was now being slowly organized into a story with a happy ending—a baby.

But Zoe's story struck me as a dreadfully familiar saga: induced labor, which then contributes to unnaturally strong and painful contractions, combined with high-risk accoutrements like fetal monitors and IV leads that confine the mother on her back, in bed. It made it more difficult for her to change position, walk around, or labor actively. Then, exhausted from hours and hours of fruitless labor, craving unconsciousness and relief from pain, she ended up going through a C-section she could still feel. This can happen; each person responds differently to anesthesia, and while most women in labor consider their anesthesiologist a shining knight, he is not infallible. And then the mysterious whisking away of her baby.

Twenty-three percent of births in California are now done as C-sections. Zoe's was circumstantial, not her choice, but birth by appointment is more and more popular, both for the convenience of physicians and because it offers the illusion of control. Scheduling birth is a last stab at autonomy for some women. And in our pain-blind, pain-obsessed culture, we are frightened by the idea of un-medicated childbirth. This is ironic, given that doctors resisted the introduction of anesthesia to childbirth in the nineteenth century. The idea of using ether to make labor less painful was thought at first to be unhealthy—and un-Christian, too. Luckily, Queen Victoria used chloroform for the deliveries of several of her nine children, which helped promote the idea.

The ideal, it seems, is the well-targeted epidural early in labor, to take the edge off the contractions without keeping the mother too numbed-out to be part of the actual birthing. Otherwise, the baby has to be fumbled out, like a pickle in a jar. Some women are happy without any anesthesia at all, but this sets the bar rather high for everyone else. The last thing a woman needs is more pressure to tough things out.

As Max nursed, I looked at the pile of snapshots taken in the hospital. Everyone else in the pictures looked thrilled, and Zoe's face said "How could you?" "I don't really like to look at the hospital pictures," she said, gazing at the baby in her arms instead, who was sated and sliding off into sleep. "Max the pearl," she crooned. "Yes, you're my pearl."

Birth stories. They are as perishable as tulips. New mothers tell them compulsively, lavishly, often in hilarious detail, for two or three or four days, to whoever will listen. They talk about their second-degree episiotomy, the strange urgency of pushing, the fabulous labor nurse, the bruises on their partner's arm, the horrible things that came out of their mouth during transition. Then a week or two later, the memory fades. The narrative seals over and becomes a set piece, reduced to a phrase: an easy birth. A breech, with back labor. A crazy cesarean. And a good thing, too, or the species would grind to a halt. The pain gets filed away in some archive of the body, as knowledge that isn't needed anymore.

THE NEXT MORNING, I was back at UCLA, looking through the transcripts of the oral interviews with some of the pioneers of pain research. The writer who came as a revelation was Dr. William Livingston—an American surgeon and pain specialist, Ronald Melzack's postdoctoral tutor, and someone who struggled to place the science of pain in a narrative, humane voice in his book *Pain and Suffering*. He died in 1966 with the manuscript almost complete. The unpublished book was packed away with the rest of Livingston's papers until

1998, when the IASP providently brought it to light again. This was the scientific voice—humane, curious, and creative—that I had been waiting to discover.

IN JUNE 1920, Bill Livingston had just started his surgical internship at Massachusetts General Hospital in Boston. He was a "Pup," the lowest on the intern ladder, and every day he took his list of duties—usually a long and unsavory one—from an older intern known as "the Junior."

One morning his Junior gave him an order he didn't understand: "Open colostomy."

The patient, a man, had been admitted a few days before with severe abdominal pain. When they operated, they found a cancerous mass in the lower colon, which (as Livingston picturesquely wrote) was "blocking the fecal stream." They would have to do a second operation to remove the mass. In the meantime, they had to create a detour, so the surgeon brought a loop of the transverse colon up and left it protruding outside the belly wall. Livingston's morning chore was to open the exposed colon.

He admitted to his Junior that he didn't have a clue how to proceed. "'There is nothing to it,'" the Junior said, "'all you have to do is to burn a good hole in the loop.'" The blowtorch was kept in the broom closet, he explained. Which operating room should I use? Livingston ventured. "'Just do the burning right there in his bed,'" the Junior answered. What anesthetic should he give the patient? The Junior was now getting exasperated with his sensitive-plant underling. He won't need any anesthetic, the Junior explained, "'because he won't feel a damned thing.'" Livingston describes the encounter in *Pain and Suffering*: "Junior went with me to the closet to get the blowtorch. He lit it and started the soldering iron heating. It was beginning to glow a dull red when we walked into the patient's room carrying the blowtorch, roaring full blast, between us. The patient reared up from his pillow."

They told him to lie back, and the two men took off the dressing, to find the colon loop exposed "like a red rosette." The patient looked on in horror. Then they went to work.

"The contact of the hot [soldering] iron with the moist flesh gave rise to a sizzling sound. A thin wisp of smoke rose from the iron and the room began to fill with the stench of burning flesh." But as the burning progressed, the patient almost relaxed. He lay back on his pillow, smiling. "I was as surprised that he felt no pain," Livingston recalled. "The patient had smiled while the wall of his colon was being destroyed by a red-hot iron."

Although Livingston had witnessed other gruesome procedures before, this one made a deep impression. The image stayed with him, and the implications led to a "period of real mental distress." Even though he had been taught in medical school that internal organs can be cut, crushed, or burned without causing a conscious person pain, he was now faced with a contradiction: He had assumed, along with the science of the day, that the man's original pain had arisen from specific "pain fibers" in his colon. "The presumptive evidence was that the patient's colon DID contain pain fibers." And those pain fibers had alerted him that something was wrong down there and sent him off to the hospital.

But then comes the obvious question: Why did the pain fibers fall silent while the colon was being burned?

Perhaps, Livingston thought, he was wrong to assume that internal organs possessed their own pain fibers. But then, how do you explain the patient's original cramping pain?

Livingston had been tutored in the push-button concept of pain. This theory claimed the existence of specific pain fibers that are activated by any stimulus "of sufficient intensity to threaten damage to tissue cells." The pain was always directly proportional to the stimulus. But the effect of the hot iron seemed to contradict this notion.

Livingston got a bit steamed up about this, to the indifference of his fellow interns. "I wanted to know WHY this patient had felt no sensation of any kind while his colon was being burned." He went off to the medical library. "I think perhaps this was the first time in my life that I went eagerly to a library," he said. He felt it was information he thought a surgeon ought to know.

"But I did not find the information I sought in my first session in a medical library nor in many subsequent sessions."

THIS STORY APPEARS IN the first chapter of *Pain and Suffering*, a book that Livingston toiled away on from 1956 to 1966, the year he died suddenly of a heart attack. The manuscript went into storage with the rest of his papers until a strange and fortuitous trail of events led to its publication in 1998. It's a little-known landmark in the study of pain—and a remarkable book, both for its vivid personality and for its creative originality. Fifty years ago, Livingston understood more about pain than most scientists do today. He also managed to develop his ideas when Descartes and the dualists still ruled the world of pain.

Livingston was a Renaissance man who pursued many undoctorly interests—playing the clarinet in a chamber music group, archery, fishing, horsemanship, gardening, and ceramics. After retirement, he became an expert in ceramics, creating his own glazes from local stones. He was good at most things he undertook, and hands-on in them all.

In 1943, Livingston had published a more conventional but equally farsighted book called *Pain Mechanisms*. It was well reviewed, but so far ahead of its time that his ideas went unrecognized. So a dozen years later, Livingston decided to take another crack at a pain book for a wider audience. "I wished to avoid any pose of authority," he said. This time he wanted to write accessibly, even personally. "I wanted to deal with pain not as a scientifically established entity but as an 'evolving idea' that could be expected to evolve still further as we learned more about how a brain can function as mind."

This is exactly what has happened. Livingston's ideas still lay in the future.

But his efforts to find the right narrative structure for the book kept frustrating him. He didn't want to be too medically esoteric; on the other hand, a personal ramble about his own pain hunches wouldn't count as science. Using the grammar of science, he wanted to sketch a more human, shaded picture of pain.

Finally, when he was about to rip up his efforts yet again, a friend suggested that he just write a "simple story of my own efforts to formulate a concept of pain," a story that would include conjecture and experiments. And this is what he tried to do.

"I thought it might be rather fun and relatively easy," he writes, "but all the fun went out of the task long ago and now, years and barrels of discarded manuscript later, I am not pleased with what I have written. As I reread parts of the story it seems to me that I alternate between sounding hopelessly naïve and sounding like a stuffed shirt, and I seem to be unable to modify either impression."

Livingston discovered what I was learning. The reason there are so few good books on the subject of pain is that when you try to isolate or pin it down, you begin to misrepresent its very nature, which is inclusive and mercurial.

LIVINGSTON MIGHT HAVE BEEN lost to us if it wasn't for that bright postdoctoral student who came to study with him—Ronald Melzack. It was a chance remark Melzack made to John Liebeskind, when he was starting to compile the History of Pain Project at UCLA, that led to the publication of *Pain and Suffering.**

From 1954 to 1957, Melzack worked with Livingston as a post-doctoral fellow, a period he calls "the most exciting of my career." Livingston's approach to pain—a synthesis of clinical work, fearless experimentation, intellectual curiosity, and a concern for what the patient had to offer, unusual for a surgeon—informed Melzack's own thinking and the development of the gate-control theory of pain, which utterly changed the field in 1965.

At the time, Livingston was chair of the Department of Surgery at the University of Oregon Medical School, where he encouraged original research into pain mechanisms and held rambunctious weekly seminars on all sorts of pain-related topics. "New ideas thrilled him the way new toys thrilled small boys," Melzack wrote. "His grin, his

---

*After Livingston's son Kenneth died, his daughter-in-law was sorting out the family home when she came across the manuscript. She donated it, along with Livingston's papers, to the Oregon Health Sciences University Library, where the book lay safe but largely forgotten. Then, in the 1990s, the psychologist John Liebeskind began to assemble the History of Pain Project at UCLA. During an interview, Melzack wondered if a manuscript of Livingston's book might still exist, and that remark led Liebeskind to track it down. The Oregon library arranged a loan to UCLA, where the book was edited by Howard Fields, another prominent pain scientist, and published by the IASP Press.

laugh, his enthusiasm were infectious." Livingston established one of the first formal pain clinics at the university hospital. "It's time for scientists to get out of the laboratory and see what pain is really about," he told Melzack.

"Livingston treated those patients with a special compassion and kindness," Melzack recalled, "and his brilliant questions . . . revealed to me what he knew so well—that prolonged pain is debilitating, demoralizing, devastating. It grinds people down and makes life a burden."

In his first job as a state medical officer on workers' compensation cases, Livingston spent his days listening to people in pain who didn't necessarily show any sign of injury or damage—people with whiplash or other sorts of "invisible" pain conditions. Then, following in the steps of his great hero Silas Weir Mitchell, he joined the navy during World War II and began to study peripheral nerve injuries, becoming head of this division at the Oakland Naval Hospital. Like Mitchell, he understood the importance of voice and narrative to a full understanding of pain—true pain, he believed, did not belong to any particular nerve or center in the brain. Pain is a "transactional process involving continuing interactions and feedback loops among all parts of the nervous system." Livingston had a cyber view of pain long before the conversion to computers.

In 1965, Livingston finally stopped rewriting his manuscript. "I am unable to decide how to wind up a story that is so far from finished," he complained. "I am sorely tempted to stop right here." And, he added, "I am beginning to wonder if our whole concept of pain may not need a careful review . . . though I dread it, this is what I shall try to do . . . in the closing chapter."

But Livingston had heart problems, and he wasn't able to put the finishing touches on his manuscript before he died in his sleep.

Melzack remembered visiting him on a Friday afternoon. "He had been writing since 5 A.M.—his usual routine—but had decided the material was bad and had torn it all up. He was wistful," Melzack wrote, "and a little depressed." Melzack, on the other hand, had had a great week, and he told Livingston about his new evidence for the descending signals from the brain that affect pain input. This cheered up Livingston. He had no time for the territoriality and competition that are now as much a part of scientific research as knockout mice. What excited him was the search for an answer that was different for each person in pain.

IN *PAIN AND SUFFERING*, Livingston starts with the obvious—that pain is hard to study. "Pain represents a dynamic transaction occurring in that mysterious embodiment of brain activity that is called the 'mind.' You can no more easily locate the transaction than you can pin down 'mind.'"

No one could agree on a definition of pain in Livingston's day. In medical school, Livingston had learned that "the sensation of pain will be an exact replica of the external stimulus configuration. Thus, the severity of the pain is always directly proportional to the stimulus intensity." There was an important "side effect" of this definition: "Any apparent deviation . . . must be attributed to the person's psychological reaction to the pain." If no organic causes can be found for pain, then you're simply having a "reaction," and a psychologically suspect one at that.

Livingston admits to having passed judgment on some patients as a result of this training. "It was easy to assume that these patients must be neurasthenic, hysterical, or malingering." He would "talk too glibly of such things as 'psychogenic pain.'"

What changed his mind was eight years as a medical caseworker in workmen's compensation, when he saw people with chronic pain problems that defied diagnosis or treatment. He saw how other doctors dismissed their pain. "I found repeated denials of the reality of the patients' pains and recurring diagnoses of hysteria and malingering in cases in which I felt sure such diagnoses were not justifiable."

Finally, Livingston decided that "there must be something wrong with the concept of pain we doctors acquire in medical school and that ANY mechanistic concept of pain might handicap a physician's efforts to understand . . . the most serious human pain problems." To support these "speculative and unorthodox" notions, he organized a pain team to look into pain problems in the lab and in the clinic. Eleven years of experiments and work with patients followed, which deepened his conviction that pain is a fluid transaction that varies from one individual to another.

For some time after his traumatic encounter with the colostomy patient, Livingston studied the mystery of visceral pain. In fact, he developed quite a little arsenal of experimental tortures for the colon. He would talk patients into being blindfolded, so that he could conduct his experiments. This included using acids and alkalis on the exposed colon, crushing a "huge area" with forceps, and pricking the surface of it. For this he invented a special device, a piece of hard rubber through which he pushed fifty needles. He then used this "hair-brush" on the surface of the colon. One wonders what nurses blundering into this scene—the blindfolded colostomy patient, the doctor with his acids and brushes—must have thought about Dr. Livingston.

But none of these ingenious tortures caused any pain. That was the point. He only found one way to cause visceral pain—and this involved the equally ingenious experiment of inserting a balloon up the rectum of a seventy-two-year-old woman, whom he called "my favourite collaborator." (Many a mouse has experienced rectal distension in pain experiments as well.) She was an "exceptionally intelligent woman who was delighted to take part in the experiments." Livingston found that when he inflated the balloon, the woman reported a vague, deep ache. This and other studies led him to believe that visceral pain might originate in peripheral blood vessels. This pain behaves differently from the sort that arises from injury to the skin or limbs, and it is also processed in a different part of the spinal cord. Livingston did further studies to show that visceral pain interfered with other reflex mechanisms, indicating to Livingston the "dynamic plasticity of neural functioning." (Plasticity has since become a buzzword in brain science.) He recorded peculiar examples of this "neuronal plasticity" in some of his patients.

Livingston described a lumberjack, a timber feller, who had cut off the tip of his left thumb with an axe. The wound healed, but the scar remained so sensitive he couldn't work. Another operation removed a chunk of the remaining thumb, after which the stump was even more painful. Doctors were at a loss to treat him. Livingston took the case on, hoping to at least ease the man's pain for brief periods with a local anesthetic. He found that when he injected the man's thumb with a local anesthetic, he suddenly felt his arm "relax" for the first time since the accident. After a series of injections, the lumberjack found he could finally put on a glove and eventually use an axe. Livingston felt it wasn't the procaine that "cured" his condition, but the interruption and reorganization of the stimulus in the area. The injections seemed to reboot a nervous system that had become stuck in an old modality.

Another odd phenomenon that Livingston encountered in his practice was something he called the "mirror image"—cases in which long-standing pain would inexplicably "jump" from one foot to another, or from one limb to its twin. He collected thirty cases of mirror-image pain, including the story of one man who was referred to him from a veterans' hospital. The chief of the hospital had written to him about the case, saying, "I have seen a lot of screwballs in my time but this man tops them all. Come as soon as you can." The man was thirty-two, tall and thin, with a personality that drove people away. He complained bitterly of a cold, painful left foot. The injury dated back to a time when he was exercising at a gym. Nothing special had occurred; his foot just started to hurt. Over the years, the pain increased, and the foot became cold to the touch, atrophied, and constantly wet with sweat. The patient said it was like "walking on a chunk of ice." The only thing that helped him were hot baths and quantities of whiskey.

Livingston examined him and warily began treatment. He tried a procaine block in his back, which helped; the foot warmed up, and the pain disappeared. This was followed by an operation on certain nerves, which was also a success. And off the patient went to live his life.

Years later, the man showed up at the vets' hospital again. This time he wanted the same operation, only on his right foot. He explained that the pains had "been going over into the right foot" for several years! Livingston did not doubt him. He simply operated on the nerves related to the right foot, and the man got the relief he was looking for.

Livingston offers no explanation for these mirror-image cases. But he doesn't file them under "hysteria," either. He understood that psychic states can mimic organic disease, pain and all. There is no deception or faking involved. "There are psychic factors involved in every patient's complaint of pain," he wrote. He tells a story of one midnight emergency to illustrate his point.

A woman called him to report that her husband had just had a "massive bowel hemorrhage and was in a state of collapse." Just before bed, he had felt some cramping pains and hurried to the bathroom. Then she heard him calling her name, followed by the thud of him falling to the floor. She found him unconscious, white-faced, and covered in sweat. And in the toilet there was a quantity of bright red blood.

Livingston told her not to flush the toilet and rushed over. He found the man lying on the bed, conscious, but in pain. Where does it hurt the worst, Livingston asked. "All over," the man whispered. He went on groaning as his wife said that he had been in fine spirits and good health, until he had gone to the bathroom.

Livingston examined him, to no avail. Then he went into the bathroom and inspected the alarming-looking contents of the toilet. Beets. Lots of beet fragments. It turned out that her husband had eaten beets for lunch, and little else. Livingston decided that this accounted for the "hemorrhage" and that the man's state—the pallor, the sweating, and the "all over" pain—had been entirely caused by fright.

The two of them walked back into the bedroom with smiles on their faces, which annoyed the husband, who was languishing on the bed. But when Livingston gave him his diagnosis, the man's condition improved rapidly. "Within half an hour he was moving about in his usual energetic fashion and offering to pour me a drink if I would stay and chat."

For Livingston, this was a demonstration of how "descending signals" from the brain, as Melzack would later characterize them, can radically alter our perception of pain. In this case, an alarming image triggered a line of thinking that led to a biochemical drama that concluded in pain—which could be reversed by a new and more logical line of thinking. As Ramachandran's experiment with phantom limbs and mirrors also demonstrated, when it comes to pain, sometimes seeing is not just believing: Seeing is feeling.

Livingston had a kind of mad-scientist eagerness to conduct experiments in pain perception, but there was the problem of getting people to volunteer. So he often used himself. He was also intrigued by treatments that were considered unscientific at the time—relaxation strategies and the use of hypnosis to anesthetize.

He once offered himself up as a subject to Dr. Meares, an Australian psychiatrist who practiced hypnotherapy. Livingston sat himself in a large leather armchair and let Meares lead him through the familiar routine ("Your eyelids are getting heavy . . ."). Then, with Livingston's prior permission, Meares made a deep cut on his forearm with a razor. "I didn't think I was hypnotized but he evidently thought so," recalls Livingston. Although he didn't move, Livingston "definitely felt pain," but the observers—two neurosurgeons—were convinced that he was indeed hypnotized; otherwise, how could he have tolerated a cut that ended up leaving a permanent scar?

Livingston responded by telling them that for many years he had practiced the set of relaxation strategies which enabled him to tolerate more pain than usual. Since his friends were skeptical, he offered to demonstrate this in a nonhypnotized state, if they would only give him a few moments to prepare. Then, he said, they could make an equally deep cut in his left forearm. That cut would also leave a scar, "but they could observe no visible response as the razor blade was dragged slowly through the skin."

This convinced Livingston that "pain relief, no matter how it is induced, is always dependent upon an interaction between many neural forces and is usually RELATIVE rather than absolute."

He couldn't resist competition, either. When he was in India, Livingston observed a young yogi who was having his alpha rhythms monitored as he kept his hands plunged in a huge dishpan filled with ice cubes (the famous "cold pressor" test, which is supposed to cause a normal person so much pain that he has to take his hand out within two to three minutes). The yogi kept his hand happily immersed for forty-five minutes. So Livingston rolled up his sleeve, took a few minutes to relax, and then put his hand in the pan for more than fourteen minutes. "Naturally the hand felt painfully cold," he felt duty-bound to add, "but not unbearably so."

Although he offered these stories merely as anecdotes, Livingston was convinced that hypnosis, yoga, and progressive muscle relaxation were capable of reducing pain perception and thought "all three claims are worthy of serious study by qualified neurophysiologists." Not many scientists were prepared to agree with him back then.

Livingston also experimented, rather stealthily, with nitrous oxide and its effects on pain perception.

He describes having the tanks of nitrous oxide and oxygen delivered to his offices on a Saturday, when no one was around. "I could not resist the temptation to try a few simple experiments on myself," he confesses, and he set up the heavy tanks for a try. "I laid a sharp scalpel on the window ledge where I could easily reach it while sitting in my swivel chair," he wrote. He breathed in the gas mixture through a mask, then cut himself with the knife.

It was still painful. He worried that putting the mask down and picking up the knife had interrupted the effect of the gas. "I then tried biting one of my hands to test for pain sensation because I only needed to tip the mask slightly in order to bite myself." Still no good. Finally, he rigged up a mask that fit over his nose, leaving both his hands free to mildly self-mutilate.

He found the gas working, but not enough, so he "sweetened the mixture and picked up the knife. As I went on breathing the gas I seemed to forget what I was supposed to be doing, for I laid aside the knife and just sat staring at the machine for a time. I recall thinking what a pretty machine it was and how brightly its metal and glassware sparkled." Vaguely, he thought he ought to turn it off, but he found he couldn't reach the valves on the tank. The next thing he knew, he woke up lying on the office floor, in a puddle of saliva. Luckily, the tube connected to the mask had become disconnected, otherwise he might have slumbered on indefinitely.

"That was my last solo effort in experimenting with nitrous oxide analgesia," he wrote, "and one I was careful not to mention at home for a long time."

He did conclude, after further tests using nitrous oxide during surgery, that the pain perception was "selectively suppressed." But there was only a very narrow zone, before analgesia deepened into a "stage of excitement" that could lead to confusion, violent behavior, and unconsciousness.

PAIN AND SUFFERING proceeds in a zigzag, hypothetical, digressive fashion—something that, as I wandered from pillar to post, I was glad to encounter. A too-linear approach doesn't do justice to pain. In fact, half of Livingston's most successful hypotheses were the result of digressive accidents in his clinical practice. He once injected a man suffering from phantom pain with too much procaine. At first, the patient seemed on the point of collapse, but afterward, he made a peculiar discovery: his phantom hand, which was always clenched painfully tight, suddenly relaxed, grew warm, and became less painful. The operation was a failure, but the side effects were great.

It's tempting to say the same about Livingston's book. *Pain and Suffering* is in some ways a magnificent and invaluable failure—too technical for lay readers and far too lively, witty, and ahead of its time to join the sober ranks of medical literature. Livingston was a natural storyteller who never quite escaped the surly bonds of his profession.

Livingston's discouragement surfaced in a chapter that attempts to pull the whole picture of pain together: "In dealing with so many different subjects that have no obvious connection," he wrote, "it might appear that I had forgotten the evolving ideal that was supposed to be the central theme of this narrative. On the contrary, it has been there in the background all the time, serving to hold these subjects in context and evolving under their influence." He went on to list some of the conclusions he and his pain team had arrived at.

They amount to a rough sketch of pain as science understands it today. "We also agreed that what was most important to the patient was the severity of the pain he felt as opposed to what we thought he ought to be feeling." He also touched on what would become a vital issue—the effect of early experience on an individual's vulnerability to pain: "An earnest effort should be made to determine the pain-controlling influence of various forms of conditioning, progressive relaxation training, hypnotism, etc. (Personally I believe that the conditioning a child receives from parental influences can change the severity of the pains he will experience for the remainder of his life.)" Also, the team agreed that "the brain exerts a 'downstream' influence on all sensory input." If a patient fears that his pain "implies some threat to his life or health and he focuses his attention on it, the pain not only seems worse, it is worse! If he decides that it is safe to ignore the pain and turn his attention to other things, the pain not only seems less, it is less!" Despite Livingston's exclamation marks, the manuscript was received with a kind of exasperated caution by his first readers.

"Whom is the book for?" responded one weary editor, Leon Virsky, at Basic Books in New York, who was also Livingston's informal agent. "Parts of the book sound as if you are talking to a group of your colleagues, parts as if you are addressing the medical profession and parts as if you are speaking to the general public."

Livingston wrote back to say, "I sincerely doubt that you would be interested in the manuscript if I ever finish it. . . . [T]he form the book should take and whom it should be addressed to has never been decided. Since my retirement in 1958 I have been writing and re-writing the Preface and Introduction—which would set the tone for the book to follow, but damned if I can do it satisfactorily."

He adds an afterthought about his wife. "I think her secret wish is that I forget the damned manuscript and have fun making ceramics."

But as a thinker, Livingston remains known, if at all, only within his profession. This is a loss. *Pain and Suffering* falls into the great tradition of humanist science writing, along with the work of Oliver Wendell Holmes and Silas Weir Mitchell. They have much to teach us. Livingston was a scientist with an artist's sensibility and humanity. He wrote in the age of the Skinner box and cold-blooded behavioral experiments on humans and animals, but despite surgical training and the mechanistic mood of the time, he remained open-minded and compassionate. The title of his manuscript says it all: He refused to sever his ideas about pain from his patients' experience of their suffering.

MY LAST MORNING IN L.A. was Easter Friday. Our pain holiday. It was Christ's willingness to suffer the agony of crucifixion that defined him as a citizen of earth as well as the Son of God. To forgive is divine, but to suffer, apparently, is human. In Christian terms, we can look for and find meaning in pain, but in our drift away from theological views of the self, pain has become something more secular, pathological, and empty.

I had a few hours to kill before my flight, so I checked out of my friendly ruin and went to the Farmers Market for breakfast. Being among fruits and vegetables always calms me when I'm on the road. It was a gloomy holiday morning, and there were few others wandering around through the aisles. I came upon a food stall that featured only hot sauces. Shelves and shelves of small bottles featuring death's-heads and pain symbols. The labels favored images of the devil or hookerish women in high boots, with fiery mouths. Taped to the shelves was a "pain meter" for the sauces, which were rated, almost like the McGill Pain Questionnaire, in terms of pepperosity. Another archive. In memory of William Livingston, I bought a little brown vial with the label "Pain and Suffering," and headed for the airport.

21

THE NURSES: "LET US LEAVE THESE JARGONS"

> *My night nurse—*
> *Oh gosh, the pain is getting worse . . .*
> *I don't want to see no doc,*
> *I need attendance from my nurse around*
> *   the clock—*
> *She's the one, the only remedy—night nurse.*
>
> —GREGORY ISAACS, "Night Nurse"

NURSES IN GENERAL, AND TWO OF THEM IN particular, have taught science more than it has cared to know about the nature of pain and suffering. Although Florence Nightingale wasn't focused only on pain, her attention to the patient and his experience, rather than the disease process, would become the heart of modern pain treatment. And in the twentieth century, one of the earliest champions of the use of opiates to ease the pain of dying was Dame Cicely Saunders, a nurse who later became a physician, and the founder of the modern hospice movement.

I had taken home a transcript of John Liebeskind's interview with Saunders and soon fell under the spell of her voice. And after so much sojourning in the male-dominated science of pain, it was a relief for me to come across the utterly pragmatic words of Florence Nightingale. The two women enter the cloistered rooms of pure science, throw open the windows, and let in the fresh air. And they shared other qualities.

Both were polymaths, gifted writers and committed Christians who disappointed their rich families by taking up nursing instead of something more seemly. Saunders, now in her eighties, has also lived with chronic back troubles, and Nightingale—well, her assorted ailments are still being debated and diagnosed.

There really should be a Broadway musical (*Flo!*) about the founder of modern nursing. She was so many things—an adventuress, a thinker, a tyrant in love (so they say). Nightingale was not just a long-skirted saint bustling among the wounded soldiers of the Crimean War. She was a gifted scientist ex officio, whose farsighted ideas have been overshadowed by her image as the Lady with the Lamp. She reinvented the idea of hospitals and helped revolutionize public health care in nineteenth-century Europe. She was also an early environmentalist who wrote passionate essays on subjects like irrigation, drainage, and "rural hygiene." Her writings, on a dizzying range of subjects from Egyptian mysticism to military hospital design, still have a visionary ring. And in a sense, pain consolidated her place in history (nurse-modest as it remains), by forcing her into a more reclusive, educational role after her war years.

After two years nursing in the battlefields of the Crimean War, Nightingale returned to England with her health ravaged. For the next twenty-five years she more or less stayed in bed, where she suffered from headaches, fever, nausea, anorexia, bad nerves, spinal pain, depression, and "feelings of failure." Her condition has been variously diagnosed as "Crimean fever" (something like typhus), post-traumatic stress syndrome, fibromyalgia, the ever-popular neurasthenia, and more recently, in the *British Medical Journal* (1955) as brucellosis, a chronic cluster of symptoms triggered by bacteria. Several biographers have portrayed her as a neurotic malingerer who had to be carried from room to room but could still manage to bully her aunt, who took care of her for decades, and to pepper the authorities with her thoughts on public health issues.

Nightingale was rich. She paid for all her publications—a good thing, since a work such as *The Zemindar, the Sun and the Watering Pot as Affecting Life or Death in India* might not otherwise have seen print. In later years, her health improved; she gained weight and lived until the age of ninety. There is no question that the war broke her health, but invalidism was also a useful fate for Victorian women who wished to break the mold: Taking to your bed was one way to lead an adventurous intellectual life. Without pain, Nightingale might have nursed many more men back to health. But as an "invalid," she was able to nurse her own thinking and writing instead, reasonably free of the social conventions of the day.

Both Nightingale and Saunders were in their early thirties before they were able to extricate themselves from their families and get down to work. Saunders studied politics, philosophy, and economics at Oxford, but the arrival of World War II allowed her to pursue an earlier "calling," as she described it, to nurse. A bad back forced Saunders to leave active nursing and turn to research, administration, teaching and writing. Pain took both women out of the trenches and into a more educational role—all the better for us, since medicine is still catching up to their radically progressive ideas about health care and the treatment of the dying.

Their first radical move was to choose nursing, a profession that in Nightingale's time was more or less reserved for aging prostitutes. The public attitude toward nurses was reflected in the fictional character of Sairey Gamp, the vengeful old hooker who sat about ignoring her sick patients in Dickens's 1844 novel *The Life and Adventures of Martin Chuzzlewit*.

But Nightingale and Saunders saw that nursing offered an education that medical training couldn't deliver. It permitted compassionate care. In the world of the hospital, where specialists come and go focused on this organ or that X ray, the nurse is often the one person whose job it is to pay attention to the person in the bed.

This brilliant arrangement—seeing the whole person—would

become the first prerequisite, a century later, for understanding pain. John Bonica may be considered the father of the multidisciplinary pain clinic in North America, but nurses have taken the "multidisciplinary approach" to pain all along. They're the ones who become familiar with the particular body, the family situation, and the moods of the patient. ("He's in good spirits this morning.") They're around. Nurses observe how people respond to medications and how attitude affects recovery long after the doctor has come and gone.

Of course, as everyone who has spent any time in hospitals knows, there are good nurses and bad ones. The bad ones are janitorial and brusque. Perhaps they take their cues from a senior surgeon, who has made it clear that detachment spells professionalism. A few even develop a kind of contempt for the vulnerability of the sick and are in a splendid position to be mean. But most nurses offer what the rest of the medical system rarely does—not just knowledge but a reassuring human presence.

The patient in a hospital bed has already forfeited his dignity when he puts on the open-backed gown and the plastic ID bracelet. Joining the assembly line of the sick nicely completes the mortifying process that illness began. Then comes loneliness and fear.

But a patient who lucks into an attentive nurse, someone who hasn't lost his or her human touch through overwork, feels less alone. A nurse who can make a patient feel less fearful is like a shot of morphine. Nurses observe what the rest of science has ploddingly discovered: When you reduce fear and anxiety, you reduce pain and suffering. A reassuring presence has a measurable analgesic effect on the body. Nurses were unofficially working the placebo response long before it ever had a name.

The good nurse takes in all of the patient, not just his chart. "He ate every scrap of his lunch," she will say to the visiting wife. Or, referring to someone who is lost in a coma, "She seems to like the blinds open." In the current system, in which nurses are overworked and underpaid, ordinary kindliness has atrophied, because it isn't valued as part of medicine. It smacks too much of housekeeping, of aunts at the bedside with mustard plasters and special teas. In a word, kindliness is too female.

Nurses in North America receive three or four years of training in subjects like physiology and anatomy. They graduate with a considerable amount of medicine under their belts. But the most useful part of their training may be the emphasis on care rather than cure. It's part of their job to lay hands on their patients and make small talk. Often this human touch is trained out of doctors. Medical students can start off determined to be warm and personal, but grueling internships amount to a kind of deprogramming. Residents go on hospital rounds and see that the head of the department doesn't play it warm and fuzzy. And a certain amount of emotional distance is necessary in the face of daily misery. But for some doctors, both male and female, coldness becomes part of their professionalism—their science.

Nurses have more freedom to be themselves with patients. Fewer people care how they go about their job. They also belong to an endangered occupation now. What little funding there is flows to technology or research; public health care has not been a political priority for some time. In 2001, the American Nurses Association released the results of a survey of the profession. Seventy-five percent said that the quality of care in their institutions had declined in the past two years. Nurses are either threatening to strike for better wages or leaving the profession in droves.

When my husband was in the hospital recently, I noticed a distinct "old nurse/new nurse" split. The new nurses breezed in and emptied first the wastebasket, then the catheter bag, without so much as eye contact. They were cleaning ladies, and the sick were dusty furniture. The "old" nurse (only in her forties, but of the old school) spoke to my husband, reassured him, explained all the tests and procedures to him, and seemed truly interested in his urine output—exactly what you want in a post-op nurse. She has become the exception.

The best thing a medical student could do to prepare for studies in the pain field would be to take a break from the neurology textbooks and turn to the ideas of history's revolutionary nurses.

FLORENCE NIGHTINGALE IS KNOWN, of course, as the founder of modern nursing: She started the first modern training school for nurses at St. Thomas's Hospital in 1860. Her droll little 1859 booklet *Notes on Nursing: What It Is, and What It Is Not* ("Oh, let us leave these jargons, and go your way straight to God's work, in simplicity and singleness of heart") is still part of the curriculum at nursing colleges. She has also been enthusiastically adopted by mystics (based on her semimad diaries from a voyage down the Nile), lesbians (she rejected two suitors and pursued her female cousin, Marianne Nicholson, but the evidence is thin regarding actual affairs), military nuts (she designed military hospitals), environmentalists (she thought pig manure superior to cow), and medical sleuths, who are still trying to diagnose her medical complaints. She wrote often about public health. One of her booklets, *The Sepoy Rebellion,* offers a scheme for sanitizing India.

Nightingale began to put her ideas about patient care into practice as supervisor of the Harley Street Hospital in London, where she insisted that prostitutes receive proper care. Then, in 1854, she led her cadre of thirty-eight nurses into the battlefield at Scutari, Turkey, to care for soldiers wounded in the Crimean War. Sidney Herbert, the secretary-at-war, had asked her to "improve conditions" at Scutari. (Her offer to volunteer crossed his letter in the mail.) The nurses arrived to find bare dirty floors, no bandages or latrines, not even knives or forks. The mortality rate was over 50 percent. Nightingale focused on hygiene and nutrition and gave morphine injections to ease suffering. Under her direction, the death rate at Scutari came down to less than 2 percent. We know this from her careful record of statistics, a science she was most enthusiastic about. "To understand God's thought, we must study statistics, for these are the measure of His Purpose," she wrote, not entirely persuasively.

As a result of her war work, Nightingale became a popular hero who was celebrated in songs and broadsides ("They keep up their spirits / Their hearts never fail / Now they're cheer'd by the presence of sweet Miss Nightingale"). But she was celebrated more as a ministering angel than for what she really was—a revolutionary thinker.

The Crimean episode gave the profession of nursing a kind of heroic halo for a time, but it was Nightingale's emphasis on cleanliness, fresh air, and the psychological aspects of healing that would profoundly change the way patients were treated. Pain experts have only recently come round to her belief that you can't treat pain without tackling the big picture. She understood that the world outside the patient is as important to healing as the internal narratives.

At the time Nightingale went to work, the sick, who had previously been cared for at home, by the women in the family, were in the process of being segregated from society and hidden away in hospitals that resembled almshouses. Hospitals in her time were last-resort refuges for the poor, unlike the high-tech corporations they aspire to be today. A committed Christian, Nightingale believed that medical care was for everyone, regardless of class.

She also believed in the curative powers of pets (long before our "discovery" of how pets can ease depression), visits from friends, and the enlivening presence of children in hospitals. On the other hand, she was strict about imposing peace and quiet. "Unnecessary noise is the most cruel absence of care which can be inflicted," she wrote, adding pointedly that "a nurse who rustles is the horror of a patient, though perhaps he does not know why." (It's a good thing Nightingale never had to spend the night in a modern hospital.) Patients need not only air and light and people, according to Nightingale, but also space and a view. "One window for every two beds," she wrote in her book *Notes on Hospitals,* with "the window to be not less than 4 feet 8 inches wide, the sill within 2 or 3 feet of the floor, so that the patient can see out."

This was what Nightingale's experience as a nurse taught her: You do not "fix" people; you try to create the conditions that will allow them to heal themselves. The patient whose comfort and dignity are attended to may come through better than the person who has a half hour of technically brilliant surgery from a doctor who then disappears.

A good nurse sets up certain expectations, even if they are the oldest ones in the book: "Are we feeling better today?" More than a hundred years before endorphins were discovered or named,

Nightingale knew how to put them to work. A nurse who believes that her care contributes to healing has already begun the recovery process.

Nightingale was innovative in small ways, too. One of her inventions at Harley Street was a call bell that let the nurses at their stations know who was ringing. She introduced a system of dumb-waiter lifts, so that hot meals could stay hot. She bought hospital supplies and food in bulk—an obvious bit of economy unheard of at the time.

But for most people, Nightingale's da Vinci brain is still hidden under her nurse's cap. One unlikely fan who is doing his bit to restore her place in history is Country Joe McDonald of the Woodstock-era antiwar rock band Country Joe and the Fish. He maintains an impressive website devoted to Nightingale's life story and writings, which he discovered through his antiwar work with Vietnam nurses. McDonald has even recorded four "nurse songs" (two with the late Jerry Garcia), and he boasts a private collection of "nurse dolls," including a troll in a white nurse hat. You can also order a beer stein featuring a cameo portrait of the not-quite-attractive Florence.

This convergence of an activist sixties rock star ("and it's one, two, three, what are we fighting for . . .") with a Victorian nurse is not as strange as it might seem. Nightingale was, in her germ-chasing way, a social reformer whose ideas still have a subversive sting to them. The idea that everyone deserves compassionate health care was as novel then as it has become fragile today. "There is no great hospital today which does not bear upon it the impress of her mind," said Lytton Strachey in his description of her as an eminent Victorian.

Despite her focus on institutional care, she saw beyond that to something better. "I look to the abolition of all hospitals and work-house infirmaries," she wrote in an essay about the future, "but it is no use to talk about the year 2000." (Little did she know.)

In the nineteenth century, Oliver Wendell Holmes wrote a poem called "The Morning Visit" about the relationship of doctors and patients. It already reflected some of Nightingale's ideas about the importance of a calm surrounding and simple kindness.

KINDNESS, *untutored by our grave M.D.'s,*
But Nature's graduate, when she schools to please,
Wins back more sufferers with her voice and smile
Than all the trumpery in the druggist's pile.

Once more, be QUIET: *coming up the stair,*
Don't be a plantigrade, a human bear,
But, stealing softly on the silent toe,
Reach the sick chamber ere you're heard below. . . .

Spare him; the sufferer wants of you and art
A track to steer by, not a finished chart. . . .

Each look, each movement, every word and tone
Should tell your patient you are all his own;
Not the mere artist, purchased to attend,
But the warm, ready, self-forgetting friend
Whose genial visit in itself combines
The best of cordials, tonics, anodynes.

DAME CICELY SAUNDERS WAS a nurse (and later became a doctor) who set up in London, England, the first system of research-based hospice care for the dying. This provided the model for what North Americans (with their customary fear of the D-word) have since renamed "palliative care." Personally, she doesn't mind what it's called, as long as somebody gets around to doing it.

What Dame Cicely calls the "halo effect" around the whole subject of hospice care has made her another sainted Lady of the Lamp, an image that overshadows her tough intellectual contributions as a scientist and educator. She was, and remains, way, way ahead of her time.

Saunders's first hospice opened in 1967. St. Christopher's House in southeast London is a community-based facility that combines teaching, research, and care for the sick and dying. New visitors to the hospice expect a hushed, somber ward with nuns gliding about. They are surprised to find a busy center with a nursery attached (many of the nurses are young married women), which welcomes nondying locals and visitors with dogs. Saunders saw that the process of dying can accommodate a great deal of life and went about unsequestering death.

Dame Cicely—the title was bestowed when she was eighty-two—was born in England in 1918, to a family who expected great things of her. She went to Oxford, but when World War II broke out, she left school to train as a nurse at St. Thomas's Hospital's Nightingale School of Nursing. She worked as a nurse in a cancer ward, until a lifelong back problem forced her to quit. It was around this time that her Christianity deepened and began to shape her ideas about how to go about her work. She went back to Oxford, where she studied public administration, and got a degree in medical social work. But a friend advised her, quite rightly, that she would find it hard to achieve her goals as a mere nurse. So, at the age of thirty-three, she got to work on her biology and chemistry and earned a medical degree. (At one time she also considered a career in music.) All of this—nursing, doctoring, politics, spirituality, philosophy, economics, social work, her first experiences with dying patients, and her studies in public administration—came into play in her concept of what hospice care could be.

By the time I came upon Saunders in my research, I had spent quite a bit of time reading about men whose theories of pain required them, however reluctantly, to saw off the tops off monkey skulls or to take penknives to their own arms as part of their experiments—strange, lonely labors, most often in the service of pure ideas. I missed the presence and voices of patients, the people for whom all this pain research was intended. In her writings and teachings, Saunders restores the role of the patient, just as Nightingale always tried to take the patient's-eye view. In her interview with John Liebeskind for the History of Pain Collection at UCLA, she constantly refers back to the person in her care who inspired her to take a new direction in her work.

"In the first ward I took over [at St. Thomas's Hospital]," Saunders said, "there was a patient—this by now is 1947—there was a young Pole, a Polish Jew originally from Warsaw, though not from the uprising in the ghetto—he'd left before then, aged 40, with an inoperable cancer. And I knew he had no relatives and very few friends. I followed him up in Outpatient; so when he collapsed a few months later, his landlady got in touch with me while he was waiting to go to hospital and I went to see him, and then I followed him and visited him about 25 times during the two months that he was dying in a very busy surgical ward. And he was David Tasma, and he is really the founder of the modern Hospice movement.

"When David died he . . . left me this legacy. He said 'I'll be a window in your home.' The legacy turned out to be five hundred pounds. So that's why we have a commitment from the beginning [in hospice care] to openness—openness to the world, openness of course to patients and their families, but openness among ourselves. . . .

"But two other things he said, or one he said and one I knew about him, were equally important, sort of pillars of Hospice, and the first was 'I only want what is in your mind and in your heart.' " When Saunders had asked if he wanted her to read to him or say the Psalms, this is how he replied. "But thinking about it afterwards I began to realize this could mean constant learning and increase in understanding, but it had to be given with the friendship of the heart. . . . And so the openness, of the mind and the heart and the freedom of the spirit, were built in Hospice in 1948, and then it took me nineteen years to build the home around the window."

Tasma was an "ordinary fellow," a waiter, dying of cancer in a busy fifty-bed cancer ward. "But he had a sensitivity . . ." Saunders said. "The idea of home came out of our conversations together. But I mean, he was obviously . . . I mean, that's a very poetical thing to say, 'I'll be a window.' He was special, David. I was very fond of him."

After Tasma died, Saunders volunteered as a nurse in a ward for the dying. "And there I met the regular giving of oral morphine . . . balanced to a patient's need. It was given regularly; the nurses didn't wait for pain to happen, for the patients to earn their morphine." She said that the matron had come to the hospital in 1935 and the regular giving of morphine had been in operation then, something she called a "nurse's view of pain." "Because a doctor will write up something for pain and come back tomorrow and see how it worked. Whereas a nurse is up and down and beside the bed all day and wants to see a patient comfortable, not either stuporous or anxiously waiting for the next dose."

(Liebeskind, who is interviewing her, interrupts at this point to say that "nurses are always riveted by the discussion of the topic of pain. They really do understand it!")

The usual procedure for the administration of morphine is for the doctor to prescribe "PRN"—*pro re nata,* to be given as needed. Saunders decided that this insightful matron had probably said to herself, "Well, it's *needed* to stop pain ever happening, so let's give it regularly." Which is how "ATC," or around-the-clock, medication slipped in.

On a clinical research fellowship to look at pain management in terminal illnesses at St. Joseph's Hospital, she initiated a schedule of pain medication, and it "was like waving a wand over the house. One of the sisters wrote to me not very long ago, saying 'I well remember those days and the change from pain-full to pain-free.' "

"It's so simple, and in a way so obvious," she said, referring to a consistent schedule rather than the traditional as-needed regime. "But I mean, a lot of important ideas are sort of around, and ideas find people just as much as people find ideas."

One of the ideas that found Saunders, just after the war, was Christianity. "I was searching hard all through the time I was nursing and then at the time of the surrender of Japan I went on holiday with a group of keen Christian friends and it sort of came—fell into place—and I made a very strong commitment. And I've been traveling on ever since. I'm no longer particularly an evangelical . . . I'm rather a liberal, I think. But it has been very much a vocation to do something about pain."

Saunders is credited with inventing hospice care, but she is meticulous about tracing hospice back to the early Christian era, and the refuges known as *zenadokia,* which carried out the "seven works of mercy," including caring for the poor and the sick. "The word 'hospes' started by meaning guest, but came to mean host as well . . . 'hospitium' meant both the place where they met but also the relationship between the two, which is a very important part of Hospice later. After that a large number of hospices were opened up all over Europe as Christianity spread. . . . They welcomed pilgrim travelers but they also welcomed the sick locals and so on. But they were never specifically for the dying.

"The first person who ever used the word for care of the dying was a Madame Jeanne Garnier in France, who opened the Hospice of the Dames de Calvare in Lyons in 1842. And she opened about seven homes altogether. But hospice isn't such a very acceptable word in Europe, and palliative care unit is much more acceptable. . . . I never obviously said we were the first hospice. What I did say was that we were the first research and teaching hospice. . . . We started doing evaluative research from the beginning. We were also doing drug studies—it was very important to do the comparison between morphine and diamorphine [heroin], for a start, because I had been using diamorphine at St. Joseph's, I'd introduced it. And I had the clinical impression it was the better drug.

"I did know we were getting better at everything. And also it's very important to test your own enthusiasms. And if you turn out to be wrong, it's ever so nice that you actually did it yourself . . . and of course we found out that there was no clinically observable difference [between morphine and heroin]."

Anyone who knows a little about early hospice care has heard of the famous Brompton Cocktail, a painkilling brew of morphine, heroin, cocaine, alcohol, sometimes marijuana, "and honey to disguise the taste." As Saunders said, it was "very much for people dying," and the cocaine was also a soothing topical painkiller for people with sore throats. It was first developed at the Brompton Chest Hospital in the early 1930s to treat people dying of tuberculosis. "But we did a study on cocaine and found it really made no continual difference, so that came out. We took the alcohol out, because some patients didn't like the bite of it . . . we were left really with the active ingredient only, the oral morphine. So we never call it the Brompton Cocktail now, and in fact we didn't call it that from early on." Dame Cicely is a stickler for historical accuracy.

She went on to explain how, in 1970, she invited Dr. Robert Twycross to work at St. Christopher's. Now the lecturer in palliative care at Oxford, Twycross was instrumental in bringing Saunders's ideas about caring for the dying to the World Health Organization, which formalized and standardized what Saunders practiced at St. Christopher's. Since world travel was out of the question for Saunders because of her back, Twycross became a sort of ambassador for her vision, and he acknowledges his debt to her. The other doctor who helped put Saunders's ideas into action in America was Vittorio Ventafridda, a professor from Milan who visited St. Christopher's. She took him into a ward where a woman with very difficult neuropathic pain was painting a picture. She was on a huge amount of medication and still managed to focus on a "beautiful blue line across the horizon of the landscape she was painting." Saunders thinks that this patient, who was young and pretty, had an important effect on Ventafridda. "I think Mrs. Hughes probably impressed him and got, you know, under his skin and thus into the WHO more than anything else. . . . I mean, when other people start using your ideas as if they were their own, you've really won, although it may be quite difficult to stomach it."

Saunders is always bringing history back to patients, reminding students that Ventafridda would not be who he is in the world without Mrs. Hughes. "But then," Saunders added, "I'm not basically a researcher. . . . I'm much more the impresario for research."

One of the research projects she did oversee was a study that demonstrated that pain patients who received morphine didn't normally require escalating dosages in order to get the same effect. Tolerance didn't develop. "It's iatrogenic if you produce tolerance, I think, by giving lots of doses . . . but if you use orally and regularly and prevent pain escalating, patients will reach their own optimum plateau." This idea was not easily accepted then, and still isn't today.

During a pain meeting, a professor working on endorphins heard Saunders claim that morphine doesn't cause tolerance. "And he would say, 'I don't believe it . . .' and we said, 'No, clinically, it is true.'

"Pain itself," she added, "is a strong antagonist to painkillers."

Liebeskind and Saunders discussed the resistance to ideas about pain treatment. "Education is a terribly slow process," Saunders said. The hospice movement has gained widespread approval, Liebeskind agreed, "but it's not all the way there, is it?"

"In the States it's much less medically respectable than it is over here," Saunders said. "It hasn't been accepted by the great bulk of medicine in the States, I don't think, from what I keep hearing. And it doesn't have enough medical input. Elizabeth Kübler-Ross did a huge amount of public relations for the dying, but in a way hampered it by making stages and things which I think were on the whole a bit of a pity, and that also got up the noses of the medical establishment."

Memorial Sloan-Kettering Cancer Center in New York City developed pain services under the direction of Dr. Kathleen Foley and started the first hospital palliative support team, a peripatetic one with no beds, at the end of 1974. In the same year, Dr. Bal Mount, a Montreal surgeon, did a sabbatical at St. Christopher's. He then went back to Montreal and set up the first palliative care unit in a general hospital, at the Royal Victoria. In fact, it was Bal Mount "who put the word 'palliative care' into the scene."

So hospice in North America was launched in 1975, even though the word itself lapsed. There is still no special care for the dying in sixty countries.

"The American hospice scene has been more a consumerist movement. I think what is sad in America is that the pain lot and the hospice lot and even now a growing-up palliative care lot don't really meld.

"You have to see pain as a whole experience. The person who gave me the concept of total pain was a lady we treated called Mrs. Hinson, in 1963. And I said to her, 'Tell me about your pain.' Without any more prompting, she said, 'Well, Doctor, it began in my back, but now it seems that all of me is wrong.' Talked about all her symptoms. 'I could have cried for the pills and the injections, but I knew that I mustn't and it seemed as if nobody understood how I felt and that the world was against me. My husband and son were wonderful, but they were having to stay off work and lose their money, but it's so wonderful to begin to feel safe again.' So she's talked about physical, psychological, social, and the spiritual need for safety, security, to be herself—and that's pain. So I've endlessly lectured, saying it's these areas, and tried to cover them. And that was thirty years ago."

In his memoir *Experience,* the hugely unsentimental essayist and novelist Martin Amis describes going to visit his old and ailing father. Kingsley Amis had just been moved from a private hospital to the Corner in Phoenix Ward, a national health hospice.

"This is the Corner," Amis *fils* writes, "and this is public transport: one-class. . . . But this is all right and I would like to die here. [V. S.] Pritchett has a bit about hospitals making the body 'feel important' because you are bringing your 'talent of pain' to the total. I very much like talent of pain.

"What surrounds me now, though," he writes, "and fills me with awe, is talent of love. Of supererogatory love. That's what the nurses here, who are of all colours, suffer from: supererogatory love."

Amis may have assumed that women are sometimes over-equipped with kindliness and must find patients in hospitals to soak up the excess. What he was seeing was not womanliness, really, but a kind of care that women only invented.

22

HOW I HURT MY DENTIST

*I advise dental patients to keep their eyes open during the procedure.
It frees you, just a little, from internalization. The dental patient
must have something to stare at—the panels of the blinds, the
framed certificates . . .*

MARTIN AMIS, *Experience: A Memoir*

MY RELATIONSHIP WITH MY DENTIST—AND people always talk about it as a relationship —has been remarkably free of tics and phobias. Many people (15 percent of the "dental population," apparently) are afraid of their dentists. Despite the fact that their profession knows more about pain and pain relief than most doctors, a trip to the dentist is still associated with being afraid and being hurt.

I tend to see my routine visits as a little caesura in the day when I get to lie down and let someone else do his job. My anxiety level on the way to the dentist is somewhere down around the professional manicure level. Or it was, until recently.

I was lying in the big chair, with the overhead TV muted and tuned to a cooking show that featured calamari. Uncooked squid looks remarkably like tooth pulp, but never mind. Swimming right over me was the big blue eye of my dentist, made huge by the magnifying glass he wore. (My dentist, now retired, is an endearingly furry man. I associate this with the probing, primal patience he brings to his job, like a gentle ape searching for mites.)

On this visit, Dr. Conway was excavating a lower molar, in preparation for installing a temporary crown. An assistant stood on the other side of me, vacuuming up my saliva. The high-pitched drill bore down. *Neeneenee!* I wore clear plastic glasses in case bits of old filling flew out and blinded me. Once again, I had forgotten my own CDs, and had to listen to the morose selection of office tapes: Moody Blues, Jethro Tull, or Celine Dion. But I only used the music as white noise, so it didn't really matter. My hands were folded on top of my paper bib. Every once in a while, they would lay a little tool on the bib.

Then something peculiar happened: The freezing in my lower jaw and mouth began to wear off. I could feel my tongue. Then I could feel my lips, and then the drill penetrating the awful little hole in my gum.

"*Ish naw frozenh!*"

"I was afraid that might happen," Dr. Conway said grimly. I had asked him to use an anesthetic that didn't have adrenaline. "Without the adrenaline, the freezing dissipates into the system more quickly. But I've already given you five vials of it, and I don't want to give you any more. We're going to have to keep going, so just hang on. I'm very sorry."

My dentist is a low-voiced man with a Yorkshire accent who seems to have a genuine horror of inflicting pain on his patients. This is a good sign in your dentist. I've been going to him for twenty years, and I trust him completely. So when he suddenly seemed to turn into Laurence Olivier in the role of the dentist-sadist in *Marathon Man*, I was taken by surprise. The high, hot pain was intermittent, but searing. I began to arch and writhe in classic phobic-dental-patient fashion, clamping my hand on the upper arm of his nurse with a pincer grip. The paper bib went up and down as I breathed fast and hard.

He had used the new anesthetic on me because I am one of the 10 percent of dental patients who react badly to adrenaline. Even though there were only a few parts per million of adrenaline in the anesthesia, I could feel it hit my system—my heart raced, my hands went cold, and my chest felt tight. I'd rather have my teeth removed with pliers than go through the anxiety and tachycardia again.

This meant that Dr. Conway had to resort to a higher dosage of a more short-lived anesthesia. He stuck the big needle in my jaw, four, five times, sliding it through the tough band of muscles at the back of my mouth. A woody sensation. As we waited for the anesthesia to take—that companionable lacuna of time called "Waiting for Numbness"—we chatted about the vagaries of dental anesthesia.

"I've seen it many times," he said. "I'll give a patient all the freezing he can take, and nothing happens. Then I'll say, 'Okay, that's it, you might as well go home,' and as soon as they leave the room, the freezing will take effect. It must have something to do with hormones triggered by stress."

Then he sent me out to the waiting room to wait. I think this was also a strategy on his part to avoid the dental-chair heebie-jeebies. After ten minutes, my mouth and jaw were more or less frozen, although not to the usual, pork-chop-in-the-freezer level. We decided to go for it anyway. And halfway through, the feeling in my mouth began to come back.

Dr. Conway began to work fast; I felt the urgency in the way he reached over me to grab a tool, when the assistant wasn't quick enough. What's the big rush, I wondered. Then I felt the drill hit the nerve, a riveting sensation. An image of Satan's pitchfork sprang to mind. Now I know why Satan carries a pitchfork: He's waiting for someone with an open tooth socket.

"How are you managing?" my dentist said with concern. "I'm so sorry, but I really have no choice. Just hang on, it won't be long."

Dentists are more knowledgable and aware of pain, and fear of pain, than most health professionals. After all, if a dentist gets a reputation for hurting his patients, he won't have any. This incentive, along with new developments in drills and drugs, has made it possible for modern dentists to eliminate all but the most fleeting discomfort. There's even something called a "DentiPatch" that delivers a hit of lidocaine to the gums, so that the needle can slide in unfelt. Nevertheless, people still associate dentists with pain, and fear, and vulnerability. There is now a booming industry in spalike clinics that deal with dental phobias.

Patients have very comprehensive fears when it comes to dentists: they fear everything from the needles, to the sound of the drill, to the sensation of being tipped horizontal in the chair. For most, it's the result of lingering trauma from being hurt by a dentist in their childhood. Early pain is permanent pain, as far as the body is concerned. You can teach the body all sorts of cognitive tricks to dismantle the alarm system, but it will still go off when the dentist looms. Dental fears and phobias are evidence of how crucial conditioned expectation is to our experience of pain—and how distressing even the expectation of pain can be.

Back in the chair, the unfreezing continued. With my tongue, I felt an awful pit, the space where my tooth had been. Into this space came and went the high-pitched drill. *Neeneeneenee!* It's just the sound, I told myself, that nasty sound. But then the drill would touch the nerve, or the pulp, or whatever lived at the bottom of the space, and I would fall into a narrow crevasse of pain, hang upside down in it for an instant, then clamber out again. The sensation was intermittent, and (I reminded myself) nothing like my own personal pinnacle of pain, twenty-five hours of unmedicated childbirth. I did all my usual Zen things and applied myself to bearing it.

I took deep breaths. I imagined myself with my coat on, walking out the door and into the elevator. Part of the problem was Celine Dion on the earphones singing "My Heart Will Go On." Maybe not! My husband, who shares my dentist, always brings a Rolling Stones CD when he gets work done—"perfect for drilling"—and he routinely takes the nitrous oxide beforehand, too. But nitrous leaves me with a headache, and it's not without its dangers, either. You can't tinker with consciousness without taking all sorts of risks.

On the overhead TV, the cooking program wrapped up and I watched cable feed from Parliament, captioned for the hearing-impaired. I glommed onto the words. Good old print. I think my brain has more print receptors than opiate sockets.

Meanwhile, Dr. Conway was sweating bullets. It was an insult to his perfectionism, to be hurting me in this fashion. It didn't just offend him, it *afflicted* him. Five long minutes passed, and the work was done. He stripped off his gloves, and sat down on a stool, looking drained.

"If you ever have to have work done on that lower jaw again, we'll have to give you a general anesthetic, or find another way around this freezing problem. It's just too traumatic. I don't want to put you through this again."

Frankly, I was fine. When you're dealing with pain, you're utterly engaged, and then the moment is gone.

"Good work," I said, refraining from patting him on the shoulder. "That must have been rough for you."

"It was! You know, it's hard when somebody is in pain and you can't do anything about it."

"Don't worry. I'm sure you did the best you could."

My reassurances were somewhat undermined by the fact that I had flakes of blue cement on my face, from the impression mold.

"You might want to freshen up," Dr. Conway said, a dental phrase I have come to understand means "You look grotesque, go to the washroom." (The last time I heard this phrase at the dentist's was when I had two wisdom teeth extracted. I was writing out my check at the reception desk, and my mouth was still frozen. "You might want to freshen up," the receptionist suggested. I went into the washroom, looked in the mirror, and saw a twisted rictus of pain on my face. My face had felt the pain, but "I" didn't—yet.)

My next appointment was for the installation of the crown—the coronation. Both my dentist and I were upbeat and jovial this time, because there would be no freezing or drilling. Our little bond of agony was over. And so we had a conversation about the relationship dentists have to their strange professional role, that of someone who both inflicts pain (or represents that potential) and rescues people from it.

"I felt terrible about last time," he said, "but there was nothing more I could do. It's such a helpless feeling, especially when the technology is there to prevent the pain. I don't like it when things don't go the way I want them to."

"I'm sure that's a dentist thing."

Then he went on to talk about what seemed like unrelated matters—sad news from some colleagues of his, who had been through personal tragedies.

"So many have gone through terrible times recently. It's strange."

"Maybe the people around dentists absorb some of the pain, too," I ventured, "just as dentists absorb the trauma of their patients. The echo effect. Perhaps dentists bear a burden of pain from all the fear and anxiety that people bring to the dentist's chair. Then that affects the people around them. Maybe pain has its own little ecosystem."

This seemed to strike a chord with his nursing assistant, who perked up and agreed with me.

"This may sound like a wacky theory," I went on, "and pardon me if I compare dentistry to the Holocaust, but the first generation of Holocaust survivors are sometimes the ones whose job it is to *not feel too much*. Otherwise, they'd fall apart. Their job is to survive, and perhaps even to forget, in order not to go mad."

Dr. Conway was not looking too comfortable with this analogy, but he let me continue.

"I've been reading about Holocaust survivors, and how the pain moves down through generations. People on the front lines of suffering become conductors of pain, regardless of how well or how badly they cope with it themselves.

"That's the problem with being 'frozen,' or going under general anesthesia," I went on. The assistant had now lost interest and was rinsing things in the sink. "The body has still been wounded. The fact of the pain is there, even if the consciousness of it is missing. Just like when I had my wisdom teeth extracted. 'I' felt okay afterwards, but my face in the mirror was in anguish."

"I don't think it's a wacky theory at all," he said. "It's taken me years to learn how to deal with the aftereffects of my work. For me, the only answer is to go to the gym. I really hate it, but it works. It's almost as if you have to wash it all out of your body. And yet I have friends who are brain surgeons, who deal with life and death every day in a way that I don't, and they don't seem to have this problem, of taking on their patient's fear and pain . . ."

"Well, their patients are unconscious, and the bodies are draped. This slab of flesh is wheeled into the OR, and they get to work on it. With you, everyone who walks in the door arrives with some level of anxiety. They bring a lot of baggage. And you have to deal with all that, as well as doing delicate, technical work in a tiny little space."

Conway looked thoughtful. I felt my dental support session was going quite well. Then he told me about the number of people who begin to cry in the chair, when the pain brought up memories of bad dental experiences in their childhoods.

"It's amazing how many people have been hurt by dentists when they were little, before they could understand what was happening to them. And they always mention this." I didn't go into the obvious sexual subtext of a visit to the dentist. The vulnerability of lying there immobilized, mouth open, as someone hovers over you.

In neuroscience, the homunculus has big gorilla hands, a giant toe, looming genitals, and huge lips and tongue; these brain-areas lie close together, or even overlap. Anything that happens to the mouth might as well be happening to the genitals, too, which is why kissing is integral to sex. By this logic, and according to the homunculus, dentistry could be considered the antikiss. If there is incest or other dark sexual trauma in someone's past, dental work can stir up those memories, too.

Or, as Conway forlornly put it, "It's never just about the tooth."

I remembered someone I knew who had just gone through several weeks of caring for a mutual friend, who was dying of cancer. For weeks, she was a rock. Even at the funeral, she didn't fall apart. "Then I went to the dentist, crawled into the chair, and began to bawl." She was relieved when I told her that this was not the least bit unusual.

Dentists soak it all up, just like the gauze pads they pack into the mouth. And perhaps the high levels of stress, depression, and suicide that accompany this profession have something to do with the fact that dentists are haunted by their patients' pain.

> *I know all about the expert musicianship of toothaches, their brass, woodwind and percussion and, most predominantly, their strings, their strings (Bach's "Concerto for Cello" struck me, when I recently heard it performed, as a faultless transcription of a toothache—the persistence, the irresistible persuasiveness). Toothaches can play it staccato, glissando, accelerando, prestissimo and above all fortissimo. They can do rock, blues and soul, they can do doowop and bebop, they can do heavy metal, rap, punk and funk. And beneath all this anarchical stridor there was a lone, soft, insistent voice, always audible to my abject imagination: the tragic keening of the castrato.*
>
> MARTIN AMIS, *Experience: A Memoir*

FOR MOST MEDICAL PEOPLE, pain is a non-life-threatening symptom that can be put aside. For dentists, pain is front and center. In the history of pain, dentists have played a crucial role.

It was a pair of dentists, in fact, who discovered modern anesthesia—a story as rife with greed, competition, and turf wars as any modern medical saga.

Before anesthesia, surgery was a brief and barbaric undertaking accomplished with speed, whiskey, and nerve, mostly relegated to lopping off limbs and extracting teeth. Barbers doubled as tooth extractors. Indeed, the origins of the Royal College of Physicians was in the Barber-Surgeons School of the nineteenth century. Neurosurgeon Frank Vertosick Jr., author of the book *Why We Hurt*, reports that a French surgeon named Dupuytren had an especially unusual approach to sedating his patients. "He once insulted a woman until she passed out, then proceeded to operate."

The two drugs associated with the modern history of anesthesia, ether and nitrous oxide, were known long before they were used to put surgical patients to sleep. Both ether and nitrous oxide started out as recreational drugs—early Ecstasy. The chemist who discovered oxygen, Joseph Priestley, first synthesized nitrous oxide in the late 1700s, when "laughing gas" became popular at parties among the rich and the restless. Another chemist, Sir Humphry Davy, noticed that people who were giggling about on nitrous oxide didn't seem to notice when they fell all over the furniture. He thought it might be useful as a painkiller in surgery, and he even did a few experiments with it himself, but at the time nobody took it further.

Ether—"sweet oil of vitriol," or sulfuric acid—had been around for centuries before several enterprising chemists and dentists plotted to unleash it on the world. Valerius Cordus discovered ether in 1540. As Vertosick mentions in his book, the great alchemist Paracelsus, in the same year, added ether to his chicken feed and was amazed to see all his chickens pass out. In the late 1700s, doctors used ether to treat colic and learned that inhaling ether can put someone to sleep. But both ether and nitrous oxide at high doses can be toxic, so they didn't want to use it.

In the early 1800s, medical students began holding ether parties—"ether jags"—and one of the doctors who attended was a country surgeon from Jefferson, Georgia, Dr. Crawford Long. He noticed that people high on ether didn't seem to feel any pain, literally. In 1842, Long agreed to give a friend some cut-rate surgery if he would try ether inhalation. Long successfully carved a growth out of his friend's neck and then used ether on other patients, too. But he lived in the country, didn't report his findings, and never got credit for his discoveries.

It took a rivalry between dental partners, Horace Wells and William Morton, to turn two party drugs into the most important breakthrough of modern medicine.

Dr. Horace Wells was a dentist in Hartford, Connecticut, in the 1800s, when his profession was basically a matter of potions, promotion, and extraction. He happened to come across a demonstration by a roving chemist named Gardner Colton, who charged people a quarter a head to try laughing gas. Colton was a kind of carny who warned his audiences that people under the influence of laughing gas could become violent—he employed a few muscular men to hold down the paying customers. Wells was watching, in 1844, when a young man took the nitrous oxide, started to struggle, gashed his leg, and didn't notice the wound until the gas wore off.

Wells was intrigued. He put himself to sleep with the nitrous, and then used it the next day to have one of his own teeth extracted, as Colton dosed him with laughing gas. It was painless. Seeing a rich future ahead of him, Wells organized a public demonstration of this new "painless dentistry" at Massachusetts General Hospital in Boston, in front of medical students and professors.

But the demonstration was a failure. The patient was having a tooth extracted. Unsure of how much nitrous oxide to administer, Wells didn't give his patient enough of it, and he began to scream in pain. Ironically, the man later claimed that he never felt a thing, but in the chair he gave every sign of being in agony. The assembled audience booed and hissed as the man struggled. Wells never recovered from this humiliation. He abandoned dentistry, became addicted to chloroform, was charged with throwing acid at a prostitute, and killed himself three years after his disastrous experiment.

In the audience during Wells's mortification was his former partner, Dr. William T. G. Morton. He was a second-year medical student at the time who practiced dentistry on the side. Morton had been experimenting with ether, putting his own dog to sleep, and on another occasion using ether on a patient with an infected tooth. He decided to repeat Wells's demonstration—only this time, he would use ether for a surgical procedure, not just a tooth extraction.

Morton managed to persuade a Harvard surgeon, Dr. John Warren, to attend the demonstration, which took place in the "Ether Dome" of Massachusetts General Hospital in 1846. Once again, professors and students gathered to watch some poor sod being cut open while breathing a strange gas. Warren was punctilious, and Morton was late, held up by an instrument maker who was helping him fashion a mask to deliver the ether. He arrived just as Warren was about to make the first cut without him. Morton fitted the mask on the patient, a twenty-year-old man named Abbott with a tumor in his jaw, and in seconds he was asleep. Warren cut the tumor out as Abbott lay motionless. The whole room fell silent, awaiting cries and screams that never came. Abbott awoke, and Warren turned to give the world's first physician endorsement: "Gentlemen," he said, "this is no humbug."

Ah, but hubris lay in wait for Morton, too. Greedy to profit from his discovery, Morton tried to patent this sleeping gas as "letheon," disguising the fact that it was simply our old friend ether, plus a little oil of orange to mask the awful smell. When the secret of letheon became known, others contested his patent, including Crawford Long, the Georgian surgeon who had used ether years before, and Morton's chemistry professor at Harvard, Charles Jackson.

Jackson's story is sad. He claimed to be the one who gave Morton the idea to use ether in surgery, although Morton fought him to the end, claiming Jackson was nothing but a fraud and an opportunist. Morton somewhat restored his reputation by administering ether to Civil War soldiers before he died, embittered, embattled, and poor, at forty-eight. His tombstone read THE INVENTOR AND REVEALER OF ANESTHETIC INHALATION. BEFORE WHOM, IN ALL TIME, SURGERY WAS AGONY. . . . When Jackson read the inscription, legend has it he went insane. He later died in an asylum.

But Colton, the freelance chemist and carny, never gave up on nitrous oxide, and eventually he introduced it into dentistry, where it is still used today. Ether fell out of favor when electricity came into the operating room, because the smallest spark around ether vapor could lead to an explosion.

The two squabbling dentists, Morton and Wells, managed to revolutionize modern medicine just the same. Life expectancy before anesthesia was thirty-seven years. By the end of the nineteenth century, it would rise to fifty. The ability of surgeons to work inside the body and the head, unheard of before ether, would become a commonplace miracle. The irony is that the birth of anesthesia should have left the dentists responsible for it in so much personal pain.

23

TWIST AND SHOUT:
BLOWING A DISK

ALTHOUGH THE REST OF US WERE BRINGING food to help celebrate my father's ninety-third birthday, my mother had put out dips anyway. Endive spears and tapenade. She worked around a slight tremor in her hands and a bunch of other things people get at ninety, but she looked very well. Her broken shoulder and wrist had healed. The day before, my father had precision-raked the yard, harvesting, as he was quick to tell us, "ten garbage bags of pinecones." No, this time it was my younger sister, Jori, who couldn't walk. She had hurt her back. And because she couldn't sit up to drive, either, they were chauffering her to physiotherapy appointments—proof that parenting never ends.

The youngest and by far the fittest member of our family, Jori had herniated a disk two months before and was still flat on her back. She made it to the family party, but she had to lie on the broadloom while we sat around her like a centerpiece and ate buffet-style. She looked beautiful, as usual, but the weeks of bad sleep were beginning to show. You could see the pain in her eyes.

A herniated disk is an especially immobilizing form of agony. Between each vertebra is a kind of natural goo-filled gel pack that cushions the bones. With wear and tear or injury, sometimes the walls of the disk weaken and begin to bulge. The bulge might retreat again, like a snail's foot, or it might tear, letting the cushion of gel, the *nucleus pulposus,* ooze out. The herniated material, which one back expert charmingly compared to "lump crabmeat," can end up pressing on spinal nerves or, in the case of disks in the back, it can cause referred pain in the legs. Which is what happened with Jori—she had pain mostly in her hip and down her leg, along with lost reflex in one ankle and a numb heel.

This event is usually the last little catastrophe in a long period of disk degeneration, which can happen undetected over years. (And many people with lousy-looking disks on MRIs suffer no pain at all.) The pain arising from disk problems has generated a multibillion-dollar liability industry in North America.

Hundreds of therapies, painkillers, and devices exist for this sort of back crisis, but the truth is that nothing will fix it. It is broken. If the disk has herniated in such a way that it involves nerves that affect the bladder or other organs, an operation called a diskectomy may help. But in most cases, resorting to surgery for back pain is pointless. A herniated disk will heal, but it takes a combination of rest, just the right level of activity, and time. Lots of time. Most cases of back pain resolve in two to three months, no matter what you do to "cure" it.

Four weeks after the disk blew, Jori could be vertical for only five minutes at a time. At six weeks, her maximum upright time was about two hours. Meanwhile, she had fashioned various nests around her house, where she spent most of her time lying down, being patient.

At the birthday party, she was stretched out on a sheepskin she had brought along, with her ice pack beside her, a pillow under her knees, a heatable bag filled with buckwheat under her neck, and her "Dr. Ho" pain reliever—a remote-controlled TENS device—attached to the small of her back. She had ordered this muscle-twitcher from a TV infomercial, in which the exuberant Dr. Ho tirelessly demonstrates how his gizmo delivers a mild electrical stimulus to sore or injured muscles. It's the gate-control theory of pain in action, sending an alternative stimulus to the brain. (It also makes the muscle jump around like a dead frog being probed in biology class, but they didn't feature that in the ad.) Jori found it helped; so did ice packs on her back, biweekly visits to her chiropractor, and a good physiotherapist. Not a fan of pharmaceuticals, she took only Tylenol 2s when the pain became unbearable. Since she is already on medication for a thyroid condition she is wary of drug interactions, too.

In keeping with our family's slightly freakish genes (witness my parents) Jori has always seemed immune to age. She pursued ballet well into her forties, when she took up kick-boxing instead. Since she works as a hairdresser, in her own home salon, she is doing physical work on her feet most of the day, on top of which she has a son in school, and two rangy, exercise-hungry dogs. She also loves to paint, and not always on canvases. She's forever crawling around the house on all fours, painting trompe l'oeil borders on the hardwood floors, or green lizards on the walls of her workroom. Just as my mother can't not prepare food, my sister has a hard time not painting.

Both painting and cutting hair require long periods with your arms raised and extended. As a result, Jori developed tendinitis in her shoulder, for which she was already seeing a chiropractor. To anchor all that upper-arm activity, she had started going to a gym, working on the machines, doing lots of leg and ab work. She liked what exercise did for her mood. There's nothing wrong with having the body of a twenty-two-year-old at forty-eight, either.

Her back had been vaguely bothering her for a while. But the real damage came one day when she was down in the basement, cleaning up. The moral here is that no one should ever clean a basement alone. To begin with, it's maddening, so you tend to mow through the job as quickly as possible, slinging rolled-up rugs about. (I have a friend with a treacherous back whose last crisis was triggered by sweeping the basement floor. This constitutes a statistic, as far as I'm concerned.) In any case, Jori was down in the storage room, hoisting heavy bins. This required her to reach, lift, and twist her body at the same time. All this despite a nagging pain in her back that she had decided to ignore, and "work through."

Then she felt "something happen" in her back. The pain wasn't bad at first, but sharply escalated over the next few days, until walking or sitting became excruciating. Life on the floor began. She installed herself on a mattress in the rec room, where the fireplace could keep her warm. The dogs kept her company, and her son and husband waited on her, for a change. At first it wasn't too bad. She did her taxes, finished a painting, and propped herself on her elbows to do whatever legless chores she could manage. Then her elbows got sore. Being on her stomach so much eventually hurt her neck. Soon everything was out of whack.

Nights were bad. And the minute she felt even faintly better, she would get up, move around too much, and be down for the count again. After a couple of weeks, it sank in that this back thing was going to take a while. She finally saw her GP and made an MRI appointment, although everyone agreed that this pain was behaving exactly like a herniated disk. But an MRI would show the extent of the damage, and any nerve involvement, which can interfere with bladder or bowel function. Luckily, that wasn't the case. By the time the family birthday arrived, two months later, she could stand up, but walking was still tough. "Now it's like going through the day with a bad headache," she reported. "It's manageable."

What was more difficult to accept was how an isolated "mechanical" problem like a herniated disk can pull the carpet out from under your whole life. Living on the floor can be refreshing for a few days—you get to drop out of your usual responsibilities. But soon the strain on the other parts of your body begins to surface, and the pain erodes your sleep, which wears down your defenses and spirits. Everyone else in the family has to take up the slack, while not understanding how it feels to be the person lying around doing nothing. It was hard for her husband, Wayne, to leave on unavoidable business trips. Pain's costly ecology set in.

Since the world's top experts on back pain (as I had heard at the World Congress in Vienna) agreed that nobody knows anything about fixing backs, I will chime in here with my own diagnosis. I think that my sister might have become too strong for her own back—that is, she had terrific muscular strength and used it beyond the limits of what her particular spine (she is small-boned) could tolerate. And I think her age was a factor, too—forty-eight, the year when things start falling apart. With women in particular, everything radically shifts in the late forties. A previously iron stomach becomes touchy, dormant allergies flare up, energy levels plummet, and suddenly you can't handle stress the way you used to. It's sneaky, because this all happens before anything obviously menopausal (like the end of menstruation or hot flashes) signals a change. It's all very new and strange, like adolescence in reverse.

Once women manage the long curve of menopause, however, they can accelerate down the next straightaway. But early on, the pavement can run out abruptly with a dive in mood, or something blowing—a disk, a gallbladder, a rotator cuff. I'm convinced it's not just wear and tear (which is part of aging, after all), but a corporate downsizing in the body connected to the hormonal shift of menopause.

Since she was already having back pain before her accident, Jori thought, reasonably enough, that strengthening her abs would help. What she didn't know was that she had a "hot disk," and that the workouts only made the damage worse. Then she went from the very highest level of physical activity to next to none. A back episode like this is a sobering rehearsal of invalidism. The hardest thing about having a back problem is the enormous patience and capitulation required. There's no point negotiating with your back; you have to surrender totally. Regardless of how you treat back pain, with surgical fusions or muscle relaxants or massage by trained tarantulas, it will probably get better. The current wisdom is to stay as active as the pain allows, to use mild painkillers, and to let time pass. Total bed rest (a popular prescription in the past) is not a wise option, nor is surgery, although for an injury that is clearly visible and diagnosable on an MRI, a specific surgical procedure might be helpful. Newer approaches such as thermal therapy—"cooking the disk"—may help relieve pain. But the days of fusing vertebrae as an expensive shot-in-the-dark solution are over.

What does help are anti-inflammatory painkillers (injections of local anesthetic can also get people over the hump); a supportive physician; a gentle, monitored program of exercise; the occasional martini; and patience. Patience is the hard part.

More or less on schedule, three months after she "went to the floor," my sister's back was well enough for her to be active. It's been almost a year now, with no further problems, except she doesn't ever bend over and pick things up. She does the stewardess dip-and-bob. She used all the right technology: a good chiropractor, two warm dogs, and an ability to live with the maddening pace of the body's own healing. Pain and injury teach us to balance strength with flexibility and to tune in more closely to how we move and exercise and work.

Luckily, Jori had a son and a husband to help her out, as well as parents still willing and able to drive her (slowly, carefully) to the physiotherapist. It's a different story altogether when you live alone in pain.

24

STELLA

ANOTHER FAMILY DINNER, THIS TIME WITH Stella, my eighty-two-year-old great-aunt. She lives alone. I hadn't seen her for half a year, and I could see the change in her. Usually, Stella is energetic and up for a good time. Until this summer she played golf, traveled twice a year on holidays, and stepped out with friends to the theater regularly. But this year has been different.

She began to have problems with back pain—intense spasms that would settle in for a week or two, peak, and then subside—when she was in her late seventies. Heat helped, lying down helped, but mostly she just had to wait for the cycle of pain to run its course. After a while the episodes came more frequently and grew more severe. She was taking muscle relaxants and Tylenol, but they didn't help. Her family doctor didn't have much to offer, so, with her usual enterprise, Stella sought out chiropractors and other therapists. She went to an acupuncturist—it gave her relief once or twice, but the effects didn't last. She found a wonderful massage therapist who made her feel better but still couldn't get at the root of the problem. When she was finally sent for X rays, they discovered she had osteoporosis, and a small hairline fracture in one of her vertebrae. Her doctor put her on medication for the osteoporosis, but nothing seemed to help the pain.

Stella is a tough, resilient, self-sufficient woman who loves to walk for miles. She has no children, and since her husband died five years ago, she has lived alone quite comfortably. The small town where she lives is an hour and a half from Toronto, and we tend to visit only in the summer, when the drive through the country is more appealing. On one particular Sunday, we came around the garage into her deep, lovely backyard, with its manicured lawn like the green baize of a pool table. Stella was sitting under the patio umbrella with her sunglasses on, wearing yellow Bermuda shorts. She looked both sporty and elegant as usual, but seemed subdued. Her hand kept going up to the back of her neck. She didn't care to talk about the pain or make a fuss. But clearly it was always there, dominating the day.

The next week, I persuaded her to make an appointment with a hospital pain clinic in Toronto, where they started her on the usual staged regimen. She began by taking half-dose Percocets, eight times a day, which muted the pain somewhat but didn't keep her comfortable. Her GP seemed resistant to the pain-clinic approach and told her that they would just give her some injections and send her back home. He must have assumed she was going to a private pain clinic, where temporary "nerve blocks" of local anesthetics are often administered. He also didn't like being told what to prescribe by another doctor. On top of that, Stella believed in toughing things out and didn't want to "get dependent" on a drug. But she was clearly putting up with too much pain, and it was changing her world, her spirit.

We paid another visit. She looked a bit clouded this time. "Well, the doctor has changed my prescription, but it doesn't seem to be doing too much," she said, with a bit of a laugh. We took a look at the bottles. Her GP had switched her to a time-release version of Percocet, which she took only twice a day. Twenty milligrams. Same daily dose, different delivery system. But she was still discouraged and depressed by the pain.

"I went for my usual walk this morning," she said, "but I felt awful. I was never so glad to get back inside my car."

Taking the weight off her spine made the pain go away, but she hated the idea of having to lie down all the time. "It's just no life, when you can't be active. And it's there, all the time, you can never forget it."

We all went out for dinner to a restaurant in town, and some sparkle came back into her eyes. She talked about plans for going south in the winter. But her hand kept reaching up to the back of her neck, and she couldn't get comfortable in her chair.

I persuaded her to talk to her doctor again, and to ask for whatever dosage she needed to get out from under the pain. She was stuck in the worst sort of tunnel now—taking enough medication to make her feel "not herself," while stopping short of a dose that would blunt the pain. And I got the sense that her GP was resisting treating her pain, because he didn't want her "getting addicted."

The next day, she phoned to say she had gone into his office.

"I think he was all set to give me the same prescription again," she said, with a bit of lift in her voice this time, "but luckily, I was having a bad day, and he could see that I was in pain." She wept, in other words. He agreed to increase the dose and see her the next week. Stella began taking more Percocets, but she eventually went off them. "I just didn't feel like myself on them," she had decided, and although I tried to convince her that her doctor should be coming up with alternatives, even a morphine patch, she had had enough. Whereas pain specialists know that it can take up to a year of tinkering, trying different pain medications to get it right, many family doctors will prescribe Tylenol 2s or codeine medication and then give up when that doesn't work.

Stella liked her doctor, and she wasn't about to switch to someone else after all their years together. But I was afraid that she was experiencing a typical response to pain in the elderly. The old often don't like to cause trouble or complain, and many doctors, like the rest of us, assume that a certain amount of pain automatically goes along with getting old. It's similar to the misguided notion that babies feel less pain than adults. The undertreatment of pain in the elderly is especially widespread; one study showed that almost half of the elderly who were hospitalized didn't get adequate pain treatment. If nobody asks them if they're in pain, they often don't or can't pipe up. But even with someone independent and otherwise healthy, like Stella, there are the usual fears on the part of both patient and doctor of causing drug dependency. Most GPs have not been trained to treat pain properly and confuse physical dependence with true addiction. And it takes a fair amount of trial and error over time, with different drugs and dosages, to balance off pain relief with livable side effects. Both Stella and her doctor may just think, Who has the time?

You have to go back a few centuries to see how long narcotics have been part of medicine, and how recently they have acquired their bad reputation.

25

SMOKE AND PILLS

*Is there anything emptier
Than the drawer where
you used to store your opium?*

LEONARD COHEN, "The Drawer's
Condition on Nov. 28, 1961"

*Whan the payne is grete, then it is nedeful to
put therto a lytell Opium.*

JEROME OF BRUNSWICK, *1525*

OPIUM IS THE HORIZONTAL DRUG. I KNEW this from pictures of opium dens where smokers lie about bonelessly, like fresh cod in the fishmonger's window, and I discovered it the one time I tried the drug myself.

It was the end of the sixties, needless to say. I was just out of college and in London, staying with friends who were more bohemian than me. Hippiedom was peaking in England then. We rolled our own cigarettes, ate only bowls of brown rice covered in droopy vegetables and tahini, and shopped for long flowing things in the Portobello Road market. My friends had just come back from India. They liked to smoke hashish, and, on the rare occasions it came their way, opium, too.

Opium's effect on me was immediate and imperative: *I must get horizontal now.* I oozed onto the floor and stayed there enjoying myself for some time. The Turkish rug had much to tell me, as I recall. Its pattern was intricate and conspiratorial—bottomless, in fact. My companions drifted nearby inside their own happy patterns. After a while, I propped myself up on one elbow and spent a long time drawing a picture of a penis-mushroom entity, from the head of which spewed most of the contents of civilization. I was quite pleased with this. The angles of the room and the corners of my personality had dissolved into a round, warm feeling of immense repose. "An opium high can be described in one word," writes the novelist Eric Detzler, "comfortable."

It was only in the early twentieth century that opium became associated with drug fiends, crime, and moral turpitude. In the nineteenth century, it was a regular ingredient in patent medicines as a "stimulant to health," and for centuries before, it was used by physicians to treat diarrhea, insomnia, stomach problems, nervous disorders, and pain. Of course, it is, and always has been, addictive—or, as they used to say, habit forming.

Opium is the mother drug of nearly all our painkillers: Morphine, codeine, and heroin are all derived from it (although heroin, a semisynthetic, requires a tweaked molecule). Aspirin and ibuprofen go to work on damaged tissue and help block the inflammatory process, but opium and other narcotics affect the central nervous system and the brain. They head straight for the spine and the midbrain, where pain becomes pain. And miraculously (or tragically, depending on your relationship to them), the chemical structure of the opiates are like custom-made keys to protein receptors on the nerve cells involved in pain transmission. They hit the spot. This is because opium and its offspring so beautifully mimic the brain's own painkillers. In fact, opiates improve on them—hence the popular phenomenon of drug addiction. It's like your very best day, squared.

For 150 years, science has been madly looking for an analgesic that will work like an opiate without narcotic side effects, addictive or otherwise. The slogan for the Eighth World Congress on Pain was "Beyond Morphine," but at the ninth congress, they admitted that this had been premature. Morphine remains the gold standard of pain relief. As it has been for several thousand years. Opium is just an herbal remedy with a bad reputation and a passkey to the brain.

Don't bother putting your red backyard poppies through the juicer, however. *Papaver somniferum,* the opium flower, is one of almost a hundred different kinds of poppies, and it still grows best where it originated, in the Middle East, India, Egypt, and China. When the ripe pods of the *Papaver* are slit, they exude a milky white latex—the poppy juice that Shakespeare described in *Othello* as "drowsy syrup." Air-dried, the juice becomes a brown paste that can then be further refined into opium powder—medicine as old as medicine itself.

A passage in Homer's *Odyssey* is often cited as one of the earliest written references to opium. To help his friends forget the loss of Odysseus, Helen of Troy spiked the wine with "nepenthes," a drug "with the power to rob grief and anger of their sting and banish all painful memories." (Drug scholars, a populous and suitably obsessive club, still debate whether this was cannabis, opium, or some stupor-inducing combination thereof.)

Opium contains about twenty alkaloids, the most important of which is morphine. (Derived from plants, other alkaloids include atropine, which comes from belladonna; cocaine, from coca leaves; the nicotine we suck out of burning tobacco; and mescaline, which is extracted from peyote. Alkaloids and the human brain have a long, intimate history.) Aspirin and opium provide the raw material for more than 95 percent of our modern analgesic medicine.

Named after Morpheus, god of dreams, morphine was isolated in 1803 by Friedrich Wilhelm Sertürner, who described this element of opium as the "Principium Somniferum," the sleep-making principle. But morphine didn't really enter medicine until the hypodermic needle was developed in 1853 by Dr. Alexander Wood. Although Cecily Saunders would popularize the use of oral morphine for the terminally ill, injecting the drug directly into the veins has a faster and more powerful effect. (And for some addicts the business of fixing with a needle is as habit-forming as the drug.)

The synthesis of heroin began as a rather bad joke. Heroin is the result of altering one molecule in the chemical structure of morphine; it was first developed in the 1870s and then put aside. Heinrich Dresser, a chemist for the enterprising Bayer Company of Germany (of aspirin fame), took it up again. Dresser decided that heroin—originally and optimistically dubbed "heroine"—not only was a potential remedy for TB, coughs, and laryngitis, but could become the perfect cure for morphine addiction. This turned out not to be the case.

Something similar happened with Sigmund Freud and cocaine, which was first purified from the coca plant in 1860. In 1880, Freud and Carl Koller, another young Viennese doctor, began experimenting with the anesthetic properties of cocaine; Koller used it in eye surgery, while Freud preferred to tinker with its effects on behavior, and his own nose. (Freud, his nose, and his nose-obsessed friend Dr. Wilhelm Fliess are the subject for another tome altogether.) Freud tried to use cocaine to cure his patients of morphine addiction but only succeeded in creating the world's first cocaine addicts. Cocaine and heroin both entered the culture's bloodstream with the best of intentions, and the blessing of science.

Historically, even the side effects of narcotic drugs have been harnessed as remedies for other complaints. Opium stalls the gut and tends to produce constipation, so for centuries it was used in remedies for diarrhea. Narcotics at high levels can also depress respiration—so a weaker morphine compound, codeine, became a popular ingredient in mixtures used to suppress coughing. Opium also eases the mind and triggers vivid dreams. Artists liked the visions it unleashed. But in the nineteenth century, opium use wasn't restricted to bohemians. British officers busy colonizing India would relax in the evening with a pipe of opium instead of a martini. All along it was no secret that opium could be habit forming, but until the twentieth century there was no public campaign to demonize it. Some dabbled and escaped addiction while others who could afford a habit had one.

Each physician had his favorite concoction, as Martin Booth notes in his engaging book *Opium: A History*. Laudanum (meaning praiseworthy) was usually red wine or port with powdered opium dissolved into it. One popular recipe called for two ounces of opium and an ounce of saffron, with a pinch of cinnamon and cloves dissolved in a pint of canary wine. The medieval physician Paracelsus was so impressed by the remedy that he more or less branded it as "Laudanum Paracelsi." In the seventeenth century, opium found another great champion in Thomas Sydenham, the father of clinical medicine, who wrote that "medicine would be a cripple without it and whosoever understands it well, will do more with it alone than he could well hope to do from any single medicine" (hence Sydenham's nickname, Opiophilos).

A remedy for depression in Robert Burton's *Anatomy of Melancholy* was more toothsome—almost a side salad: Combine laudanum with roses, lettuce, mandrake, henbane, and nutmeg or willow, and toss. (Willow bark is the herbal antecedent of aspirin.) Iced poppy tea, according to Booth, is still served to mourners at funerals in the Middle East.

Not everyone enjoys the effects of opium or its hangovers. Sir Walter Scott took six grams of laudanum a day while writing *The Bride of Lammermoor,* although he disliked how he felt on it, as well as the "accursed vapours" that beset him the day after indulging. But the list of writers who fell in love with opium is much, much longer. Samuel Taylor Coleridge, who took opium for his back pain and sore joints, found the visionary aspect fed his poetry ("In Xanadu did Kubla Khan / A stately pleasure-dome decree . . ."). Thomas de Quincey will always be known first and last as the man who wrote *Confessions of an English Opium-Eater*. (Despite the pleasure he found in opium he loathed being addicted and finally broke free of his habit after seventeen years.) Many nineteenth-century writers and painters either experimented with opium or became dependent on it. Even upright Ben Franklin was rumored to have been an opium addict in his later years, and Florence Nightingale may have brought back a discreet little morphine habit from the Crimean Wars.

Thomas Shadwell, the Restoration dramatist and poet, was so well known for his opium appetite that it ended up in John Dryden's mock epitaph: "Tom writ, his readers still slept o'er his books, / For Tom took opium, and they opiates took."

Biographer James Boswell noted the casual acceptance of opium among the pharmacopoeia of the day: "On Sunday March 23 [1783] I breakfasted with Dr. Johnson, who seemed much relieved, having taken opium the night before." Edgar Allan Poe was first and foremost a hopeless alcoholic, but his writing also betrays the spectral visions and gothic gloom of the opium dabbler. "I had become a bounden slave in the trammels of opium," he writes in the short story "Ligeia," "and my labors and my orders had taken a coloring from my dreams."

Sir William Osler, one of the most influential doctors in North America a century ago, called opium "God's own medicine," and at the other end of the social spectrum, comedian and unrepentant heroin addict Lenny Bruce said, "I'll die young, but it's like kissing God." He died at forty, of a heroin overdose. The poet Baudelaire was addicted to laudanum (indeed, he was a walking toxic spill, knocking back quantities of digitalis, valerian, and quinine, until he finally toppled over at the age of forty-six). Jean Cocteau, author of an optimistic treatise called *Opium: The Diary of a Cure,* described it as "the ultimate siesta." (While exiting the clinic where he was "cured," Cocteau mused in his journal, "Shall I take opium or not?" His reasoned answer was "I will take it if my work wants me to. And if opium wants me to." Opium did.)

Women are conspicuously absent from these literary references to opium. Colette mentions visiting a fashionable Parisian den once, but presumably opium smoking was too time-consuming and clubbish to include most women. The "smoking room" has always been a place to which the men retire, alone. Many women developed their own covert and solitary addictions—to laudanum, usually, in remedies for menstrual cramps or "neurasthenia," or to chloral hydrate, and sometimes to "morphia," too. Women used ether for childbirth and opiates for physical pain, "hysteria," and depression, whereas men were more likely to take narcotics to unblock the imagination. Or for fun.

As Barbara Hodgson writes in *Opium: A Portrait of the Heavenly Demon,* Cocteau claims to have overheard Pablo Picasso remark that "the smell of opium is the least stupid smell in the world." Sometimes compared to roasting peanuts or to a "pleasant creamy odor," the Black Smoke seems to have left an olfactory imprint on anyone who tried it. Novelist Graham Greene wrote in his diary that the smell "was like the first sight of a beautiful woman with whom one realizes that a relationship is possible." Greene also described his first experience with opium smoking in a letter to his mother, oddly enough, saying that he "rather liked it."

Although China is associated in the public mind with the spread of opium, it was the British who first enjoyed a brisk trade in opium, buying it in India and selling it to China. By the middle of the nineteenth century, alarmed Chinese officials tried to cut off the trade, which led to the Opium Wars. But the efforts of the Chinese to stop the opium trade were defeated, and the levels of addiction in the East skyrocketed. By the time the drug had made its way to North America, the toll of addiction was harder to ignore, and a somewhat racist reaction to the drug's association with China, along with a new streak of prohibitionist puritanism that arose in the early twentieth century, meant that opium's heyday was over. Narcotics like opium and morphine lost their original medical aura and became the work of the devil instead. The irresistible nature of addiction, along with the opium smoker's single-minded pursuit of pleasure, became emblematic of the body's carnal appetites. To fall prey to opium was to become a slave to sin.

Sure I like to watch. Sure I like to see it hit. Heroin got the drive awright—but there's not a tingle to a ton—you got to get M to get that tingle-tingle.

NELSON ALGREN, *The Man with the Golden Arm*

In America, the Harrison Act of 1914 outlawed opium-based home remedies and began the strict regulation of narcotic drugs that is still in place today. Doctors and pharmacies had to acquire a license for writing prescriptions or selling medicines. Opium-based potions were out, and over-the-counter aspirin was in. This was the beginning of the criminalization of narcotics—a movement that would end up costing Americans $40 billion a year to prosecute and jail drug offenders.

I do not recommend spending much time in the opium aisle of your local reference library, however. Books on the subject tend to be written in the sort of mad-paisley detail of someone a little too obsessed with the wood grain on his desk. Martin Booth's history of opium and Barbara Hodgson's illustrated book are the exceptions. But perhaps the least judgmental, most succinct essay on narcotic drugs is the ratherly scholarly appendix to *The Naked Lunch*, by William Burroughs. (His nonfiction book *Junkie* is another remorselessly honest portrait of addiction.) Originally written for publication in the *British Journal of Addiction* in 1956, Burroughs's essay goes overboard in praising the potential of methadone, but his portrait is still accurate, not to mention a remarkable one-man home study in the addictive powers of dozens of narcotics.

"Over a period of twelve years," he writes, "I have used opium, smoked and taken orally . . . heroin injected in the skin, vein, muscle, sniffed (when no needle was available), morphine, dilaudid, pantopon, eukodol, paracondine, dionine, codeine, demerol, methodone. They are all habit forming in varying degree. Nor does it make much difference how the drug is administered, smoked, sniffed, injected, taken orally, inserted in rectal suppositories, the end result will be the same: addiction. And a smoking habit is as difficult to break as an intravenous injection habit."

Burroughs goes on to formally describe ten different cures he tried as an addict, as well as the rigors of withdrawal. Then he offers a cameo of the morphine addict, which is inextricably linked, in his view, to its painkilling powers:

"[Neurologist] Sir Charles Sherrington defines pain as 'the physical adjunct of an imperative protective reflex,' " he begins. "The vegetative nervous system expands and contracts in response to visceral rhythms and external stimuli, expanding to stimuli which are experienced as pleasurable—sex, food, agreeable social contacts, etc.—contracting from pain, anxiety, fear, discomfort, boredom. Morphine alters the whole cycle of expansion and contraction, release and tension. The sexual function is deactivated, peristalsis inhibited, the pupils cease to react in response to light and darkness. The organism neither contracts from pain nor expands to normal sources of pleasure. It adjusts to a morphine cycle. The addict is immune to boredom. He can look at his shoe for hours. . . . Morphine may relieve pain by imparting to the organism some of the qualities of a plant. (Pain could have no function for plants which are, for the most part, stationary, incapable of protective reflexes.)

"Scientists look for a non–habit forming morphine that will kill pain without giving pleasure, addicts want—or think they want—euphoria without addiction. I do not see how the functions of morphine can be separated, I think that any effective pain killer will depress the sexual function, induce euphoria and cause addiction. The perfect pain killer would probably be immediately habit forming." ("If anyone is interested to develop such a drug," Burroughs adds helpfully, "dehydro-oxy-heroin might be a good place to start.")

"The addict exists in a painless, sexless, timeless state. Transition back to the rhythms of animal life involves the withdrawal syndrome. I doubt if this transition can ever be made in comfort. Painless withdrawal can only be approached."

He concludes by describing morphine addiction as a "metabolic illness," and heaps cold scorn on the psychological treatments popular in the fifties. After this little foray into medical publishing, Burroughs went back to a life of judicious drug consumption and writing fiction. His theory of addiction as a "metabolic illness" was farsighted, now that genetic factors of addiction are coming to light. Too bad he was never motivated to open the Bill Burroughs Rehab Clinic, with its simple, one-step program: Kicking the Habit.

As Booth notes, opium has been smuggled into the language via slang as well as literature. The word *yen* comes from the Chinese word for opium, and the longing for it; phrases like *yen sleep* refer to withdrawal. The term *cold turkey* is said to originate with the goose-flesh that an opium addict develops during the chills and fevers of kicking. (In fact, *kicking the habit* originally referred to the involuntary jerks and foot twitchings that accompany withdrawal.) And the all-purpose twentieth-century adjective *hip* has been traced back to

American addict slang of the nineteenth century—perhaps a reference to smokers who ended up with sore hips from long hours of reclining on opium-den bed boards.

Come to think of it, everything hip and American, from jazz and the Beat writers onward, arrived in a cloud of illicit smoke. Although nobody likes to admit it, opium dreams have always been part of the visionary vitality of the American dream.

Half a million of America's 2 million prisoners are currently in jail for drug offenses, and 700,000 people each year are arrested for marijuana possession. This amounts to quite a public tab. The costly and futile drug war has ended up punishing many, at great expense, while failing to address the roots of addiction. (Only a quarter of the budget for federal antidrug money in the States goes to prevention.) Addiction runs much, much deeper than issues of accessibility, crime, or punishment.

The most recent controversy over "street diversion" of a narcotic drug has arisen around OxyContin, sometimes called "hillbilly heroin" because it first became popular in Arkansas and a few other rural states. OxyContin is a synthesized relative of codeine, only more powerful. One of the reasons it has caught on as a street drug is that it is often prescribed in a multidose time-release tablet that can be crushed and injected or snorted for a powerful rush. Both Barbara Walters and the *New York Times Magazine* have already set up OxyContin as the next scary villain in the drug wars—illegal use of the drug is widespread—while little has been said about its legitimate role in relieving pain. Tougher regulation of narcotics has not been shown to prevent addiction, but it will clearly penalize people in pain.

ANOTHER PAINKILLER WITH A long pedigree (though a better reputation than opium) is the anti-inflammatory aspirin. Despite hundreds of modern competitors, aspirin remains a potent analgesic—especially in the treatment of rheumatoid arthritis, a source of daily pain for one out of ten people in the population. The use of aspirin to relieve arthritis goes back to 1876, when the *Lancet* published a paper called "Treatment of Rheumatism by Salicin." Salicin was an extract of willow bark, which physicians had been prescribing for cases of "aigue" and fever since the days of Hippocrates and Galen. Anyone who assumes that herbal remedies are in a different class from corporate pharmaceutical products should remember that aspirin began as a tree. The tree was the white willow, *Salix alba,* and the chemical extract of acetylsalicylic acid has since become the world's most consumed drug—forty tons of it a year in America—not to mention the first patented player in the modern pharmaceutical industry. Bayer lost its monopoly around the beginning of World War I, when the U.S. Supreme Court, in a trademark infringement case, ruled that the company had marketed aspirin to the point where it was a generic term.

In the 1890s, Felix Hoffman, a German chemist employed by Bayer, was experimenting with sodium salicylate in an effort to find something to help his father, who was crippled with arthritis. Rummaging around in the company records, Hoffman came across the formula for aspirin and tried it on his father, with good results. His employer saw the potential in this new drug and put aspirin on the market in 1899. Originally sold as a powder, the familiar round white tablet of aspirin went on sale in 1904 and launched the era of mass-marketed pharmaceutical products. There's no ceiling in sight for pharmaceuticals, it seems. In 2001, the *New York Times* reported that spending on prescription drugs in America was up by almost 19 percent from the previous year, to $131.9 billion a year. Among the top sellers were two pain drugs for arthritis, Vioxx and Celebrex. In the number one position are antidepressants, followed by prescription drugs for ulcers and heartburn. Pain, pain, pain.

However, in a familiar sequence of events, aspirin became a success before anyone understood how it worked. It wasn't until 1971 that scientists finally discovered that the drug prevented the synthesis of a key inflammatory cytokine called prostaglandin E. Aspirin works to reduce pain, swelling, and fever, as it says on the side of the box. For all its homey connotations, it's a remarkably effective drug, especially for the pain and swelling of arthritis.

Aspirin's ability to prevent blood clotting may also help prevent coronary artery disease, although this has recently been questioned. Its anticoagulant powers have a downside, and large dosages can lead to serious bleeding in the stomach.

Aspirin belongs to a larger group of anti-inflammatories called NSAIDs (nonsteroidal anti-inflammatory drugs). These include naproxen and the more familiar ibuprofen, the main ingredient in Advil. Another painkiller is acetaminophen (Tylenol), which was also discovered in Germany in the late 1800s. But after its accidental discovery—a patient was misprescribed acetaminophen instead of another medicine, but it turned out to relieve his pain—the drug fell off the map until the 1950s and only went onto the market as a serious competitor to aspirin in 1960. Acetaminophen is a pain reliever that also reduces fever, and it is easier on the stomach than aspirin. But it does little to reduce inflammation, and it can damage the liver, especially when mixed with alcohol. Tylenol 2s and 3s are just acetaminophen with caffeine; people in severe pain try to stay on these rather than "move up" to opiates, when in reality prolonged use of acetaminophen is much harder on the liver.

In the 1990s, scientists became excited about the prospects of a new breed of superaspirin, the so-called COX-2 inhibitors. (Vioxx and Celebrex, prescribed for arthritic pain, are the best-known examples.) They held out the promise of pain relief without hurting the gut. These new painkillers were developed to target only the cyclooxygenase-2 enzyme, or COX-2, while not interfering with the COX-1 enzyme, which helps protect the stomach. The COX-2 drugs enjoyed huge popularity until the news that Vioxx seemed to increase the risk of heart attacks. This is the problem with all painkillers. Basically, any drug that reduces inflammation is going to interfere with an otherwise protective process.

Also, treating the pain of arthritis with any sort of anti-inflammatory doesn't get to the root of the problem. Rheumatoid arthritis is an autoimmune disease, possibly triggered by infections, and the real future for tackling it may lie in drugs that suppress the immune system. But immunosuppression amounts to waging war on the body's own resources and could entail the same risks as using chemotherapy to wipe out cancer cells. The line between just enough and too much artillery in these skirmishes is difficult to draw.

In the meantime, aspirin, the first branded painkiller, and morphine, the aging monarch of pain relief, have yet to reach their expiry date.

26

THE HANGOVER

A WEDNESDAY MORNING. MIDWEEK, NOT officially a hangover day at all. But here it is. My head is in a concrete bootie. I have spent the night flipping around the bed at the mercy of my thoughts, lying in that fretful, twilit-sleep that alcohol induces.

Hangovers are so humbling. The thing you were never, ever going to endure again in your life, six days or six months ago, is back.

This morning's hangover was incurred at a literary fund-raising event. I was uncharacteristically wearing stilettos and a feather boa, which predisposed me to drink in the first place. These evenings involve talking to other writers, who are inevitably drinking at a brisk clip. After cocktails, you are seated at a large table of strangers, while unseen waiters stealthily top up your wineglass with wine that is free but often of headache vintage. The trick, of course, is to drink ice water all night. Or alternate: wine, water. The trick is to slam your hand over the glass before he pours. . . .

Oh, never mind. I drank too much.

The trouble was, I drank just enough to incur a medium-grade, work-shredding hangover, but not enough to have a fabulous time. I had a pleasant evening. I had substantial conversations. I remembered to congratulate people. People who had written, completed, and published books. ("Waiter, another glass of red.") I floated home to bed, noticing how deliciously soft the bedclothes felt after a night of standing up on high heels. I congratulated myself on a well-behaved night out and fell asleep.

An hour or two later, I swam back up to the surface, surrounded by gargoyles—the smiles and faces and jackets and gestures of the night before. Snippets of conversation, a few ill-considered sallies of my own, random glimpses, jittery, like footage from a security camera. It's as if alcohol removes the discriminating filter that keeps out the irrelevant. My mind whirled with garbage.

Three A.M. It was all there, demanding a rerun: the glint of gold ribbons on everyone's name tag, the new hair highlights on the gossip columnist, the way a friend's face looked too pink and post-facial, the tired yawns of the pretty young magazine editors across from me after a long day at work, the look on a man's face as he told me about his wife's breast cancer, a glimpse of my imperfect jawline in the gilt mirrors of the ballroom where the function was held, my conversation with not one but three editors about their back problems—an occupational hazard.

All of it swam around in my head like postcyclone debris.

To ward off a cold I had also gone to sleep sucking on a zinc lozenge. I woke up with the most dreadful taste in my mouth. My head felt like a cantaloupe that had been poked, smelled, and then dropped, once, on the way to the cashier. The technical term is brain edema—the swelling and lurching of the tapioca with which you think.

With a hangover, the brain gets bigger and presses against the cage of the skull. The brain, fortunately, cannot feel pain itself. You can slice into the brain of a person under local anesthetic, just as if you were cutting a pound of butter. (I did think longingly of trepanning.) With a hangover, your brain has grown, but your mind feels like a dwarf.

I was thirsty. On top of the pain was the scuzz of unfocused remorse that always accompanies a hangover. Interestingly, I had not a thing to apologize for. But I felt steeped in regret, a dark, tea-colored medium.

Hangover logic is self-critical and merciless: When I so warmly congratulated that friend and writer on his "good loss" of a recent prize, was I being unconsciously vindictive, or frank and convivial? Who knew?

I lay in bed comforted by the snufflings and sudden gasps of my husband beside me. I love it when he sleeps and I don't—when he's there, so proximal and innocent, and I'm awake, thinking. I love the way he breathes in and out, and how I don't have to worry about him at all. I can just inhale his warm, solid presence. I could really enjoy "sleeping around" in the literal sense—lying beside people I like, when they're asleep. It's so calming. I could be a sleep vampire.

At four A.M., I calibrated the seriousness of this hangover. Bad. But no nausea, thank God. Nausea is the worst. No throwing up, something that as a Scottish Presbyterian I do only once a decade, anyway. Cantaloupe head. Too Many Thoughts. The headache will last into the afternoon, but I can function. And by four o'clock, I will be mistaking an absence of active hangover for downright well-being. I make a vow to drink only ice water, for the rest of my life.

I know some people who are improved by hangovers. They become chastened, soft, and open. With a hangover, the whole world appears much more clever and scintillating. The first bit of print you read in the morning seems like a work of genius; the party rubble lies about with Cézanne beauty. Meaning lurks everywhere, ready to pounce. Art vibrates. Perhaps so much of the body is called upon to process the guck of a hangover that the senses are left unpoliced, and the world streams in, uncensored.

I got up, thrusting my feet into sandals so I didn't have to bend over to put on shoes. Poured out cereal for my son. Noticed his new haircut. Fed sullenly on the newspaper for a while, like a fish loitering in weeds. My Teflon spouse, who drank heartily, strode into the kitchen refreshed by a night of socializing. He was off to work. My son shouldered his backpack and left for school. In pajamas I climbed up to my office and turned on the computer, hoping that the reluctant whirr of the hard drive booting up would be a signal to my brain that the party's over.

27

HOMEGROWN MORPHINE:
THE PLACEBO RESPONSE

THE JITTERY DEPRESSION OF A HANGOVER may be caused by a sudden plunge in serotonin and other chemicals related to both mood and pain perception. It feels as if some protective chemical tide has receded and left a very nasty stretch of beach exposed. The brain is in deficit mode. Intoxicants have a powerful grip on us partly because they go hand in glove with our biochemistry.

Morphine molecules perfectly fit certain chemical sockets in the brain. The presence of these opiate receptors suggests not only that the body can produce painkilling substances on its own—there are several kinds, although we tend to call them all endorphins—but that it may do so for a good evolutionary reason. Endorphins help explain pain.

In a life-and-death situation, the body is able to call on resources that let us override pain in order to act and avoid further injury. When a tiger clamps his jaws around our arm, instead of falling about and shrieking in agony, we can calmly, numbly, think, A tiger is gnawing on my arm, and this must stop. Escape and survival are the first things on our mind, not the pain of the attack. Then, if we don't bleed to death or go into shock, soon enough we move into the agony phase. Agony is good. It means we're still alive, and the pain forces us to keep the injured arm immobile and to rest, which speeds recovery.

This mysterious ability to endure horrible tissue damage without a corresponding intensity of pain is related both to our chemistry and to the role of emotions in pain.

"Strong emotion can block pain" was the conclusion reached by Lieutenant Colonel Henry Beecher, an army anesthesiologist during World War II, who later headed up the Department of Anesthesia at Massachusetts General Hospital. Beecher studied the reactions of 215 badly wounded soldiers and wrote up his findings in 1946. Later, he published the results of a larger study in a landmark 1955 article, "The Powerful Placebo." He found that roughly 35 percent of the patients in the study showed a response to a placebo "treatment." Many other studies have since put the percentage higher, up to 60 or 70 percent. Beecher's was the first study to demonstrate the effect on the body of our expectations and beliefs.

Curious to find out whether there was a relationship between the intensity of the pain the soldiers felt and the severity of their injuries, Beecher talked to them in a combat hospital within thirteen hours of their being hurt. Although these men were not in shock and were mentally coherent, they had suffered terrible wounds— gunshots to the abdomen or head, compound fractures, and other grievous damage. He was amazed by what he learned. Out of the 215 men he interviewed, 48 reported that they were in pain and wanted morphine. But an astonishing 157 reported that their pain was "only slight," and they didn't need medication. As Scott Fishman points out in his book *The War on Pain,* "a full 75 percent of these terribly wounded soldiers reported that their pain was not just tolerable but *insignificant.*"

Since the same men were also capable of moaning and groaning about getting a needle, Beecher couldn't account for this amazing stoicism. He finally concluded that the *meaning* of their injuries had led to powerful emotions that actually diminished their perception of pain. Their wounds meant they were going home. Normally, pain signals a situation that is potentially threatening. But in this case, the soldier's pain meant release from the danger of combat.

"Consider the position of the soldier," Beecher wrote in 1946. "His wound suddenly releases him from an exceedingly dangerous environment, one filled with fatigue, discomfort, anxiety, fear and real danger of death, and gives him a ticket to the safety of the hospital. His troubles are about over, or he thinks they are. He overcompensates and becomes euphoric. Whether this actually reduces the pain remains unproved."

But after his soldier survey, Beecher continued to wonder if perhaps he had only stumbled upon a side effect of war. Could he produce the placebo effect under gentler circumstances? Ten years later, he undertook another study, involving more than a thousand patients who had been given drug trials comparing certain active treatments to placebos. The patients were suffering all sorts of things, from headaches and seasickness to acute postoperative pain. Some took pills; others were given injections. And Beecher found that about 35 percent of the people in the study responded to the placebos. Not only that, but the more seriously ill they were, the more relief they experienced. His subjects came from a range of educational and professional backgrounds; gender and intelligence were found to have no bearing, either. Beliefs and emotions were calling the shots.

The role of emotion in pain says to Descartes, "I refute you thus." The impact of a placebo demonstrates some of those "descending messages" that influence pain—anxiety, fear, or joy. In fact, there can be no pain without emotion, as the currently accepted definition recognizes ("an unpleasant sensory and *emotional experience* associated with actual or potential tissue damage, or described in terms of such damage"). The growing acceptance of the placebo response has helped bury old dualistic notions such as the distinction between "psychogenic pain" and "real pain."

Beecher's was the first of hundreds of studies into the placebo effect and the largely unrecognized role it plays in every sort of treatment, from shaman rituals and "psychic surgery" to "take two of these and call me in the morning." If medicine could fully understand and harness the power of the placebo, we would finally get somewhere in the pain game. Indeed, the National Institutes of Health in the United States are on the case, with numerous conferences and publications devoted to the subject, including reports of a Beecher backlash.

In the spring of 2001, a flurry of scientific articles appeared that questioned the placebo response. In the *New England Journal of Medicine,* two investigators conducted a study of more than eight thousand people. Instead of comparing an active treatment to a placebo—the usual scenario—they compared patients who received a placebo to those who had no treatment. They found "little evidence in general that placebos had powerful clinical effects." Effects on disease, that is.

The problem with this study is that they *did* find that placebos had a measurable effect on pain. The effects on pain weren't dramatic, but they were consistent and real. They categorized this as one of the "possible small benefits." You could, however, turn the study inside out and say that, in fact, the one area where placebos *do* work is in pain treatment. Another article in the same issue concluded that "the evidence that placebos might contribute to pain relief may merit their continued therapeutic use."

But what about all those sheepish research volunteers whose back pain evaporated after swallowing a sugar pill? People who respond to a placebo naturally feel like imposters for doing so—and some doctors assume that a placebo response only unmasks people who are faking their condition. In his book *Pain: The Science of Suffering,* Patrick Wall describes the sequence of events nicely. "A trusted, impressive physician prescribes the very latest analgesic for your pain and the pain disappears. Later, you learn that you were a guinea pig in a trial and you were in fact given a blank tablet. You are angry, cheated, embarrassed and shaken. I have responded to placebo trials and I am always mortified and ashamed of myself. The pill could have had no action on the reality of my injury and yet my sensation changed.

"Some physicians think that anyone who responds to a placebo did not have a 'real' pain. They are wrong. Some physicians think that a placebo is the same as no treatment: they too are wrong. Some think that only weak-minded, suggestible people in minor pain respond: they are wrong. Even physicians respond to placebos!"

Many sizable studies since Beecher's have shown than anywhere from one-quarter to three-quarters of patients will respond to a placebo. And the more we learn about the placebo effect, the more ammunition it gives to the pharmaceutical companies. They now have evidence that round white pills are less effective than a colored tablet with corners, and that certain colors have more powerful associations. Red suggests power, green and blue are associated with calm, and the most promising pill is a capsule with lots of colored beads inside. (Witch doctors with feather anklets may have the right idea.) Also, a patient is more likely to respond to an injected placebo than to a pill, because we have learned that injections are serious medicine. And an intravenous placebo, with a nice little hanging bag attached, is the best of all. As Wall writes, "The placebo response is the fulfillment of an expectation. Expectations are learned by individuals and if enough individuals share the same expectation it is called a culture. . . . [O]n the Zambesi, the belief may centre on the shaking of bones; on the Seine, on the power of Vichy water; and on the Hudson River, on a psychoanalyst." The placebo could even be described as culture in pill form.

The important thing to remember about the placebo effect is that the magic is not in the pill. A placebo will only work if the person receiving it has *already had* the experience of relief. If someone has never been free of pain, being given an injection of saline solution and told that this will cure his pain will do nothing. The placebo effect is a learned cognitive response that triggers a complex physical reaction in the body. But first we must know what to expect.

I HAVE MY OWN version of the placebo response. I don't even have to swallow anything—I simply decide to pursue treatment. Many people share this. I call it the "receptionist response." All I have to do is make a doctor's appointment (grueling in itself, given the air-traffic control of incoming calls at clinics), and my symptoms start to back off. The "wallet cure" works, too. Just buy an expensive herbal remedy and leave it unopened on your kitchen counter for months. It often works like a charm (literally). Recovery seems to kick in the moment I open my purse.

There is a fascinating negative side to all this—the nocebo response. This is an inert substance or treatment strategy that you are told will make you feel worse. Merely reading the list of possible negative side effects that come with a medicine can induce the nocebo effect; people have been shown to experience not just a placebo cure but the expected unpleasant side effects as well.

I began to wonder if the nocebo effect might not have a larger insidious presence in the culture. For instance, our elderly population, who are more or less expected to live sickly, passive, unproductive lives, are being fed a sour diet of expectations that steers their health down a certain road. The nocebo effect may already be at work on us in ways we don't realize.

The more we learn about the placebo response, the more our focus is beginning to shift from drugs, technology, and medical intervention to the role of culture and the relationship between healer and patient. Just as pain arises from the pinball interplay of mind, body, and spirit, the ability to treat pain depends on a science broad enough to look at the rapport between doctor and patient, and the impact of fears and beliefs on our flesh and blood.

But what are the neurochemical messengers of the placebo effect? How does the body tell itself to ignore a bullet in the gut?

In 1973, two American scientists, Solomon Snyder and Candace Pert, announced that they had discovered opiate receptors in the brains of mice. A race was under way among American, Swedish, and Scottish scientists to locate these binding cells in the human brain that respond specifically to molecules like the ones that make up morphine. And in 1976, Scottish scientists found and named the opioid chemical *enkephalin,* a Greek word meaning "from the head." The body makes three natural opioids—endorphins, enkephalins, and dynorphins—but eventually the American term *endorphin* caught on as a blanket term. It was the start of a new approach to pain treatment that looks into the body's own painkilling resources rather than depending on surgery or on pharmaceutical intervention.

WHY ISN'T EVERY DEATH bathed in this elixir? Since we have innate analgesic powers, what has kept us from harnessing endorphins more efficiently? Why do some people die serenely, while others go through agony?

In *How We Die,* the surgeon and medical teacher Sherwin Nuland offers some dramatic examples of the natural opiates at work. He begins with the horrendous story of a mother who was forced to witness the murder of her nine-year-old daughter. The mother and her two daughters were wandering through the crowd of a small-town fair in England when one of the little girls—enacting every mother's nightmare—was snatched away by a stranger and brutally stabbed to death, in front of dozens of witnesses, who first froze in horror and then retreated. The murderer was a man who had killed before, a schizophrenic off his medication and freshly released from an institution. The girl's mother, twenty feet away across the street, was at first "rooted there by disbelief and horror. She would later remember that the air seemed too thick to let her move through it— her body felt warm and benumbed, and she was enveloped in a dreamy mist of insulation."

Then several men intervened, prying the man off the girl, and the mother went to her daughter, holding her in her arms as she died. She would never forget the look in her daughter's eyes—not terror or pain, but a tranquil look, with a glimmer of surprise. " 'Do you know what it looked like?' " said the mother, months later. " 'It looked like a release. After seeing him attacking her that way, it gave me a sense of peace to see that look of release. She must have released herself from this pain, because her face didn't show it . . . she looked surprised but not terrified—as terrifying as it was for me, it wasn't that way for her.' "

Nuland then quotes a passage from the French essayist Montaigne, describing an experience when he was violently thrown from his horse. Battered and bleeding, Montaigne was sure he had been shot in the head, but he felt nothing but a sense of tranquillity. " 'My condition was, in truth, very easy and quiet, I had no affliction on me, either for others or myself; it was an extreme languor and weakness, without any manner of pain.' " Fully expecting to glide away into death, he passed "a serene two or three hours," until " 'I felt myself on a sudden involved in terrible pain, having my limbs battered and ground with my fall, and was so ill for three nights after that I thought I was once more dying again, but a more painful death.' "

The sense of serenity, languor, and comfort, the oblivion to pain—just what an injection of morphine delivers to somebody in pain. "It is not farfetched to believe that the human body itself knows how to make those morphinelike substances and knows how to time their release to correspond with the instant of need," Nuland writes. "The 'instant of need,' in fact, may be the very stimulus that sets off the process."

Endorphins are generated by the pituitary glands, the periaqueductal gray matter, and the hypothalamus. They work with ACTH, a hormone that affects the adrenal glands. The endorphin molecules are able to bind themselves, just like narcotics, onto the receptors of nerve cells, to modify both sensitivity to pain and mood. When our homegrown opiates are exhausted, this is when morphine can step in and take over. In some ways, morphine used for pain relief can be said to compensate for a natural deficiency, just as synthetic insulin compensates a diabetic for what the pancreas can't produce.

Nuland goes on to hypothesize that acupuncture needles might stimulate the production of endorphins, making it a useful alternative to anesthesia during surgery. The only problem with the endorphin effect is that it is short-lived and capricious—we still don't know how to turn it on or off.

Although endorphins have only had a name for thirty years, the nineteenth-century explorer David Livingstone observed their effect in an account that Nuland relates in *How We Die.* Livingstone was in South Africa when he was attacked by a wounded lion, who clamped its jaws around his left arm and shoulder and shook him "as a terrier dog does a rat. The shock produced a stupor similar to that which seems to be felt by a mouse after the first shake of the cat. It caused a sort of dreaminess, in which there was no sense of pain nor feeling of terror, though [I was] quite conscious of all that was happening. It was like what patients partially under the influence of chloroform describe who see all the operation but feel not the knife. This singular condition was not the result of any mental process. The shake annihilated fear, and allowed no sense of horror in looking round at the beast. This peculiar state is probably produced in all animals killed by the carnivora; and if so, is a merciful provision by our benevolent Creator for lessening the pain of death."

Nuland includes a cartoon example of his own endorphin experience. Confessing to a mortal fear of drowning in deep water, he describes a freak accident that befell him on a trip to China. He was making his way in darkness down a path, beside what he took to be a wide, shallow pool of water. Then he took a step off the path and found himself plunging straight down in murky water. This was his worst nightmare, but at the time he felt only a vague sense of irony, as if he had attempted a silly stunt and not quite pulled it off. Then his feet touched bottom and like an umbrella, he bobbed back up again, where he was rescued by his horrified Chinese hosts.

His Chaplinesque calmness, Nuland observed, probably saved his life and prevented him from inhaling stagnant water or hurting himself on the jagged rocks that lined the edge of the pool. Thinking about it would have caused far more terror than the actual experience. This may explain the biochemistry of bravery, or those stories of a mother who can lift a car off a child pinned underneath. Fear and pain can be overridden, temporarily at least, when it's a matter of life and death. Before we learned how to extract morphine from the white sap of the poppy, we were already making our own.

28

THE POLITICS OF PAIN

DR. FRANK ADAMS IS A NEUROPSYCHIATRIST who specializes in brain disorders and the treatment of pain. Although he has worked in a number of hospitals and medical centers, including the world's largest cancer center, the M. D. Anderson Cancer Center in Houston, he now practices in a private clinic in Kingston, Ontario. Or rather, he did, until The College of Physicians and Surgeons of Ontario (CPSO) charged him with "medical incompetence and a failure to maintain the standards of his practice" and suspended his license on October 6, 2000.

The inquiry began in May 1998. Acting on a complaint that no one has been able to track down, since it didn't arise from any of Dr. Adams's patients, inspectors from the CPSO showed up at his Kingston office with a warrant for twenty-five patient files. Six days of hearings followed in August and September, during which a four-member panel reviewed Dr. Adams's case. The panel only considered eight patient histories in particular. In their statement, the CPSO said that "the Committee was concerned that Dr. Adams, who is a psychiatrist, had been using substantial quantities of narcotics on a long-term basis to treat non-malignant pain problems without adequate history-taking or physical examination." At issue was Dr. Adams's history of prescribing high doses of narcotics such as morphine, Demerol, and especially Dilaudid. In the case of one patient, he also prescribed up to 9 grams of acetaminophen, which the committee believed had put the patient in danger of renal damage.

But what really rattled them was one case in which Dr. Adams let an individual patient, a diabetic accustomed to injecting herself with insulin, take her pain medication home and inject herself. This sort of thing should be "strongly discouraged and abhorred," they concluded (using the impassioned, if dated, words of the 1983 *Alberta Guidelines for the Treatment of Chronic Pain*).

He was found guilty by the CPSO panel of medical incompetence and professional misconduct. Dr. Adams appealed the decision. His license to practice medicine was suspended until he underwent a program of "re-education," and agreed to practice only under certain restrictions. He would not be able to do the things he used to do for people in severe pain; for instance, patients would not be allowed to inject themselves, and Dr. Adams could not prescribe the high doses of injected opiates that some people in pain require—up to thirty times the conventional dose.

Dr. Adams, a youthful sixty-four-year-old who drives a black Porsche, dismissed his patients and shut the clinic—but not his mouth. He condemned the decision in no uncertain terms. "What the college has done with its poor judgment and its vicious war on pain doctors is to set up a medical crisis at least as dangerous and potentially more tragic than Walkerton [where contaminated water in Ontario had caused seven deaths that year] because we can have a higher death toll in a situation that was completely avoidable."

Dr. Adams is an outspoken pain activist, and his case makes an important point: Withholding treatment for people in nonmalignant pain by refusing to prescribe narcotics, or by prescribing them in doses too low to be effectve, may represent a greater risk to health than the dangers of overprescribing these drugs. It's not a popular view, but he's sticking to it.

Born in Hamilton, Ontario, Dr. Adams was originally a journalist for the *Globe and Mail,* covering the race riots in Detroit and other major stories. When he won a Southam fellowship to study sociology and theology for a year, he enjoyed it so much he was inspired to leave journalism and study medicine. He acquired his medical degree at McMaster University in Hamilton, where he specialized in psychiatry and neuropharmacology. In 1983, the M. D. Anderson Cancer Center in Houston asked Dr. Adams to come down and set up its first neuropsychiatric department. There he found that before he could get down to treating brain injuries—his particular focus—he was constantly having to deal with the pain that patients were in. Gradually, his interest switched to treating pain, both in cancer patients and in people with nonmalignant chronic pain.

What he discovered after a certain amount of trial and error was that some people could get relief only with levels of opioids that were much higher than the federally approved standards. The U.S. Drug Enforcement Administration (DEA) eventually got on his case for what they called "nontherapeutic prescribing," and Dr. Adams was charged in Houston with exceeding the limits in his prescription of narcotics for pain patients. He spent two brief periods in jail before being cleared of the charges and fully exonerated by a medical board. He decided to look for friendlier conditions in Canada. He worked at several hospitals in eastern Ontario and held assistant professorships at Queen's University and the University of Toronto, until he decided to pursue his own practice in the lakeside city of Kingston. He opened a pain clinic and was treating a caseload of about two hundred patients, some with serious brain injuries, when the inspectors from the CPSO came knocking.

To the CPSO, cracking down on Dr. Adams was intended to discourage "drug diversion" to the street and addiction among pain patients. But to Dr. Adams, the withholding of opiates in these cases signals a "human rights issue" and a new form of malpractice—the undertreatment or mistreatment of people in terrible pain. "The textbooks tell you to use the least amount of medication needed," he said in an interview with *Macleans* newsmagazine after the investigation was under way, "but in treating pain, I say, use the maximum necessary dosage that can be tolerated by the patient."

Each province in Canada and every state in America has laws regarding the medical use of narcotic drugs. Doctors must report all opiate prescriptions to the appropriate agencies or regulatory board, and if a physician shows a history of "overprescribing," he runs the risk of being investigated by the DEA or other authorities and being charged with a crime, disciplined, or having his license revoked. When Dr. Adams left Texas and came back to Canada, he hoped Ontario would be more enlightened about pain treatment. It has turned out not to be the case.

BY THE TIME I went to talk to Dr. Adams, he was fulfilling the terms of his "retraining program" at a Kingston pain clinic. He explicitly requested a nonsmoking rendezvous, so we met for lunch at The Sleeping Goat, a local vegetarian restaurant. At first Dr. Adams unnerved me a little with his jewelry—a gold chain around his neck and a gold pinkie ring and his cool leather windbreaker. But several things quickly became clear in the course of our conversation. He is extremely intelligent and a self-declared "medical elitist and reductionist" who has no truck with psychological models of pain. He's strictly a science guy who cares about "outcomes"—that is, safe pain relief in his patients. At the same time he came across as being passionately involved in his patients' well-being, angry at the politics surrounding pain treatment, and intellectually engaged in the complexity of pain. The only sign of fallout from his recent embattlement was his colorful vocabulary. "My wife says I swear a lot more now," he said.

Dr. Adams is married, with five kids, two of whom are in the health care profession. "But my wife is dying for me to get out of medicine. She's seen me through all this, of course. She says she's never seen me as happy as I am now, not practicing."

"So who blew the whistle on you?" I asked.

"I have no idea. The medication I prescribe is expensive, so I wasn't popular with the insurance companies, who have their own investigators. Or it could have been the police. One of my patients, a very devout woman in her sixties, attended a church meeting in jail and was so impressed by this one inmate that she eventually married him. He was a lifer in for murder, but she married him. Unfortunately, coming out of church one day, she slipped and fell, cracking her skull open. She ended up with a fairly powerful memory loss, as well as a concussion headache. I treated her with some Dilaudid, and her husband was stupid enough to announce this in jail to his buddies. Some of their friends on the outside jumped her on the street and said, 'Sell, or your husband's in trouble.' The cops found out about this, set up a sting operation, and nailed her. And they may have turned my name over to the insurance company's internal drug squad. I don't know."

"So it wasn't hostility from the college, then."

"Oh, things were already brewing with the college. But they operate behind a veil of secrecy and aren't accountable to anyone, so there is no way of knowing what provoked the investigation. And they were really vicious about it, fast-tracking my case and going at it hammer and tongs. After the first day of the hearing, I told my lawyer, 'Don't worry, you're going to lose. Clarence Darrow couldn't win this one.' "

"But if the college guidelines don't work, how would you define sensible restrictions to avoid the abuse of opiates? What about all this OxyContin abuse we hear about?"

"Let me object first of all to the use of the word *abuse*," he said. "It's totally impossible to abuse an inert substance, and the real issue is misuse. Obviously, the word *abuse* is too well entrenched in the literature and in the culture for it to change, but we're talking about misuse. It tends to mean that the patient wasn't educated in [the use of] the drug, or wasn't being followed up and counseled. That's where misuse comes in. The safeguards are already there. What it really means is that physicians must become acquainted with how opiates work. GPs don't normally have the experience to use them properly. My background is in intensive care units, in a big cancer hospital, so I know what toxicity looks like."

"Aren't doctors just worried about the side effects that opioids can have, like causing breathing problems? Or something worse?"

"Well, if you're opioid-naive and your brain stem has never been exposed to it, if we give you a big dose it will stop your breathing. But the brain stem adapts rapidly, literally in hours. I've seen patients who crash on two milligrams of morphine, but the next day they're up to sixty-four to one hundred milligrams a day, tolerating it very well—the brain stem has adapted. The rule is 'start low, go slow.' It takes time, and tinkering with different combinations and lots of monitoring. You can't just push it in and disappear."

As we started to talk about customizing pain medication to each person, Dr. Adams began to get animated.

"Custom-tailoring, yes . . . I mean, I just love drugs. You're like Michelangelo. You're not painting a barn, you're painting the Sistine Chapel—a tincture here, a splash there . . . you blend them into the perfect picture. It's gorgeous when it's finished, and it takes months to get it right. It takes about a year for most patients to achieve effective results. Most doctors don't know this. If they don't get results overnight, they bail out. Or they say, 'Aha, I know what you want; you're addicted now and you just want drugs.'

"But most doctors don't know what the hell they're doing around pain. People don't have a model for pain. If you have diabetes, I have a model—I know your pancreas isn't producing enough insulin. What do I do? I give you an external source, insulin, to inject. In other words, I'm supplementing what that deficient organ is unable to do. We give thyroxin to people who don't produce enough. Thyroxin is a peptide, just like the neuropeptides that our bodies produce in response to pain. Insulin is a neuropeptide, too. When pain is inflicted on the brain, it ultimately diminishes the capacity of that organ to respond. . . . I mean, it's only three pounds; it has limited production capacity. With people in chronic pain, all we're doing is replenishing that painkilling substance from an external source.

"Doctors don't do enough cognitive testing of their patients with pain. Almost every patient who has severe pain has a memory disorder. How do I know that? Because I do a one-hour battery of cognitive functions. These GPs . . . they put a stethoscope on your chest, they tap your knees, they look into your ears, and they give you opiates, but they don't look at the target organ, the brain. They don't look to see if you have significant memory and concentration problems. If you're female, and you complain about your memory, and you're thirty-five, they'll say, 'You're premenopausal.' Well, I mean, so are sixteen-year-olds, they're premenopausal, too."

It's very easy for Dr. Adams to get worked up about the benightedness of other doctors. Somehow it doesn't come off as hostility, though. It's just that he can't be bothered to be diplomatic. He talks like someone completely convinced that history will bear out his ideas.

"Ten years ago, I actually published some guidelines to pain treatment. I said that it should be mandatory, if you are giving somebody opiates, to do a mental status on them every time they come—to test for alertness, speech clarity, things like that. I've got data on all my patients and I graph them. Then you follow them, and over a period of about a year, you will start seeing changes. At the end of a year, if you have been successful in sufficiently alleviating, although not necessarily ending, the pain . . . you have a patient who is so phenomenally different you wish you'd videotaped them. It's like someone who becomes hypothyroid. There's a tremendous delay between the time you give them thyroxin and the time their cognitive functions recover. And it's the same with opiates. We can't get doctors to think about that."

The CPSO accused Dr. Adams of not doing a proper physical examination of his patients, so I asked him what his procedure was for new patients.

"I spend two to two and a half hours when they first come. Then I have them come back for another couple of hours for cognitive testing. When they come back a third time, they must come with family. Because the family's been devastated—I always want to get a feel for what the hell the family's been thinking, and what kind of support is there.

"A lot of doctors are quick to diagnose depression and push antidepressants, but I don't. Depression is totally overdiagnosed. I say treat the pain, then see what's left over. The occasional patient is truly depressed, and then you give them something for it. I'd hate to tell you how few antidepressants I've prescribed.

"I appear to be quite cavalier about my approach, but I'm really not cavalier. I'm incredibly systematic. You talk, tell me your symptoms, and use a diagram of the body to mark where the pain is. As for undressing patients to examine them. . . . [I]f a guy comes in and says, 'I can't move my shoulder,' what do you want me to say—'Take your clothes off, we'll do a rectal'? Then look in his ear? And he says, 'Well, my rectum's fine and my ear's fine, but I can't move my shoulder.' This is what I call ritual undressing. The college got really pissed at me because I said to them, 'You know, if you stopped your doctors from taking off patients' clothes, you wouldn't end up with doctors who diddle everybody.' I undress with great caution and real reason. Otherwise, it only makes the patient more vulnerable."

It was at the M. D. Anderson Cancer Center in Houston that Dr. Adams began working with oncologists. He was frustrated using Demerol and morphine with his pain patients, and an oncologist suggested he use Dilaudid, a synthetic derivative of morphine. "Dilaudid is the preferred drug for cancer pain now. We get fewer side effects. It hits harder, much quicker, and you get a cleaner patient out of it. Morphine can be a little more sedating, with a tendency to produce more delirium, confusion, and other brain problems. OxyContin is another synthetic related to morphine. It's a nice drug. I've done a lot of nice stuff with it."

When Dr. Adams first began using intravenous injections of Dilaudid in the Anderson ICU, he wasn't sure how it was going to work.

"The nurses would be there with the paddles and the resuscitation equipment. . . ." Dr. Adams gave an almost nostalgic laugh here. "You wouldn't believe how much weight I lost during that period . . . it was terrifying. We had no idea what we were doing. But we were careful. I was there in the morning, and then late at night to check on how they responded. The thing is, most doctors give drugs, but they don't stay at the bedside. And the effects of narcotics can show up hours later, sending the patient into respiratory distress.

"For the first three years at Houston I was on call seven days, twenty-four hours a day, with an average of seven or eight calls a night. I dealt a lot with people who were dying. That's when you go in heavy-handed. The highest dose of morphine I ever used was thirty-two thousand milligrams of morphine intravenously every twenty-four hours. The woman lived for fifteen days. We were just pounding the stuff into her.

"Sometimes a GP will say, 'I don't believe in doing that.' And I will say, 'I don't give a shit what you believe—this isn't church. What is it that you *know*? Your theology doesn't interest me in the least.'"

I focused on getting my mouth around the enormous cheese sandwich that had been delivered to our table as I waited for Dr. Adams's grilling of GPs to pass.

"Dealing with dying patients is the most rewarding aspect. I mean, you go in, you say, 'What I'm going to do is to give you all the medication that you want. I will do it safely, and I will probably end up putting you to sleep . . . is that acceptable? And when I put you to sleep,' I say, 'it is entirely possible that I will put you to sleep forever.' And they grab your hand and say, 'Oh, please,' and the relatives say, 'Anything to prevent more suffering.' You say to the relatives, 'I don't think the medication will kill them, but they are dying, and there is no way of knowing.' And you make it very clear that the reason they are getting the drugs is to relieve the pain, not to harm them or to shorten their life. You should see the change in the room when this happens. You sedate them down nicely, all the writhing is gone, the nurses straighten the sheets out the way they never did before, the room becomes quieter. The whole room takes on this incredible aura of peace."

When I mentioned that using patient-controlled pumps to administer opiates to the dying sounded like progress, Dr. Adams disagreed.

"To give out those pumps and tell patients to look after their pain is negligence," he said. "It's simply a sign of lazy physicians who don't want to keep coming to the bedside every fifteen or twenty minutes, so they assign your care to you. Well, shit, they wouldn't do that with chemotherapy—'Here, take all the chemo you want.' I see a lot of patients with brain damage as a result of over-dosing themselves this way. Monitoring is one of the secrets of success in pain treatment.

"But there's one thing I should make clear, which is that I'm not a singular proponent of giving drugs for pain. My point is that they're not being given a thorough chance. All kinds of things should be tried for pain—but tried quickly, because if you're at an acute pain stage, you're going to convert to chronic, and then you're in real trouble. They say [it takes] six months for acute to turn chronic, but in two to three months, you see this happening."

We talked about the appeal of the multidisciplinary clinic, but "the problem with that approach is that it's very expensive. Besides, I want to call the shots with my patients. If they need a chiropractor or whatever, I'll refer them."

Dr. Adams then told a most colorful story about a woman in the ICU who was in terrible pain and not responding to huge amounts of morphine. He was talking to a neurosurgeon who said, "Why not get the drug right into the brain, where it can do some good?" So the neurosurgeon drilled a burr hole in her skull, and Adams delivered half a milligram of Dilaudid straight to the brain (an experiment to which she consented). "The woman had no pain for eight weeks. I was clearing the wall for where I was going to put the Nobel Prize," he said, laughing. But the responses of patients were too variable to use this method with any consistency.

Dr. Adams wasn't eating lunch. He looks like a jogger (which he is) and someone who takes care of himself.

"Do you have any pain?"

"No. None."

"Take any supplements?"

"Absolutely nothing. I don't take anything I don't know about. I had to have hand surgery about a month ago, for a genetic thing, a contraction of the muscles. I came out of the operation, woke up in the recovery room, and my hand hurt like hell. The nurse said,

'Well, we've got fentanyl and morphine,' and I said, 'Don't give me any fentanyl, morphine's plenty. I don't need two drugs, one will do.' And she said, 'Well, it's fifteen milligrams of morphine.' And I said, 'No, make it five. I know what I can take.' "

After several hours of talking pain and drugs over many decaf coffees, Dr. Adams's phone rang. His wife was on her way to pick him up. Dr. Adams's reinstatement examination with the CPSO was coming up, and I wished him luck with it. As we said good-bye, he showed me the tidy scar on his hand from the operation. It seemed to be healing nicely.

IN AN ARTICLE PUBLISHED in the *American Journal of Pain Management* in 1995, Dr. Adams offered some clinical guidelines for treating both cancer and noncancer pain. He began with a quote from Dostoyevsky: "How many ideas have there been in the history of mankind which were unthinkable ten years before and which, when their mysterious hour struck, suddenly appeared, and spread over all the earth?" In it he writes that "freedom from pain is a fundamental human right" and that "severe pain of any cause—acute or chronic—should be regarded as a medical emergency requiring aggressive opioid treatment, vigorous dose titration to relief, meticulous patient monitoring, and prompt treatment of side effects."

He also recommended that the "customary practice of describing drug therapy of pain as high dose or low dose is obsolete and unhelpful," suggesting that the term *most effective dose* (MED) replace it. The most effective dose is "the level that gives the best pain relief with the highest possible neurocognitive functioning."

Dr. Adams's perspective on pain treatment is not shared by the CPSO. In fact, if you log on to their website in order to find a doctor for a particular condition, pain isn't even listed on the menu. This suggests what the decision regarding Dr. Adams spelled out in no uncertain terms—for doctors, the treatment of pain remains optional.

Although the written decision of the CPSO makes a point of claiming that the Adams case was not about the wisdom of using opioid therapy for nonchronic pain, other experts who followed the case would disagree. Dr. Harold Merskey, the London, Ontario, psychiatrist who crafted the definition of pain now in medical use, was a witness for the appeal. It was his opinion that Dr. Adams was not overprescribing painkillers, and that there were no grounds for his being disciplined or for his suspension. Merskey obtained transcripts of the trial with facts that, he said, contradict the statements put forth in the college's disciplining of Dr. Adams. As far as Merskey is concerned, the CPSO "misstated the evidence" in its eagerness to indict Dr. Adams. Merskey and Ellen Thompson, a former council member of the CPSO and a pain specialist in Ottawa, Ontario, later published a formal rebuttal to the Adams decision.

The odd thing about the regulatory boards in the provinces and the States is how wildly they vary from one region to another. In Canada, British Columbia, Alberta, and Nova Scotia have relatively liberal policies regarding the use of opiates for pain—that is, they accept their use, in experienced hands. In the United States, as of 2000, fifteen states have passed laws that make it impossible to suspend the license of a doctor for prescribing narcotics to patients with severe pain. Oregon is one of the most progressive states, and the only one in which a malpractice suit has been brought against a doctor for failure to treat pain.

But in Ontario, according to Ellen Thompson, "The old boys still rule. And they're just pissing into the wind with this decision regarding Frank Adams. They say they're basing their decision on clinical evidence, but there haven't been enough trials to produce reliable guidelines."

The medical resistance to administering narcotics for pain relief is based on a number of concerns that have, at first, a sensible ring to them—a fear of addiction, concerns about potentially dangerous side effects of opioids in inexperienced hands, and the possibility of patients selling drugs on the street. But Dr. Adams feels that these dangers have been exaggerated, and that the CPSO decisions were based on ignorance rather than evidence. And they overlooked the damaging consequences of their own decisions, too.

The small city of Kingston in eastern Ontario is not an area overstocked with pain specialists, especially ones with as many years of experience as Dr. Adams. When his two hundred patients, some physically dependent on narcotics, were abruptly left without a doctor to oversee a gradual withdrawal, this created more unnecessary suffering. "We couldn't answer the phone," said Dr. Adams. "There would be people on the other end crying, vomiting, going through withdrawal. I wouldn't let my wife take any more calls. It was horrible."

Dr. Adams doesn't hesitate to call this sort of thing "iatrogenic pain"—pain caused by the treatment (or abrupt withdrawal of it) rather than the underlying condition. In this case, the harm was inflicted not by the doctor but by a regulatory body composed of senior physicians whose knowledge of pain treatment, in Adams's view, was dangerously out of date.

Instead of undertaking the pressing challenge of collecting clinical evidence on the kinds of treatment or drugs that do help safely relieve chronic pain, the CPSO scapegoated one physician in order to send a message to its other members: If you want to stay in business, don't count on opiates to treat your pain patients. And the unspoken corollary is just as serious: If doctors continue to neglect or undertreat pain—an acceptance of suffering in a patient that in any other context would be considered unprofessional, if not unethical—they won't have to fear investigation or expulsion.

The Adams decision will now encourage doctors in Ontario to turn their back on the most hopeless pain cases.

Disciplining Dr. Adams for his use of high dosages of opiates also ignores what other studies have demonstrated, which is that people vary dramatically in their response to narcotics. Whereas one person will get relief from 30 milligrams of morphine administered over the course of a day, another can safely tolerate 300 milligrams. The medical literature has also made it clear that although opiates will cause physical dependence and require a few days of tapering off to deal with withdrawal symptoms, true addiction develops only in a very tiny percentage of cases who weren't substance abusers in the first place—less than one in ten thousand cases. So what, exactly, is holding up acceptance of opioids?

North America seems to have a multiple personality disorder

when it comes to its drug habits. We spend billions incarcerating cannabis consumers while refusing cheap, effective, and available drugs to people in pain. We eat painkillers and antacids by the metric ton, but turn puritanical—Dr. Adams calls it "pharmacologic Calvinism"—when it comes to opiates.

This other "drug problem" in America—the withholding of safe drugs for pain—is obscured by the focus on illegal drug traffic. But the prevalence of addiction has not been solved by the costly and concentrated political crackdown on narcotics. In the meantime, we remain a drug-dependent culture in ways that could turn out to be even more damaging than the effects of recreational drugs.

For instance, aspirin at high doses can cause serious gastrointestinal bleeding. Prolonged or high dosages of acetaminophen, one of the ingredients in Tylenol 2 and Percocet, can damage the liver. But aspirin has a benign corporate image, so its potentially destructive side effects remain acceptable. Taking Tylenol 2s means you're still "above" depending on something "stronger," like morphine.

The issue of pain is also vexatious to doctors, because they feel so helpless to treat it. Managing pain lacks the presto factor of a quick fix. It requires a willingness to palliate rather than cure.

As I was slogging through the seventy-two-page *Ontario Guidelines for the Treatment of Chronic Pain,* the phone rang. It was Dr. Adams, giving me some phone numbers for his former patients and saying good-bye. He had passed the retraining program with flying colors, he said, and his license was now reinstated, but he had had it. He and his wife were moving back to Houston, where he will look for work. "The Joint Commission on Hospital Accreditation in the States has just this year decreed that every hospital has to be certified as having a program of pain treatment. American hospitals must begin to chart the 'fifth vital sign,' pain, using visual analogues, and document outcome. If they don't pay attention to pain, they can lose their accreditation now."

"When are you going?"

"The truck arrives Thursday," he said. "I can't wait to leave."

29

PAIN THAT MOVES AROUND: ADDICTION

For the past few days I've been reading a textbook for medical professionals on palliative care. There are many facts and drugs in it, but no dying voices at all. I became fascinated by the medical lingo in it and how it tends to anesthetize the reader to the real subjects of the book—death and suffering. Medical vocabulary acts like a form of technology, reframing the mess and murk of disease. It took me a while to figure out, for instance, that "extrapyramidal symptoms" have nothing to do with disentombed mummies. The term refers to the sudden, jerky movements people experience on certain narcotics. As I drowsed through the book, I kept thinking about two people I know and their relationships to drugs. One is a friend who has cancer. She is adamantly unmedical in the way she talks about this disease. She has gone through chemo and radiation and found it devastating to the spirit as well as to the body. The other person I think of when I read *Topics in Palliative Care* is a fifteen-year-old girl addicted to heroin.

One has tumor pain—a specific subspecies of pain, with its own regimen—and the other has life pain. One resists using drugs; the other really likes them. One has unrealistic worries about addiction; the other has an unrealistic belief that the rules of addiction don't apply to her. The woman with cancer has pain with an organic cause, but one on which fear, anxiety, and anger feed. The addict has been through years of family pain—causing it as well as enduring it—and she happened upon an effective form of self-medication, namely heroin.

What is ironic about this situation is that while the cancer patient must hold out as long as possible for opiates, for $20 the addict finds it wonderfully easy to get relief from her pain on the street. As long as she has the money to buy drugs and her habit is young and small, life as an addict assumes an almost reassuring routine. Addiction has that Filofax side. You wake up in the morning and know exactly what your day is going to be about: finding the drug, buying the drug, taking the drug, coming down from the drug, then worrying about where to score next.

It's as regular as a day in school, with bells between periods. Using heroin becomes the shortest, most efficient route from pain to numbness and then back again. (It's not called "a fix" for nothing.) Addiction manages to translate big insoluble problems into one that can be cured—for a while. If you're fifteen, jobless, living on the street, and your on-again, off-again romance with heroin turns into a habit you can no longer afford . . . that's when addiction becomes a pain in the ass. You need more and more heroin just to maintain. Instead of the leap from normal to high, heroin becomes the only way to get from sick to unsick. It turns into medication.

Pain can become a habit, too. Some people in chronic pain find a reassuring new identity in a life organized by doctor's appointments and pharmaceutical regimes. If you're in daily pain, it is as if you have entered into a bitter but secure marriage—there is you, and always close by there is your dependable companion, pain. Chronic pain may even replace someone whose ability to deliver suffering was unpredictable and therefore scary. A bully or a beater delivers not just pain but the anxious sense of never knowing what will happen next. But a person in chronic pain lives inside a more predictable relationship. (The treatment world sometimes refers to the upside of living with pain as "secondary gains," such as gaining sympathy or quitting work.) This is not to say that people choose chronic pain or become addicted to it. But sometimes people choose not to treat their pain.

I've been thinking about why so many people in pain hesitate to ask for drugs. Someone else I knew had metastatic cancer and at a certain stage she went through periods of excruciating pain but didn't want to ask her doctor for narcotic drugs. This reluctance seems to run deeper than fear of addiction or wanting to be the kind of person who can tough it out. Staying inside the pain may even be a necessary stage of any serious illness—but it's not a good idea to get stuck there.

Perhaps a stage of physical pain becomes a way to make cancer both real and private. A diagnosis of cancer is alarmingly objectifying, in the same way that people feel free to pat pregnant women on their bellies. You join the cancer club. But pain anchors the experience of cancer inside you, making it yours. The pain forces you to face the reality of it as well.

Most people assume that doctors are to blame for the undertreatment of pain in cancer patients, but Dr. Kathleen Foley, a leading figure in palliative pain care, agrees that it is often the patients who resist the idea of "strong drugs."

For treating cancer pain, Dr. Foley helped develop the "analgesic ladder" that was laid out by the World Health Organization in 1986. This strategy of staging was an enlightened approach to pain at the time—that is, it acknowledged that pain was a separate issue, not just a symptom. But now that the WHO staging has become the accepted regimen, many doctors and their patients still find ways to use the ladder as a way to postpone "strong drugs" until the very last moment. So while cancer pain is being addressed, undertreatment continues.

The staging works like this: If you have cancer, you start on

NSAIDs, move up to mild opiates like codeine with a little NSAID action thrown in, and then you finally arrive at the sultan of painkillers, morphine. But too many people stall at stage two, hoping that Tylenol 2s will give them relief, when they should be moving on to morphine. They fear addiction or being "out of it," they have heard about constipation, and they associate being stoical about pain with having a fighting attitude toward the disease.

Above all, what the WHO staging offers is a reassuring structure and protocol. In the face of insoluble pain and an unfixable disease, doctors are very grateful for protocol; it offers control over the uncontrollable. But too many doctors caution their patients to stay at level two as long as possible, so they end up taking too much codeine and acetaminophen, to no avail—they are still in pain, only now they're constipated, too. Stage-two analgesics will also do more damage to other organs over time than judiciously prescribed opiates. In this sense, Percocets, Percodans, and Tylenol 3s are more dangerous than low doses of morphine. So it's not necessarily healthier to stick with "weaker" drugs.

There are all sorts of reasons why doctors underprescribe pain medication, beginning with fear of prosecution, and the stigma around narcotics and myths concerning addiction. But I still couldn't fathom the reluctance of patients themselves to take opiates. Why would someone *choose* pain? Some people with cancer would rather feel the press of a tumor than endure the nausea and vomiting that can accompany the first few days of treatment with opioids. Or, I suppose, they take the vivid presence of pain to mean that they are still alive, not dying. Painlessness becomes associated with the numbness of death.

Then there is fear of dependence on a drug, which represents loss of control over one's life. For someone with cancer who is afraid she might be dying, accepting dependence on a drug represents that first crucial dismantling of individual control and power. Our deeply held fear of addiction is also about loss of control over our lives.

As for doctors, they stand to lose control in another way. Patients who find release from narcotics may shift their focus from the doctor to the drug—and with good reason, since the drug helps them get on with life. Opiates radically alter the power relationship between doctor and patient, which neither of them may want to forfeit.

The other factor is this paradigm of "fighting disease" or "winning the battle against cancer," as the obituaries always put it. But pain is more of a collaborator. It's the thing that tunes us inward, where we need to focus first. Perhaps the cancer patient needs a grace period in which pain offers up its message before she decides to turn down the volume of pain and turn outward again.

But at a certain point, pain loses its helpfulness and becomes nothing more than a thief of vitality and joy. It destroys health and compromises the immune system, interfering with sleep, love, and our connection to the rest of life. At that point, treating the pain releases someone to think about something else for a change.

True addiction, as opposed to physiological dependence on a painkiller, could also be described as one of the most prevalent forms of chronic pain. Somewhere between 5 and 20 percent of the population are addicted to one thing or another—a percentage that matches the official figures for chronic pain. And the body is so beautifully set up for addiction, with our opiate receptors just waiting for that chemical key in the latch. For some people, addiction also feels familiar. It can reproduce a pattern of being fed and then starved, loved and then hit, held and then dropped; it's a great way to perpetuate any pattern of injury in your life. The effect of alcohol, for instance, eventually mimics the lousy parent: At dinner it sings your praises, then later on it gives you a kick in the chops. Being addicted to something cleverly impersonates freedom at the same time that it digs you in deeper. Addiction is like a long, drawn-out strategy for staying in the same painful place that got you addicted in the first place.

THIS TIME I WENT to Wellesley and Church, where she was waiting for me inside the door of a bagel shop, her black sweatshirt hood draped over her black hennaed hair. She has big hazel-green eyes in a white face and enormous lips. When I first met her, at the age of twelve, she reminded me of Kim Gordon from Sonic Youth. Now she just looked rough. Although it was March and icy, her hands were curled up inside the sleeves of her windbreaker, which was filthy.

Her child-sized fingernails were bitten. Her usual nose and lip rings were missing.

"Hi," she said, softly and rather shyly. Not the usual invincible Heather. Her long hair was matted and tangled, and her skin was bad. It was the worst I had seen her.

"Did you notice I took all my piercings out?"

"So I see."

"Yeah, I'm kinda sick of that whole punk thing now."

We went to the Second Cup and she ordered tea. "I can't drink coffee on the drugs I'm on," she said. The street clinic was giving her Clonidine to help her withdraw from heroin. She sat hunched over the table and hugged her midriff.

"How are you?"

She shrugged. "I'm all right."

Heather bitched a lot about other people, and what morons they were, but she was stoical about her own life. She had grown up in a comfortable middle-class Toronto home. Her parents were separated. There had been some sketchy business involving another family member and "a little abuse" when Heather was younger, but I didn't know the whole story.

At fourteen, Heather ran away from home, and within a year she had fulfilled the stereotype, ending up in Vancouver, wired to that city's especially cheap and potent heroin. Soon she had an $80-a-day habit. She went through several overdoses, followed by a stint in the local detox and rehab. But there was nobody to care for her dog, Grimace, so she checked out of rehab early and made her way back to Toronto. Now she was fifteen. Her mother, once a runaway herself, had given up and shut the door on Heather. This wasn't the usual sort of pain, but it was an advanced case of pain-in-the-world.

It was always easy to fall back into conversation with Heather regardless of how calamitous her situation was, or how little our lives resembled each other's. Although she could be a bit of a galoot, she was smart as hell, and a good talker. She read, wrote songs, and diligently kept a journal, which she was always leaving splayed open in our house or losing. God knows she had material. She also had the addict's flair for seeing through other people's bullshit while stepping right around her own.

The guy sitting beside us in The Second Cup glanced at us and moved to another table. Heather stirred her tea without drinking it and asked after my son, who had been her friend back in the seventh and eighth grades, before she got into trouble. But even then Heather required a certain amount of rescuing and collusion. So, my son did the first really hard thing in his life and ended the friendship. At twelve, he understood the impossible dilemma of caring for someone who refused to be helped. But after she ran away, our intact family remained a fixed point on her map. Every once in a while she would call from the road, collect, and talk to me.

When I first learned she was addicted, I gave her a bunch of contacts for rehab programs and counselors. She would always thank me, put the names in her bag, and never call the numbers. Being wired to heroin annoyed her, but she was sure she could stop using on her own. And it's true, she was no waif. Heather was physically strong and mentally tough. Of course, heroin is tougher than the toughest, as many big guys have discovered. And withdrawing physically isn't even such a big deal—it's not going back that's the problem. Street life can be habit forming, too.

This time I didn't bother giving her the phone numbers, just an old knapsack with a wool hat, gloves, a sweater, a bottle of herbal sedatives, some vitamins, and a button that said "hell." I also gave her a little money. That was my first mistake.

A week later I met her on a Sunday, down near Kinko's. She helped me do some photocopying. This time her eyes were flat, her spirit had fled, and her responses to everything were slow and syrupy. Stoned.

"How's the old withdrawal going?"

"Okay. Not good. I'm always fine until the fourth day. It's the fourth day that gets me." She was like a big black hole.

The next time I saw Heather, I gave her another list of residential rehab programs, including one for teenage girls. I drove her by the place.

"It looks quite nice, doesn't it?" I said. We stepped inside. It was a narrow Victorian house with a soupy smell.

"I don't think it's for me," she said, reading a notice on the wall. "You can't even smoke."

This time I didn't give her money, I brought her groceries and a book: *The Diary of Anne Frank*. Not in the best of taste, but I thought Heather could relate, as she sweated it out in her attic room. Heather was glad to have the food, but when I accidentally left *Anne Frank* behind in the car, she looked panicked and said, "Oh, can't I have the book?" She had been through four days of withdrawal again. The worst part was over, and she was almost looking good.

"Why not take a bed in the women's detox, have someone bring you sandwiches and make sure it sticks this time?" I asked. "Okay," she said, unconvincingly. Part of the problem was her dog, Grimace. She had no one to leave him with, and shelters and rehab didn't allow pets. Grimace was her main companion in life—but on the other hand, Grimace made a great excuse.

"There's a bed at Dundas Street right now—you could phone and reserve it," I said. I balanced a quarter on the table where we were having yet another coffee. "Okay," she said without moving. Then, "I have to talk to my roommate first about taking care of Grimace."

Although she was just as happy sleeping outside under a bridge, at this point she was living with an indeterminate number of street kids in an evil-looking rented house near Spadina. The front yard was littered with stolen grocery carts and rusted bikes; the porch was a rotting slurry of sleeping bags, an eviscerated couch, and old coats. There was chalk graffiti, witless and mean, on the brick walls. The front bay window had been broken and was covered with cardboard.

"I fuckin' hate it there," said Heather. "It was okay until the French guys moved in and trashed the place. They shoot PCP in the halls and piss right down the stairs."

When I dropped her off, I decided to check out the house. A Chinese woman out front swept the sidewalk and shot me an expression that said "Nothing good goes on in there." Grimace came to the door. He is a big, gentle dog, some mix of German shepherd and Lab, with a shapely, noble head and white paws. Heather takes excellent care of him. I stepped inside to the smell of damp, mildew, and fallen plaster. The first room was a demolition zone of smashed walls and sodden couches. The PCP punks, having been given their eviction notice by the owner, to no one's surprise, were now diligently trashing the place floor by floor. It was worse than an abandoned house— it was a temper tantrum of construction materials.

Although others in the house were on methadone maintenance, Heather refused to go that route—"government heroin," she called it. She disdained PCP, too. She was a beer, pot, and heroin girl.

We went into the kitchen, which was like some kind of disgusting art installation. The sink was full of water topped with thick mold—no one would ever reach their hand in there. Month-old food sat on a cutting block.

"It used to be nicer," Heather said, like a housewife embarrassed by dust bunnies. We didn't bother going upstairs. Wow, I thought, and left.

Two days later, the phone rang.

"The police just came and kicked us out," she said. She sounded angry, which was normal, but almost scared, which was rare.

"I'm not surprised."

"I had to leave a bunch of my stuff behind," she said, "even Grimace's leash." My son passed a note to me: "If she needs to stay here overnight, that's okay." I told Heather to ask the cops to give her subway fare and said I would pick her up at the station.

It was raining, but not too cold. Heather and Grimace were waiting outside the station when I drove up.

"Look at what I had to use for a leash." Grimace wore a hot-plate cord around his neck, with his usual aplomb. "Load!" she said, Grimace's signal to jump into a car, any car. The two of them piled in with an unzipped knapsack spilling out the things she had managed to stuff into it.

She could hardly talk, she said, because her throat was so sore—from a cold and from yelling at the punks in her house to stop shooting up in the halls. "Can't you have a little respect for me, I'm trying to quit heroin," she would shriek at them.

Meanwhile, when we got to my house, my husband was cooking salmon trout and organic broccoli. The four of us sat down for a charming meal with wine. My husband was polite, but he didn't really approve of this open-door policy. He felt that Heather did quite well for herself out in the world and, in a sense, he was right. Addicts, even baby ones, are charming users. I knew that.

It did occur to me that I was in way over my head. I was neither a heroin addict, nor her mother, nor a therapist—I just liked Heather and couldn't forget that she was a fifteen-year-old girl, someone who should be cared for and protected. I also knew that some part of me identified with her, too, the lost-girl, mini-addict part. She made my heart ache. I thought maybe I could give her some help—or at least get her connected to professional helpers—while not, as they say, facilitating. To turn my back on her because my own motives were muddled seemed worse than letting her know that I cared about her and wanted to see her survive.

The next day we drove her and an even scarier girlfriend, and their two big dogs, to Kingston, Ontario, where they said they had "nondrug" friends. Everyone piled in, and a smell of wet dog and unwashed girls rose in the car. I rolled down the window a few inches. My husband gave me a look that said "You are in my debt forever." I didn't think the smell was that bad, frankly.

It was a three-hour drive. When we reached Kingston, we let the girls out near their new address, an apartment over a pizza store. It didn't look too promising. Heather didn't even have a sleeping bag—just a ratty floral duvet that trailed out of her pack. Her friend carried a big bag of kibble and a garbage bag of clothes. Heather had my old steel-frame pack and an open box of Lucky Charms, which she had bought in Toronto for breakfast.

"I can see this is what I'm going to be dealing here," she said cheerfully, shaking the box. It was a very astute take on this small, pretty university city, which was also home to the country's only prison for women.

People on the streets turned to look at the raggedy girls with their packs and black dogs and Lucky Charms as they made their way up the street. I told myself that this was a good move, delivering them to a smaller place with lots of social services. But I was also relieved to be able to FedEx the problem someplace else. Helping somebody get unaddicted is not a drive-through thing. You have to be willing to get all the way in, and they have to let you in.

KINGSTON LASTED THREE DAYS. Then they went to Montreal, where Heather was beaten up by a biker, followed by the west coast again. A few months later, she turned up in Toronto, fed up with street life, desperate to get a job. "I want to run my own business," she announced, "and have hobbies." She thought she could begin by cleaning houses, and some friends of mine were willing to give her a chance. Heather told me she was totally free of heroin, had been for three months. She did seem straight, and the tracks on her arms had healed. Then she left her journal on our couch (again). I read the last few entries, including a description of a horrible OD in Edmonton, down by the river valley. And in the clothes she left behind I came across two broken syringes. My heart sank; I felt the sucker punch that comes to everyone who interferes with the logic of addiction. I had been vain enough to think that I was someone she still didn't lie to.

We met for tea in a Chinese restaurant. I confronted her about the journal, the syringes, and her lies. She cried. They were broken old syringes she had forgotten about, she said, and Edmonton was a "stupid lapse." "You don't understand," she sobbed, "you don't understand how much I want to stop." She had been so sure that the housecleaning job would be her ticket out, and now this.

"It's different in Vancouver," she went on. "The dope's so strong you get wired faster."

"You can't just use a little heroin now and then. Plus you drink too much." I leaned in like a social worker. "Heather, you have a problem with drugs."

She wept on, silently.

"I don't go looking for it."

"I know you're not wired all the time. But you binge. And your binges have almost killed you three times this year."

"I just need a job and a place to stay, that's all. Not rehab. That whole rehab business just makes you feel more like a weak fuckup. I don't want to be around losers," Heather pleaded, "I only want to be around happy people now."

She did have a point. But people who stop using on their own tend to have money, family, or some sort of life to pick up afterward. Heather only had Heather, Grimace, me on the phone from time to time, and a network of street pals.

I gave her an ultimatum. I would only help her get a job if she checked into a residential rehab program first. She didn't have to like it, I said, she just had to do it. This made her angry and her face shut down. Yeah, she said, okay. Whatever. I could feel her adding my name to The List, all the ones who had let her down.

Street life works like an addiction in itself, organizing your days around little fixes of shelter and food. One of the many tattoos that Heather sports is on the knuckles of one hand: DAY BY DAY.

When someone grows up in pain and anger, becoming addicted to heroin is just like changing channels—with the bonus of being able to erase the misery over and over again. Addiction replaces pain with a drug. Nothing deeper shifts.

IN THE END, SHE didn't check into anything; she stayed on the street and went through withdrawal alone. Heather went west, she went south, and rode freight trains through eighteen states. She got a job mopping floors in Circus, Circus, a casino in Las Vegas. She made jewelry, and had a boyfriend for a while. The phone would ring, and I would hear her husky voice calling from Tucson or Buffalo, and once from a jail in New York City. "They arrested me for having a dog off a leash," she said with disgust. "New York sucks." But despite all this, she sounded lighter and straighter. Grimace, a veteran of freight yards all over the United States, was still with her. I have my hopes.

30

CAROLE

IT WAS EARLY JUNE. WE HAD MADE arrangements to go up north for a week, to some cabins on Georgian Bay. The plan was for me to do some work and for Carole to "lie around on the rocks." Her preferred version of chemo was to sunbathe on the whale-sized pink and gray granite of the Canadian Shield. Both of us were looking forward to escaping Toronto at the end of a long winter.

This plan was a rather gallant move on her part, because the two of us weren't especially close friends, and she was ill. Moreover, Carole was a writer, and a private one. Her world focused on writing fiction, some community work in the arts, and life with her family—her husband, Layne, an actor, playwright, and theater director, and their teenage daughter, Charlotte. But once the word was out that Carole had cancer, she seemed to want to connect with other people, and luckily I was one of them.

Carole was pointedly unmedical about her illness. A year earlier, when someone had asked how her writing was going, she alluded to "a few health problems." She had had some surgery for cancer, she said, but now everything was fine. Something abdominal, although she never said which kind. We accepted this breezy explanation, since no one could have looked healthier or more attractive. Carole was a beauty—small, slim-boned, with dark, curly hair, an expression in her light blue eyes both yearning and mischievous, and teeth that had a slight, sexy prominence to them. Her voice was low and pleasing, with a conspiratorial lilt that wanted to move toward laughter. She cut to the chase in conversation and had an edgy wit that her quiet presence didn't prepare you for. "At dinners or parties Carole never put herself forward," one of her friends observed, "but the things she said tended to stay with you."

Born in Quebec and transplanted to Ontario, Carole had a bipolar intelligence that was both passionately inside events and outside them, observing. She painted, wrote fiction, and practiced journalism. Her two novels, *Voiceover* and *In the Wings,* combined deep emotion and sensual language—a rare blend in English Canadian fiction—with comic bite. Intuitive and honest, double-natured, her voice stood apart. When Michael Ondaatje, the author of *The English Patient* and *Anil's Ghost,* received his half of the prestigious Canadian literary prize The Giller, he used his acceptance speech to commemorate Carole and her interrupted talent.

The C-word didn't spring easily to her lips, and for several years Carole dealt with her illness privately. She hated the idea of being identified first with the disease and the loss of privacy that entailed. Then, when she had to give up teaching and writing to concentrate on her health, she began to let people know in a roundabout way.

Whenever Carole and I exchanged e-mails, she was crisp and journalistic about cancer—but in person she didn't use words like *tumor* or *metastasis* or *chemotherapy.* She hated the institutional aesthetics of cancer. I don't think it was denial; she was used to facing herself on the page. I think it was a writer's allergy to ugly language. Cancer jargon is as aggressive and graceless as the disease itself. (When another friend, Ramiro, developed cancer, we agreed that the word *diarrhea* simply had to go. Too onomatopoeic. Ramiro substituted the word *cántaros* instead. It's part of a Spanish expression, *llover a cántaros,* meaning "to rain buckets.")

But Carole had a great deal to live for and eventually she tried everything she could afford in the medical and alternative spectrum, from surgery and chemo to Gershon therapy at a Mexican clinic and personal healers (the profession our generation graduates to after personal trainers).

Like an animal, cancer sleeps, prowls, hibernates, turns surly or placid. There were weeks when she had energy and optimism and almost no pain, and then stretches when all that changed. Layne would report that the pain sometimes made her pace back and forth for hours. Nights were the worst. Her doctors were doing the WHO analgesic-ladder thing, keeping her on Tylenol 2s and 3s as long as possible. It was the same story with Ramiro, who had colon cancer. The intermediate stage of cancer, before the palliative care and opiates are ushered in, is the worst for pain management. Patients can stall in this terrible tunnel, without knowing how to proceed. But when Carole and I spoke in June to plan our getaway, she was having a "good week" and wanted to take advantage of it. I had the car loaded with organic vegetables and the laptop zipped when Layne called.

"Carole can't go, she's in too much pain, and she's afraid of getting into trouble so far away from help," he said. I was disappointed, but not surprised. It had seemed too miraculous to just drive away.

"We've decided to look into this place in Mexico and maybe give that a shot," Layne went on, "so we need to get going on that this week. She's so sorry not to go. She was really looking forward to this."

I unpacked the car, put the groceries back in the fridge, and looked up the clinic they were headed for on the Internet. It focused on detoxification and a nutritional regime to undo some of the damage wreaked on the body by chemotherapy. The clinic looked too fundamentalist Christian for my taste, and it didn't bother to mention outcomes or any other sort of statistical evidence, but I hoped it would do the trick. Faith, prayer, and optimism are a cellular approach, too. Most of all, Carole wanted to be cared for, not moved through the cancer assembly line.

They flew to Mexico, and then back to the small Ontario town where Layne was working in a summer theater festival. She began the clinic's program, which involved an expensive organic diet, total bed rest, and freshly squeezed juices, every hour through the day. Carole adored food and hated the idea of downing all that carrot pulp, but she stuck with it. An old friend moved in with them to help out—the juicing schedule alone sounded exhausting. When I spoke to her on the phone, she reported that she felt "amazingly tired" but hopeful that this was only a natural stage of her turnaround. I was out of the province on vacation with my family. The next thing I knew, we were all back in Toronto, it was fall, and Carole was dying.

Layne continued to pour himself into Carole in the lightest, steadiest way possible, but he was worn out caring for her at night and trying to run a theater during the day. His sister Billie moved in to help. It was time to round up a team of people to stay with her at night. Some were old friends, and many were from the theater community. Carole did a brilliant job of reassuring her daughter that the best thing she could possibly do for her mother was to enjoy her own life as much as she could. Charlotte moved in with Carole's sister Jo-Anne and visited each day. Then the key to the back door of the house became available to a rotating team of five "night nurses," of whom I was one.

THE FIRST NIGHT, I went with Janet, who had already been broken in. Carole's first rule was no big bedside scenes. I hadn't seen her since the spring, and Janet prepped me for how she would look. "Like a skeleton, basically, except the tumor makes her look pregnant." The illness had also metastasized through the house; the entire ground floor of their house had been cleared out and a rented hospital bed occupied the bay window of what had been the living room.

A house with a sick person in it looks different at night. It's not just that the porch light is always on, or that one low light might shine through the drawn curtains. The whole house has a charged, altered look to it. On my first shift, I was nervous about how I would be with Carole—at the best of times she was a lie detector, and I had the superstition that in sickness she would see all the way through me. I wanted not to get in the way of helping her.

We arrived about one A.M. and crept in the back door. Carole's red winter coat hung in the hall, with the short, dark wig she had sometimes worn flung on the rack above it. The faintly industrial hissing, breathing sound turned out to be the oxygen tank. I went into the darkened main room, heard the smallest of sighs, and then saw the silhouette of a startlingly bony arm lifted. The arm went around someone bending over Carole—Annie, the person on the early night shift, saying good-bye. It seemed a shockingly tender, ardent scene, and I stepped back, unsure how to approach.

Finally I came close, embraced her, and in recognition Carole gripped me, apologizing for her frayed, slurry voice. "It's this thing I have to use," she rasped, sounding a bit like Brando in *The Godfather* as she touched the oxygen tube in her nose. "Oh, it's so good to see you!" she exclaimed, as if at a soirée. But then she began shifting and rearranging the bedclothes, in obvious discomfort. Time for the next injection. Janet pulled the covers back, found the plastic port taped to her thigh, and stuck a needle full of morphine into it. You could see Carole brace slightly, hand on her chest, before the downward drift of the drug in her blood. Then she closed her eyes and slept.

We turned the lights off and sat in chairs on either side of her bed for a long time. The oxygen tank hissed and sighed. It was peaceful to look across the heap of blankets and see Janet's silhouette, with her tent of long hair. Proximal silence. Easy breathing from Carole, punctuated by sudden, air-hungry sighs from time to time. I felt the same absurd sense of accomplishment that you feel getting an infant to finally surrender to sleep. Just sitting there felt like time well spent.

In fact, over the next few weeks, I became grateful that I was on the night shifts—they were longer, sometimes from one A.M. to six A.M., but they had a calm, otherworldly feel to them. After months of pain, Carole now had a palliative care routine in place and was on enough morphine to keep her comfortable. Plus Haldol, for the anxiety that morphine sometimes triggers, although the Haldol only seemed to make her hallucinate.

The pain would always surface in the third hour, making her stir, like a swimmer tiring in the water. But the nights I saw her she was lucid, often funny, and appreciative of our smallest efforts. Good company. She was on top of her medication schedule, knew where everything could be found, and enjoyed ordering us around and then making us feel like geniuses for finding the Q-tips. Janet told me about one of her early, nervous nights, when she was reaching for something on the night table and accidentally hit the remote-control button for the hospital bed. Carole shot bolt upright, much to Janet's horror, and then they clutched each other and laughed. "I could have catapulted her right across the room."

THOSE LAST WEEKS WERE when I got to know Carole as intimately as I know anyone. Each person who cared for her ended up feeling the same way—it was like falling in love, you were in way too deep before you realized it. On my second visit, I felt emboldened to give her a foot massage. Her feet were swollen and felt strangely wooden, but I tried my best to be upbeat. "They're a good temperature," I said admiringly. "Oh yeah, I'm in great shape," Carole sort of snorted, picking up on my nursey tone. It was hard for me to reconcile her ravaged body with her undiminished intelligence, but I got onto that one pretty fast.

Mostly, she exuded openness, appreciation, a heightened sensuality, and a lover's sort of tenderness—a combination of qualities that melted everyone who cared for her. She seemed to have burned her way down through the usual resentments and fears to a light, titanium core of love—the openness to others that Buddhist writer Stephen Levine describes in his book *Who Dies?*

"It is the direct experience of who we are that cuts the root of pain," Levine wrote. "It is by entering into the vastness of being that we go beyond identification with the body and mind. We don't find ourselves so contracted about experience. Indeed, we see that it is the loss of contact with our natural spaciousness that is at the root of much of our suffering. When we start to honour our original nature, no longer is a resistance to life encouraged, a desire to keep a stiff upper lip, an unbreakableness. Instead we touch on the strength of the open heart which has room for all."

The next Saturday night, I tiptoed in. Carole exclaimed, "Oh, I'm so happy to see you," and put her arms around my neck. She welcomed the fresh energy of the new shift, someone still unaffected by the room with its little vials and creams and lowered voices. Those bony arms clasping me, like a long, thin, eager infant. She was easily thrilled.

Someone had finally given her a pretty nightgown, a white cotton one with some embroidery, even though her thin arms were now exposed. She had a weakness for fashion and feminine things, and I didn't like to see her swimming around in one of Layne's old T-shirts. Tonight she was sitting up. When she had the energy, she liked to switch from bed to armchair. I hated the chair; it was stupidly designed and didn't support her at all. We swathed it in quilts and packed it with pillows, but it was never quite right. By the time I arrived for my shift, she was ready to lie down again, so I got myself in position for the delicate tango-transfer to the bed. This was hard to do without either pulverizing Carole or wrecking your back. "The trick when you move her," said Janet, "is to put her down in exactly the right spot on the bed. We should really mark it with an X."

Although her doctor came regularly, and toward the very end a palliative care nurse was on duty during the night, for the rest of the team each shift became a crash course in the thousand details of caring for someone dying at home.

The dance from the chair to the bed went like this: First, remove the oxygen tube, making sure not to trample it underfoot during the move. Then have her put her pencil arms around your neck, as you count "one, two, three," and she musters her energy to stand up. Once vertical, you dance her the few paces to the bed, scoop up her white, cool legs, and lay her gently (but never gently enough) on her side. Make sure the cotton swabs are tucked behind her ears, to keep the oxygen tube from chafing, and help her get the annoying little oxygen pincer back in her nose. Fold a pillow up against her spine, and slip another between her knees, to take the pressure off those bony places. Make sure the maroon knitted slippers are on her feet, with the pink polish still growing out on the toes. Draw up the covers, which are never the right weight.

As I got her tucked up one night, I noticed that it was getting colder outside. Late September. A draft was beginning to flow from the bay window across the top of her bed. Should we organize drapes? Or wait?

I went looking for the expensive massage lotion I had stolen from my husband and brought along the week before. Carole adored being touched and loved the way this lotion felt. "It's so amazing when you smooth it, it just goes on and on!" she said. "It must have cost a million dollars."

A massage therapist, Jane, sometimes came during the day, and Carole took a profound comfort from these sessions. She had a touch hunger that I recognized in myself. Once I was better at moving her around in the bed, I offered to give her a massage, which she was happy to accept. I think she sometimes tired of entertaining her endless round of caretakers, and hands-on stuff took care of that.

It was too cool in the room to uncover her, so I had to bend over and snake my hands up the bedclothes, which was awkward. Then there was the shock of her littleness in the bed. But I found areas of palpable tightness in her back that I could work away at. Her shoulder blades were as sharp as wings, and every time she talked, the vibration of her voice passed right up through her and into my hands. After some appreciative murmuring, she became quiet. I worked away as best I could. Massage has always been my alternate career option, if the writing caves. I did her scalp and forehead as well, pressing hard on the acupuncture points. I could tell she was right inside the massage like a landscape, like a canyon. This went on as long as my back could take it.

"Oh, I can't begin to tell you," she said when I was finished, "this was the most amazing evening in my life." "Surely not," I said, laughing. "Well, maybe not the most amazing, but it's up there." This pleased me, of course, although I didn't take it too literally. We were all the recipients of rapturous reviews for whatever we did for her.

The first night I came, I brought some lavender from our garden. Janet crushed the stems and Carole held them against her nose. "Exquisite," she murmured, inhaling deeply, "so exquisite." She could drink a glass of ice water like someone taking notes on a vintage Burgundy. It was partly the morphine, I suppose, but it was also her ability to respond to pleasure.

At the end of her bed was a table covered in the accoutrements of palliative care—little pink spongy swabs on a stick for moistening her lips; vitamin E for her thinning, dry skin; eye drops when her own tear supply waned; and other vials I never investigated. The main medications were the soon-abandoned haloperidol, for anxiety, and the premeasured hypodermic syringes of morphine, kept in the door of the fridge, ready to be injected into a capped port that was taped to her thigh. The self-administered morphine pump came later.

The business of exposing her thigh to inject her always felt somewhat invasive and illicit, requiring that junkie tap on the needle to drive the bubbles out. The injection routine was passed on from one helper to another, like a muffin recipe. We also maintained a log, in order to keep track of the medication schedule and to pass on any helpful notes. These had a touching formality. "Carole and I passed a peaceful night" or "Carole feels bad complaining about the covers all the time but the weight of them bothers her." "Seems more comfortable on her left side today."

Once I was moving her from armchair to bed when her strength suddenly abandoned her and she sagged. I almost dropped her on the floor. I don't have the know-how, I thought wildly. Why isn't there the same pressure to learn palliative care moves that we have to take driving lessons or to learn CPR? Not everybody has a car, I thought, but we are all going to die. When the two of us finally made it to the bed, the task of shifting her into position remained. But being sick had allowed the secret bossiness of the writer full rein. "Let's just sit and recoop for a minute," she would say in her frayed, cottony voice, "then we can try again."

Sometimes she slept or rested in the dark, and other times we would talk to keep the night moving along. One night I was telling her how I often took her with me in my mind, on walks down by the lake. I knew she loved the lake, from her summers on Wolfe Island, near Kingston. Then she asked me to talk about where I had grown up. I told her that I was born in Winnipeg and still had relatives on the prairies, but never got back there. She got quiet then, and finally said, "Something about the prairies hurts." Her husband, Layne, was from Saskatchewan, I knew. "It's about unlived lives," she finally decided. "Thinking about the prairies makes me want morphine," she murmured, in one of the only times I ever heard her name the drug.

It was always easy to take her places in her mind by describing them in detail. It was partly her dreamy morphine state, but her mind was also hungry for new experience and beauty. I told her about iceboating with my brother on Lake Ontario when I was growing up, flying across the frozen bay on a homemade pontoon fixed onto skate blades, which she loved. "How wonderful!" she cried.

Another time she confessed that she sometimes saw visions, and that they bothered her. "Like being pulled down into my grave," she said, sitting in the chair and gesturing toward her bed. I held her and she touched my face very, very gently, like a lover, and said, "I don't know what comes next, what do you think comes next?"

She was also hardheaded about moving through a mental list of messages that she wanted to deliver to people in her life. Some were responses to the cards and letters and stories that poured in. One friend wrote about a time when they had been going down a river in canoes. Then they tied up the canoes and just lay in the water on their backs, letting the current carry them along under trees. I could see her going right back there on that river. Another time, she remembered that she had things to tell me, hot research tips on the subject of pain. "The secret is not to dwell on it," she told me. "As soon as you start dwelling on it and letting negative thoughts take over, the pain only gets worse." This was not a scoop, but what I did notice was that she rarely used the word *pain* and couldn't bring herself to say *death,* either. She used other phrases. "If I lie on my side too long, I get into trouble," she would say. "How long did I sleep?" she would ask when she woke up, and then when we told her, she would be disappointed. "Only that much?"

Another time she was sitting up when I was in the kitchen, resorting to a hammer to break a chunk of ice into chips, and I heard her say, "Oh, I hate that." "What?" I said, coming back into the room, thinking the noise of the hammering was bothering her. "I just thought to myself that I was sitting here in my deathbed-chair. I hate it when those words come up. Why do they come up like that?" "Maybe because those words go together sometimes," I said. "Death, bed. Bed, chair. Anyway," I said, "right now you're in your sitting-up-living-room chair." "That's right," she said, "I am."

It was amazingly easy to call forth endearments. I don't know where this came from, since we weren't old friends. What we really had was a potential friendship and a long, subterranean connection as fellow journalists and mothers of teenagers. We had a lot in common, which no doubt had kept us slightly wary of each other. Two writers. She still had a great deal of pride about letting other people see her like this, weakened and defenseless—especially other healthy, successful writers. There were people she cared for whom she wasn't prepared to see. It was too hard to be plucky around someone embodying the way life might have turned out for Carole.

She told everyone who helped take care of her that she loved them, and that was certainly how it felt. There was a sense of intimacy and lightness in her presence—nothing oppressive or confining, despite the demands on everyone. This connection made me sad for the overlooked potential in every friendship or relationship to go that deep. It's always there, it seems.

For a while I was obsessed with improving her pillows and bolster system—the bed always seemed ramshackle and lumpy, despite our best efforts. I went out and bought assorted baby pillows and bits of foam rubber to try to rig up something more comfortable. The room began to fill with stuffed and quilted things.

"Please tell Marni not to bring any more pillows," Layne finally said to Janet. I had a strong urge to invent a whole new set of palliative accessories in luxurious fabrics.

Small and thin to begin with, in a matter of weeks Carole was as insubstantial as a milkweed. During the day, her doctor, a priest, and palliative care people came round. The "final stage" brochures were now lying on the kitchen table. The sight of the brochures caught me off guard.

The night before she died, I looked at her for a long time as she breathed raggedly, that irregular pattern known as Cheyne-Stokes, an appropriately strangled term. I wanted badly to sketch her. Everything about her was fleeting and in its own way beautiful, as with a newborn. I was amazed at the changes that took place in her every day, almost every hour, like the blooming of a flower in reverse. She was now becoming elemental. But there was no paper around to draw on, no camera. Was it strange to want to take a picture of her?

Her mouth was drawn back in an O around her teeth, her eyes were neither open nor closed, her skin was now whitish yellow, and her dark curly hair, which had grown in after the chemo, had lost the luster it had had even the week before. There was that mottling they warn you about in the brochures, as the circulation slows and the blood pools. She moaned with almost every breath, but it seemed more sighlike than a suffering sound. What I noticed was her ebbing presence. It felt as if she were half in the room, half not. Now and then she fiddled with her blankets or lifted her arm to scratch at one spot on her neck. Sometimes she twirled a lock of hair. The gestures were a shock, because when she was still she looked so gone.

I went back home to bed at six A.M. I didn't sleep. The next day I felt snagged, anxious, and distracted. Part of it was worry that I might be the only one there when Carole died. Which would be fine, but hardly appropriate. I called an old friend, long distance, but no one answered, and in the evening I was upset that both my son and my husband happened to be out. I wanted everybody home and accounted for.

On the last night I was there, she spent about three hours in quiet sleep. I held her hand a few times and went in and out of the room. It didn't feel so imperative to be beside her anymore. Layne, exhausted from another long day's watch, was asleep upstairs, and across the hall his sister was asleep as well. Gloria, the palliative nurse, a big placid spot of darkness in the chair, sat beside Carole's bed. Gloria, ultracalm and very religious, had a lot of years behind her of sitting up with people dying. A few nights before, she had sung a hymn to Carole, which she had quite enjoyed. "Get Layne and sing it again!" she insisted. The hymn triggered a dying moment, and everyone gathered around the bed. But it passed. Hymns will do that. "Well, I guess I'll have to try living again," Carole had said apologetically.

I stretched out in the TV room, nervous, not knowing what to expect. I kept listening for that ragged intake of breath from the next room, or for the sound not to come. Time passed very slowly. At six A.M., I woke Layne up, and we talked a bit. He said the previous day had been especially rough. They had had to give her anti-spasmodic drugs. There was a lot of agitation (which can be the result of stepped-up, "end-stage" levels of morphine), then periods of quiet, then more struggle. "It's like false labor," one of the team members said, "and we're the midwives."

I remember how, after my good shift with her the week before, I had come home feeling absolutely impregnated with her—the kind of cell-deep possession you feel after sex. I lay there in bed with my hands folded over the blankets in her gesture, moving in the same slow way. It was a very odd feeling of being inhabited by someone. She slips into other people easily, I thought, like the female hero in her novel *In the Wings* who always says "I love you" recklessly early. Someone open to seduction by the world. Of course, everybody who spends time with her is dancing with morphine, too. So we moved through the days in a slightly altered state.

All the clichés about the privilege of caring for the dying turned out in Carole's case to be true. Being able to see her, touch her, and care for her during her last weeks felt like a great gift rather than a loss. It can get confusing, sorting out the drama and the intimacy from the fact that the story is not going to turn out happily at all. There is a bubble of happiness in the middle of the sadness—the joy of a pure connection with someone else's life. It happens so rarely, and only in sex, love, or death.

The women who cared for Carole were a mixed bunch of new and old friends. The only time we saw one another all at once, in the daylight, was after Carole's funeral, when we went out for a drink. That was when it struck me that everyone, not just the actors, had low, soft voices, which Carole had, too—a melodious voice with a subversive lift in it, the equivalent of an arched brow.

The night after my shift, Layne called and left a message, telling me that Carole had died. He had been with her all afternoon, telling her once again how much he loved her and was grateful for the time he had spent with her, right to the end. It was hard to know if she took it in, but he talked to her anyway.

"Then I stepped out of the room for a minute and when I came back, she was gone." Apparently, this is often the case—the need on the part of the dying to slip away when there is no one present in the room to disappoint. Layne's message on the tape was such an outpouring of love, such a selfless witness to Carole, that I couldn't bring myself to erase it for weeks.

For a while after her death, whenever I went to sleep, I would get images of her mouth, drawn back from her teeth, which were so central to her beauty, a kind of prow to her face. I would remember a persistent, delicate gesture she had with a bunched-up Kleenex, touching the edges of her lips. I was imprinted.

IN TERMS OF HER physical suffering, Carole was better off when she was dying than in the earlier stages of cancer. One of the most advanced areas of pain management, thanks to nurse-driven progress in the palliative care field, involves the care of the dying. Pain doesn't have to be the admission price of dying. If everyone is focused only on how much the dying are suffering, the orderly progress of letting go, and the real but often lucid struggle of saying good-bye will be obscured. The goal is not to medicate the dying into some sleek designer form of death—an equivalent of the elective cesarean. The idea is to address and treat unnecessary pain.

In her testimony at the U.S. Senate hearing on the Pain Relief Promotion Act in April 2001, Dr. Kathleen Foley reported that 37 percent of children with cancer were not adequately treated for their pain in their last days of life. Nursing home studies have shown that 40 percent of elderly cancer patients have pain, but less than 25 percent of them receive any analgesics at all. And she cited one study of ten thousand seriously ill hospitalized patients in which 50 percent endured significant pain in the last days of life. Since 2.4 million Americans die each year, that adds up to a sea of unnecessary suffering.

Carole's final weeks demonstrated that the process of dying, far from involving an escalation of pain, may bring a respite from it. Once proper palliative care kicks in, the myths and misinformation around chronic pain become less of an obstacle. It no longer makes sense to raise the issue of addiction for someone who may have only days or weeks left to live. And fears about breathing problems or other side effects become merely fine print in the face of death. Dr. Foley also pointed out in her address to the Senate that people fear that relaxing the rules around opiates and the dying will allow physicians to use morphine to hasten death. This is an unscientific myth, she said. Physician-assisted suicides use barbiturates, not morphine, and studies have shown that patients on high doses of morphine often live longer rather than die more quickly.

What you want for the dying is not to see them suffer any longer. This is the job of palliative care experts, who aren't there to cure an infection or fix a fracture. Their goal is comfort, compassion, and quality of life. It's enough to make people with chronic pain wish they could check into a hospice.

Being cared for at home by her family, with her pain more or less under control, allowed Carole to shine as a person in her dying. It was a bravura performance—not an act, but a projection of spirit, which all great performances tend to be. She demonstrated dying to all of us around her with honesty, wit, and courage. Of course, *courage* is the word you always hear in the same sentence with the word *cancer*. But in Carole's case it was exactly that, a delicate bravery that characterized her writing as well.

Which is not to say that opiates provided her with a smooth, angel-with-folded-hands ride. Dying still looked to me like a case of getting through a tight, scary bottleneck—a bony birth. No one gets to practice it. Do you look behind you, or straight ahead? Try to shut down, or open up? Some drugs helped, and others didn't. Anxiety and fear often overwhelmed her. But the morphine let her concentrate on something other than pain. It also gave other people a chance to receive her gifts and see her light.

31

RON MELZACK

RONALD MELZACK HAS DEVOTED FIFTY years of his life to the study of pain. At the age of seventy-two he may well be the scientist with the broadest and most detailed understanding of this subject in the world. He and his lifelong collaborator, Patrick Wall, produced the standard book used by medical students, the *The Textbook of Pain,* as well as wrote *The Challenge of Pain,* a modern classic in its field. For some time now, Melzack has been working on a new book for Oxford University Press. (Pain books, as I have nervously noted, seem to exert a Macbeth-like curse on their authors, consuming whole decades.)

Although we had met briefly in Vienna, I put been putting off talking to Melzack for four years. After all, I was a tourist in his world, using not much more than a witching stick to make my way through this endlessly complex terrain. I didn't want to sit across from someone who might say, "Oh my, you've been barking up all the wrong trees." My ongoing confusion of the thalamus with the thymus gland could also prove to be a problem.

With any luck, he'll refuse to see me, I thought, as I called the psychology department of McGill University in Montreal to track him down. But it was Melzack himself, now professor emeritus, who picked up the phone. A book on pain, he said, lovely, let's have a chat.

So on a summer morning I made my way to the biology building of the McGill campus, on the flanks of Mount Royal. Montreal figures largely in the science of pain. Melzack's office is on Dr. Penfield Avenue, named after the legendary neurosurgeon Wilder Penfield, a pioneer mapper of the brain (we owe the little man in the brain, Mr. Homunculus, to Penfield) and founder of the world-famous Montreal Institute of Neurology. Bal Mount, a friend and colleague of Melzack's, established the first North American hospital palliative care unit at Montreal General Hospital, which also has a long-established pain clinic. The McGill Pain Questionnaire (MPQ), the most widely used pain-measurement tool in the world, was developed here in 1971 by Melzack, with the help of mathematician and statistician Warren Torgerson. Rather than burden their project with a double-barreled name, Melzack simply named it after his university.

As I hurried across the campus, the city of Montreal presented its usual schizophrenic face—ravishing beauty combined with a faint sense of ebbing or diminishment. Weeds shot up between the cracked stones of the paved square between buildings. It reminded me a little of Havana, another seductive city in decline.

Melzack was already waiting in his office, where a lovely view of the silver St. Lawrence River at the foot of the city had been compromised by two new office towers. He stood up and greeted me, revealing the slightest trace of a stammer. He has a distinctive, strong, and warm voice, and a good laugh, too, which he used strategically. Whenever I embarked on some idea he had written about twenty years ago, he would simply chuckle.

"WHAT INTERESTS YOU NOW about pain?" I asked, meaning what could possibly still interest him about pain.

"Right now, I'm interested in looking at pain in a broader sense than just a sensory system. I've become aware of how important stress is," he said. "Every time we're injured, or have a major infection or disease in which pain is a factor, obviously there is stress, and the stress system is very, very powerful. Once it's called into play, you have the neuroendocrine system involved, and cortisone. Cortisone is wonderful, because it can block pain."

I had brought along coffee and some bagels. Although I had planned to pick up the thin, glossy, irregular ones from the famous bagel factory on St. Viateur, I had to settle for some substandard English ones nearby. Melzack peered into the bag and deployed breakfast on the desk between us. He started to talk about a book, *Why Zebras Don't Get Ulcers,* by Robert Sapolsky. It explores the ability of animals to override pain in order to escape a predator: for instance, a zebra attacked by a lion. (Lion attacks seem to figure largely in pain literature.)

"But the lion is in stress, too," Melzack added, "because he's starving to death. So we have all these different control systems involved in pain. My feeling is, these control systems can run amok and become the basis of some of our chronic pain syndromes." Sitting in front of a wall of pain books, Melzack was proceeding patiently, like a professor feeling out a first-year student.

"Or take soldiers in battle," he said. "They're in severe stress, damn right they're stressed—so if they're only injured, they don't feel it.

"Now I was in an accident recently," he continued, "and the same damn thing happened. I was driving home from a music camp that my wife, Lucy, goes to every summer, up north, and on the way back I thought, I'll just get a coffee, and then go into Montreal for a Chinese meal. So I stopped at a McDonald's, got back into the car, didn't put my seat belt on, and had an accident. Went flying through my windshield. And as I was sitting there, with blood just dripping down my forehead and nose, I was worried about my clothes." He laughed and brushed a hand over the front of his nicely ironed short-sleeved shirt.

"I had no pain! For two days, I didn't have any signs of inflammation, so I felt pretty good. Well, I'd wrecked the car, but I phoned my sister and her daughter, who have a van, and asked if they would drive me the next day to pick up Lucy and her cello. And they could, sure. I woke up that morning, and I was black and blue. It had taken two days for this to suddenly appear—the inflammatory response, which is good, it's all part of the healing process. But if pain is suppressed, along with these other protective aspects, the body's reaction to bacteria and whatnot . . . well, that can kill you, too. All these mechanisms can run amok."

I never heard whether Melzack made it to Montreal or not, because he was off and running as the subject of his own little pain experiment.

"Now, I'm giving you more than you want here, but what cortisone and these other steroids do, during stress, is they try to conserve energy. So they try to prevent the replacement of calcium in bone, and they have all sorts of effects on muscle . . . and my feeling is, I bet a lot of these pain problems that involve muscle—let's say fibromyalgia or bone problems—a lot of these are perfectly wonderful programs in the brain that evolution has produced. But they just don't function right now, which could be stress-related."

This theory fit in with what I had read about Melzack's concept of the neuromatrix. This is a neural network that is laid down early in the developing embryo to prepare the brain for a certain set of responses it can expect to use. For instance, at birth the brain already "knows" and "feels" a body with two legs, even if the child is born with one leg missing. Otherwise, how are we to explain phantom pain in limbs that were never there in the first place?

"So I've been thinking a lot about stress and cortisone, and I've been thinking a lot about genetic factors. There are tremendous genetic factors involved in pain."

"Is a susceptibility to pain inherited?"

"Let's say there's a big inherited factor, absolutely. Just down the hall from me now is Jeff Mogil, a psychologist who is studying the genetics of pain. People asked me who I would like to replace me, and I said him, because I think genetics is where the field is going."

"If we start to look at pain as something that is partly rooted in our genes," I said, "then people will see that pain isn't a transient thing, but something with the potential to change us deeply, even at the cellular level."

"Oh yes."

"But what does that mean for future generations?" I asked. "For instance, can chronic pain be inherited?"

"You mean in the sense of having a sort of biased system, to overrespond or underrespond to pain? Yeah, I think that could well be. For instance, an inability to feel any pain at all is something that's inherited," Melzack continued. "There's a very readable little book"—he cast an eye over his bookshelves—"what the hell was it called—a novel that dealt with a surgeon in the seventeenth century who had this condition . . . *Ingenious Pain,* by Andrew Miller. But the argument the author makes is a terrible argument, namely, that this guy had to suffer pain in order to become a compassionate human being. I hate that argument, because it's practically a statement that pain is good. Well, it ain't good. It's no good at all."

"But isn't it true," I said, "that pain does play a protective role, evolutionarily speaking? Maybe the problem is that we've outrun some of the earlier biological functions of pain. It's as if the car alarm is being triggered now by cats instead of criminals."

"That could be. What has become evident is that pain is part of a much larger system. That's why a great many of these new drugs that work for pain, the antidepressants and anticonvulsants, are not part of the so-called pain system at all—they're working on limbic systems or other structures involved in stress."

"So now we're treating pain attitudes, too."

"We are."

"But people keep making this distinction between mental pain and physical pain, even though it doesn't exist."

"That's right. It's funny, eh?" He neatly cupped the bagel crumbs off his desk and into the palm of his other hand.

Perhaps, I said, pain is not just about private misery but about public pain and "history in the body." Pain not only goes back in time but forward, too, affecting future generations and their responses to pain. Which is why it's so important to take pain seriously, and to treat it properly—before it sends down deeper roots.

Melzack smiled agreeably and reined in the rhetoric a little.

"I think that somewhere in your book you want to say that there are big individual differences in pain. And part of those differences may be due to genetic factors. And if you have a book that we hope will be a popular book, then I think it's comforting for people to know that, gee, you know, they say I overrespond to pain. But maybe I'm not being a sissy—maybe I'm really built like that."

"You don't want to blame people for their own pain," I said, "but you can go too far in the other direction, too. People are dying to blame genes for their behavior."

"It's a fact that far more women than men have chronic pain," Melzack said. "That surely is a genetic factor."

But surely not only a genetic factor, I thought, unwilling to go careening off into the nature-nurture discussion just then. One interesting difference between us was that whenever I said the word *culture,* Melzack would talk about "the brain" rather than social forces. I tend to think of external social forces as a weather system that shines on certain ways of thinking and rains on others, whereas for Melzack, culture is part of memory and learning, which reside in the neural network. I still find it hard to locate myself on the broad spectrum that runs from pure reductionist to cultural relativist.

"But for women, the difference in pain levels off as they age, yes?" I said hopefully. "I thought women only have more pain between the ages of twenty and fifty."

"Yes. Once the hormones kick in, or out, it all changes."

TO PREPARE FOR OUR conversation, I had read the interview that John Liebeskind conducted in 1993 with Melzack for the History of Pain Project at UCLA. It's clearly a fond exchange between two peers who respected each other enormously. What was also striking was how often Melzack deflected praise to his colleagues. I noticed this as well in our conversation. He is always giving credit to other people's work, which is unusual in the competitive realm of scientific research.

Liebeskind asked him about some of the early personal factors that took Melzack into the pain field. Melzack described himself as a "very insecure kid who came from a Jewish family that was not religious." His father emigrated from Poland to Canada as a teenager, learned the "needle trade," and worked in a factory until Ron's older brother, Jack, convinced their father to open up a bookshop. Their other brother, Louis Melzack, took over the bookshop, eventually developed a chain of bookstores called Classics, and became a multi-millionaire. Jack was more of a hellraiser and less lucky. He was living in Toronto when he died at the age of twenty-six, after a bout of pneumonia. The police had mistaken him for a drunk and tossed him in jail. Ron Melzack was nine when his brother Jack died. "It was a great tragedy in the family," Melzack said, "and it had a terrible impact on me."

In school, Melzack remembered himself as an underachiever who was "almost always depressed, to some extent, between fifteen and twenty-five. I was really searching for something to do," he told Liebeskind. At McGill University he studied psychology with no great enthusiasm for two years, until in his third year he met his mentor, the behavioral psychologist Donald Hebb, and became his student. Melzack's first project for Hebb in 1949 was "an experiment on curiosity in the rat," during the heyday of Skinnerian, conditioned-response psychology. Meanwhile, his very successful brother Louis was saying, "Why don't you give up playing with rats and crap like that and come with me into the book business and do something important?"

Melzack's master's thesis was on irrational fear in dogs. "Not learned fears, but fears of things like statues of animals, or fears of skulls. Fear of that which is different and unexpected and unusual. And that brings you to prejudice, of course." It would make sense that the son of Jewish immigrants might want to explore the notion that fear of the Other is a part of our nature that we must struggle to overcome, rather than a choice.

One experiment in particular laid the groundwork for the gate-control theory of pain. It now sounds slightly barbaric: It was a project involving dogs raised in social isolation, in cages.

When they were let out into an environment they weren't used to, they didn't seem to feel pain normally—the dogs would stick their noses into a flaming match, for instance. "Everybody interpreted this experiment to mean that the dogs did not feel pain," Melzack recalled, "and that you have to *learn* to feel pain. And I knew that that just couldn't be true. I knew they could feel pain, because in their home cages, they could, but when they came out, somehow they would ignore it. And I came to the realization that the brain somehow had to receive information about what was going on in the outside world and evaluate that info. Then it would send messages down to some gating area, as I would call it now, where it would let the stuff in or keep it out.

"And pain suddenly became an interesting problem to me," he remembered. It also took him away from the world of pure behavioral psychology, which was fixated on a Cartesian model of stimulus-response. "We're not input-output machines . . . to me life is continuous action and continuous perception," Melzack said, "and what I do now is influenced not only by what happened in the past but my dreams of what's going to happen generations from now. It's concern about life long after my death." It also immersed him in the animal experiments that were uncontroversial then, but have become difficult to read about now without flinching. Nevertheless, animal experiments remain the sine qua non of pain research.

Melzack went off to Portland, Oregon, to do graduate work in physiology with William Livingston. "The real passion for the field of pain came when I worked with him. Livingston said to me, 'You know, you could work on cats from now till the cows come home, but you've got to see people in pain.' So I went with him to the clinic.

"One of the first patients I met there was a Mrs. Hull," Melzack recalled. "An amputee with diabetes, gangrene, she had lost both legs. She was a very well read, intelligent lady, and she began to describe the different pains—they were shooting, they were cramping, they were this and that, you know. . . . I began to write the words down. I felt there was something in these words that was important." He later put that list together with other terms he had come across in his work, until he came up with about two hundred words—the beginning of the McGill Pain Questionnaire.

After five more years of postdoctoral training in physiology and psychology, Melzack went to MIT and crossed paths with Pat Wall. "Pat knew my thinking pretty well, and it turned out that it was congenial to what he was thinking. We were both dead against the Cartesian, stimulus-response straight-through one-to-one psychosocial bullshit." The two of them conducted further studies on the influence of early experience on pain perception in dogs.

"It's not that the dogs coming out of isolation didn't feel pain, it was that their brains had to learn how to selectively pick the things that were important in life, to survival. And they eventually learned that a little flame can cause a big blister that will last for weeks, whereas that piece of furniture over there or that big guy in front of them was nothing to worry about. So then the question became, how can the brain know about pain and the meaning of what is coming in, before you actually *feel* the pain? Which is when I developed the idea of a system of signals that goes up to the cortex very quickly, and doesn't produce awareness of anything, but simply activates memory stores. The more slowly entering information, on the other hand, is selected and filtered by the brain. . . ."

"Just like an editor."

"That's exactly what the brain does, saying 'I'm going to pick out this stuff, and leave out that stuff.' And that's where the second great fluke of my life, and Pat's too, came in—meeting each other. There he was, working on the transmission of signals of all kinds— touch, warmth, cold, and so on . . .

"In the spinal cord."

"And here I was working on the brain—"

"So Mr. Brain met Mr. Spinal Cord . . ."

"That's what happened."

"Pain needed both of you, obviously." In the specificity theory, there was a problem with not fully understanding the mechanics of pain in the body. Then there was the problem of understanding the interaction between the brain and the spinal cord, which Melzack and Wall addressed. I asked Melzack if there wasn't a new split now, between the culture and the body.

"Well, the neuromatrix concept is slowly catching on . . . very slowly. And what that concept incorporates is that culture is not 'out there,' but something integrated into all the patterns of thinking in our mind."

"The idea of a matrix gets around the inner/outer dilemma and suggests something more inclusive—a convergence."

"Yes, a convergence of all these components of the nervous system—the cognitive, the affective, and the sensory."

"But people still make this distinction between what is scientific and mappable, and what is cultural." I didn't add that I was probably one of them.

"Well, that's dumb. To ask how the brain works is as scientific as to ask how the spinal cord works."

"I keep thinking that Freud was trained as a biologist," I said, "and that psychology now seems to be circling back to something far more rooted in biology and physiology. And that rather than being 'reductionist,' this may be a good thing. Being rooted in the body."

"This is an excellent thing."

While Melzack and Wall were developing their ideas, they were also "writing and writing and writing," Melzack recalled.

"The editor of the journal *Brain* at the time was Lord Brain," he said with unavoidable relish, "and Lord Brain accepted a paper from us about this hypothesis. I think three people read it and that was the end of it, until our article on the gate-control theory appeared in *Science* in 1965. We reversed our names. First it was by Melzack and Wall. I think the second one was by Wall and Melzack.

"That was when I realized that by a fluke I had stumbled into an area that I could make an intellectual life out of. The study of pain gave my life the meaning I had been looking for. It was useful and could be a contribution. I always had the sense that I could do something good with my life, or I could do something bad. That sense of guilt that goes along with depression was always with me. This work could take some of the guilt away." When Melzack was offered a job at McGill, he accepted, but he continued to fly back and forth to Boston to work with Wall.

"I'd usually bring a bottle of whiskey, so that's how we started, we'd argue like crazy. Pat does not like the brain. He's not comfortable with the brain, he doesn't like working with it. Pat reads philosophy voraciously. I mean, he reads Hegel and Kant and everybody, but nevertheless, in science he is a spinal cord physiologist and he thinks like a spinal cord physiologist, and he can't get away from that. So we've always fought and argued, but there was always a fundamental respect there between the two of us. No matter how mad we used to get at each other, we'd always be friends. And that friendship has survived all these decades."

In the summer of 2001, Melzack visited with Wall at a conference in Istanbul. Wall had been suffering with prostate cancer for a number of years, and was frail, but engaged, still traveling around the world to pain gatherings. "We talked for a while in his room and I said, 'Will you be going to the dinner tonight?' and he said 'I'm going to be right there for the rest of the day,' pointing to the bed." A month later, at the age of seventy-six, Patrick Wall died.

Friendship and *family* are words that come up often when Melzack talks. A brother-in-law who died of cancer in great pain inspired Melzack to connect with Bal Mount, who helped pioneer the concept of palliative care. Melzack's wife, Lucy, travels with him to the conferences her husband attends around the world, and she is his first reader as well. When his own children were young, Melzack wrote and published several books for children based on Inuit legends. He even talks about the International Association for the Study of Pain, an organization he has been involved in since it began, as a "family" of professionals.

This turns out to be one of the ironies of pain. Even though it often isolates the people who suffer from it, it has created new communities among the scientists who study it.

When I mentioned this curious side effect of pain science, Melzack agreed. "Yes, it's true, but John Bonica," he said, deftly shifting the focus away from himself, "he was the one with the passion to say, 'Look, we've *got* to stop pain, which is horrible, which destroys people and destroys families . . . so to hell with all these barriers, let's get rid of them.' And he organized the IASP, which brought together nurses and dentists and social workers and other people. Bonica said, 'Nobody can play God around here because we don't have the answers, and people are suffering.'

"Bonica was an amazing guy," Melzack continued. "He could talk about pain and suddenly begin to weep. He would tell the story of his own wife, who nearly died in labor, which is why he became interested in the whole field of obstetric anesthesia—and he would start to cry. He was just like that. He created the pain field. Pat Wall and I may have proposed the gate-control theory, but it wouldn't have taken hold if Bonica hadn't brought us together at that first meeting in Issaquah, Washington, and said, 'We've got to talk.' That was 1973. The IASP grew out of that, as well as a new journal, devoted to pain.

"A lot of people were skeptical at the time, and I was one of them. But it happened, and, boy, it's important."

He had put his finger on one crucial way that the issue of pain is changing science and medicine. It's easy for specialists to burrow into their own particular field and never think outside it. But pain requires a back and forth between the pure scientists in the lab and the doctors in the clinics. Treating pain requires communication, above all.

"It's got to be that way," he agreed. "But the scientists are now becoming overwhelmingly dominant, which I think is going backward a little."

"In your interview with Liebeskind, you said that as scientists 'we're learning more and more about less and less.' "

"Yes. Science is getting into more detail, and it's important—but you can get lost in detail and forget the larger picture of the human being who is suffering."

We talked about how long it takes for pain issues to sink in. In 1990, Melzack published an article in *Scientific American* called "The Tragedy of Needless Pain," which addressed our resistance, both as patients and doctors, to using opiates for pain. "The evidence that people in pain rarely get addicted to opiates has been around for years," I said, "but these fears and prejudices persist. Why?"

"Well, there are many facets here. One is that we all grow up in our culture hearing that narcotic addiction is terrible. And you know what? It is terrible. For people who are addicted, I mean, it's a horror. They ruin their lives. So we know this is true. And then the medical profession has to be extremely careful, because they're walking a tightrope. If they overprescribe drugs or make an error in prescription, they're held accountable and can be brought up before a board, which is what happened to this guy Frank Adams. He's a terrific example of this sort of thing. So the fact of the matter is, there is a price to pay. And then there is the great worry by most people that they will become addicted."

"But what's at the bottom of that?" I asked. "Maybe a fear of addiction is partly a fear of losing our capacity for pain—losing our emergency system. There's got to be more to our resistance than the obstacles to getting the drug itself."

"That's right, people don't want to lose something that is important for them to know. That may be part of it. Well, there are whole books on the blooming thing, but nobody has worked it out."

"People worry about becoming dependent on a drug."

"It's not only that they fear dependence but that they're ashamed. This patient I wrote about in the *Scientific American* article, he didn't want his colleagues at work to know he was on morphine because they might think he was a junkie. He kept protesting, saying the pain wasn't so bad. And his wife kept telling us, 'No, it's terrible. You don't hear yourself moaning and groaning in your sleep,' she said, 'waking us up, and the kids.' "

"It's almost a matter of changing the name."

"That's how we got him to take it. We gave the drug a fancy new name."

"We really haven't scratched the surface of the whole addiction thing," I declared, forgetting once again that I wasn't in line for the Nobel Prize.

"No," he tactfully agreed, "we have not."

PERHAPS THE MOST important quality that Melzack brought to his studies was an interest in language.

"And communication," he said. "It takes everyone, working together. I mean, Pat Wall is a brilliant neurophysiologist, but we always had great debates about me moving in just the direction you're going—the direction of culture, family, the larger picture. Because what that pain means to you is critically important. You can't just tack meaning onto the sensation. It's what it means to you that makes it a big pain or a little pain. Or an intolerable pain."

I asked Melzack what he was most proud of in his long career.

"Most proud of?" He laughed. "Gee whiz. I guess it's that I've worked with a bunch of wonderful people to bring the issue of pain forward. So that it's seen as a problem in its own right, and so that people can get proper care for their pain."

"Is that idea being taught in medical schools right now?"

"No."

We laughed.

"Well, I shouldn't say no. There is more pain teaching now than there has ever been before, sure. The message that people in severe chronic pain should be given opiates is getting across. But there are setbacks. You have to keep looking at it all through the perspective of the history of science. Galileo was stoned for supporting an idea that Copernicus had had almost a century earlier! Everything takes centuries, it really does."

I ran Jim Harrison's rain-on-the-roof theory of pain relief by Melzack, thinking it might give him a few new ideas.

"Read the section on 'audioanalgesia' in my book," Melzack said with his customary "been there, wrote about it" chuckle. "I did a study using white noise as a form of pain relief for people in the dentist's chair. But it didn't work. Wrong sort of pain. It works for slower sorts of pain, but not the sudden sharp jabs you get in dental work.

"But Lucy and I put in a skylight recently, and one of the nicest things about it isn't the extra light, but that sound of the rain. You can really focus in on it, and it could help you work up a trance-like state. So there may be something in that."

It was almost time for Melzack to leave, so I began gathering up my tape recorder paraphernalia. I asked him if there was anything more about pain that he wanted to impart. "No, I think we've covered a nice range of topics here." We stood and looked again at the St. Lawrence River gleaming in the notch between office towers. On the way out we chatted about where he thought the study of pain might be headed.

"Well, genetics, as I said before. Jeff Mogil has been doing some work recently with bee venom to produce an artificial pain, because we need good models of pain—"

"Bee venom? Really?"

"Oh, a bee sting will give you a good sharp pain," he said with the brio of someone comparing wine vintages. "It hurts enough that you worry about it, and it lasts. It also makes you think—Well, what's this going to do? Will it leave scars? A bee sting is a classic pain, the type we can learn a lot from."

Well. I had the feeling of having come full circle—from bee to bee. My inquiry had begun when a bee flew in my mouth and stung me; and now, at the end of the road, I had stumbled into bees once again.

32

THE HUMAN PINCUSHION AND
THE UNIVERSAL RAT

THE FACT THAT SOME PEOPLE ARE BORN
incapable of feeling pain seems at first glance
to be a lucky fate. Imagine: no hangovers, no
sore pitching arm, no tremors in the dentist's
chair. But congenital analgesia (as it's known)
turns out to be both a nuisance and a life-
threatening peril. In *The Challenge of Pain*,
Melzack and Wall recount how one girl with
this condition suffered third-degree burns on
her knees after climbing up on a hot radiator
to look out a window. Because there was no
discomfort to let her know when she should
shift her weight or change posture, she eventually developed an inflammation in her joints
and died at the age of twenty-seven. Another
woman with congenital analgesia experienced
nothing but a "tight feeling" when her appendix burst. She would have died, too, if her
family physician, aware of her insensibility to
pain, hadn't sent her to the hospital. When
the same woman gave birth to her first of
two children, she described the sensation as

a "funny, feathery feeling." But the best-known example of this rare inherited disorder was the first circus performer known as "The Human Pincushion," a thin young man who made his living sticking pins into his body on stage. It seems that for those born incapable of feeling pain, the career options are rather narrow, and life is short. Be glad it hurts when you stub your toe.

Congenital analgesia is at the far end of a wide spectrum of inherited pain disorders. It's impossible to sort out how much culture, family behavior, and other factors have to do with our range of pain sensitivity, but genes definitely play a role. Genetic factors are involved in 39 to 55 percent of migraine cases (familial hemiplegic migraine in particular, but "normal" migraine appears to have an inheritable factor, too), 55 percent of menstrual pain cases, half of the back pain population, and 21 percent of sciatica cases. Other gene-related differences are linked to gender, which will come as a surprise to no one. Men appear to suffer less pain but need more pain relievers. There's no proof that women tolerate pain better than men; but they are three times more likely to suffer migraines, and six times more likely to develop fibromyalgia. In a 1999 Gallup survey, 46 percent of American women said that they feel daily pain, compared to 37 percent of American men. And whether it's genetic or stiletto-induced, one in four women reported that their feet were sore.

While I was reading up on the genetics of pain, my eighteen-year-old son had four wisdom teeth extracted. This can lead to pumpkin-headed swelling and agonizing postsurgical pain, but my son took the prescribed medication and had an easy time of it—another example of pain's unpredictability. Whereas, on the day after his surgery, *I* developed a weird new pain in the head—an impressive feat, given that I've already used up a number of psychosomatic syndromes. It was an electrical tic, a small nerve-jab that jumped sporadically but insistently in my right temple. I assumed that this was the result of unconscious, sympathetic jaw-clenching, as I went about blending bananas and pureeing soups for my son, who lay about in a happy fog of Tylenol 3s. Of course, this is not at all what the geneticist means by inherited pain, but it did help me uncover one of my own. When my mother called to check on her grandson's recovery, I mentioned this strange new zapping pain of mine.

"Oh, I get that, too, and so did my sister," my mother said breezily. "It comes and goes."

"Which side?"

"The right."

"Up the temple, and behind the eye?"

"Oh yes, the eye, too."

At this point I remembered that my mother was ninety-one, afflicted by various tremors and cardiac shudderings, but very much alive and well. I was happy to inherit whatever minor tics came packaged with her genes.

I went to talk to Jeff Mogil, the first person in the world to put together training in psychology, genetics, and pain. He studied under the psychologist John Liebeskind in California and after post-doctoral training in genetics he joined the faculty at University of Illinois in 1996. In 2000, Melzack lured him to Montreal, where Mogil has just succeeded him as the new E. P. Taylor Professor of Pain Research in Psychology at McGill University. Whether this means that psychology has become more rooted in neuroscience or that geneticists are worrying more about the big picture isn't clear. But it suggests that the pendulum has now swung back: Science has moved away from seeing pain as a slippery psychological interpretation of something that happens to the body to an experience that is neural, emotional, and deeply rooted in our cells and genes.

Mogil is doing research into pain-related genes.

"For a long time, people have accepted that there are wide variations in the way people respond to pain or to analgesics, but no one ever seriously considered attributing it to genetics, until now.

"Pain genetics is where all the action is now, but it was a totally empty field when I moved into it," says Mogil, who is thirty-five. "I used to go to all these neuroscience meetings and put up my little posters. People would come down to check them out and say, 'Oh, very nice,' you know, just to be polite to one of John's students. Nobody thought that pain had anything to do with genes. But then other people started working with knockout genes in mice, figuring out what happens when you remove this protein or that protein . . . and now knockout genes are everywhere."

Knockout mice always sounded to me like something you might run into at three A.M. on an infomercial. The sea-monkeys of science. "It's the hottest technique in biology right now, and in pain research, too.

"It used to be that scientists didn't concern themselves with whatever particular strain of mouse they used in their studies. Then they discovered that the genetic background of the mouse was affecting their outcomes because some strains would react differently to exactly the same test. And it turned out that I was the only person collecting this sort of information."

When it comes to pain, he found, there is no such thing as a "universal rat." Pain sensitivity varies widely from strain to strain, and some mice are either "doubly lucky" or "doubly unlucky": Both oversensitive to pain and underresponsive to analgesics, or vice versa. Mogil was thrilled. Variability, the bane of most scientific studies, is what you want with genetics. "Messy data" also mirrors the individual nature of pain perception.

"What the study of knockout mice means for people in pain," Mogil said, "is that it helps explain individual sensitivities to pain, and to drugs, as well as the fact that while most people will recover from an injury, some five percent won't. They'll go on to develop chronic pain. Obviously, the factors that determine this are both environmental and genetic, but if we know that some people have a propensity to chronic pain, we might be able to find ways to keep it from developing in the first place. And as we learn more about pharmacogenetics, we can target the treatment with more precision. It also means that people who complain more about pain aren't necessarily whiners—they may actually *feel* more than other people.

"If humans really are like mice, then roughly half of that variability in pain response is due to their inherited genes."

Mogil has also studied the variety of ways people respond to painkillers. Indeed, the world seems to be divided into "responders" and "nonresponders," since morphine is only successful with about

65 percent of the population. This inconsistency explains why pain doctors have to fiddle around with a variety of pain medications when they treat patients. Among Caucasians, 7 to 10 percent are known as "poor metabolizers" who won't respond to codeine. Codeine is thought to metabolize into morphine, but some people don't have the genetic wherewithal to do this. They end up getting all the side effects of codeine and none of the pain relief.

"Doesn't the suggestion that pain may be partly genetic create another misbegotten magic-bullet notion that we can just zero in on the 'pain genes' and knock them out?" I asked.

Genes don't work like that, Mogil replied. "Just as there is no pain center, there is no single pain gene. But it doesn't look like there's a hundred of them, either. We're looking for a particular type of gene that exists in different forms, that can be inherited—and of those genes, there are five to ten, maybe twenty tops."

But can pain change expression? For instance, I asked (harking back to my archaeology-of-pain hunch), could depression in one generation manifest itself as chronic pain in another?

"It could," he said, "but you have to be very careful about how you frame this. Chronic pain in one generation doesn't *cause* chronic pain in the next. More likely, it has to do with the way the parents model pain to their kids and other cultural factors. But the same genetic structure that might make one generation prone to depression could make their offspring prone to a pain condition—it might end up being expressed that way."

People are eager to blame their genes for everything, I reminded him. Doesn't this new focus on the genetic aspect of pain downplay the role of culture and social forces too much?

"But that's the thing about pain," Mogil said, "the cortical stuff is really, really important." As with Melzack, Mogil automatically translates the word *culture* as "cortical activity." But I got his drift. "Cortical stuff" in the brain refers to emotions, ideas, and attitudes that are the result of our memory, learning, experience, and environment. And it's the "cortical stuff" that exerts that famous downward effect on the purely "sensory stuff" coming in. In other words, info moves up; "culture" moves down. For both Mogil and Melzack "everything is equally biological."

I was still getting used to this notion that culture may have roots in various corners of our brains, rather than being the result of a dialogue between a responder (us) and a stimulus (society). Perhaps I was the Cartesian holdout after all. Mogil seemed to be suggesting a much more incarnate interpretation of culture—one mirrored and embodied in the "cortical stuff" that helps shape our experience of pain.

It's interesting, I said to Mogil, that both you and Melzack, two pain pioneers, are psychologists, who are sometimes seen as low men on the totem pole when the hard-science boys get together.

"Pain *is* psychological," Mogil emphasized. "There's all this neural activity going on, but it can always be trumped by culture, attitudes, and behavior. The thing that being a psychologist lets me do is to work with a high level of variability in my tests. Most scientists are looking for consistency. But I get happy when I see messy data."

I TOLD HIM the story of how a bee sting had launched me on this investigation, and I asked why he was interested in bee venom.

"It's the sort of pain that really happens to animals, for one thing," Mogil said. "They get stung. The trouble with the formalin test is that injecting formaldehyde into rat tissues is not something that ever happens to rats in real life."

As Melzack had told me, "a bee sting gives you both the fast, sharp pain and the slower-acting, C-fiber pain. It's got all the dimensions." "The only problem," Mogil added, "is that there's a lot more to bee venom than the stuff in it that makes you hurt. It has a ton of active ingredients, and we don't understand much about it yet."

It turns out that a bee sting is not a simple thing at all, and the complexity of my reaction has some basis in biochemistry. The main toxin in bee venom is something called melittin (not to be confused with melatonin, the popular jet-lag supplement), a peptide containing twenty-six amino acids. In fact, the literature on bee venom therapy, or BVT, is vast. It's been popular for centuries, especially in Europe, where live bee stings are used to treat arthritis. Beekeepers, who are stung repeatedly, were found to have elevated levels of the anti-inflammatory cytokines. Bee venom therapy is also used as a protective agent against irradiation in cancer patients. But BVT is only one aspect of apitherapy, which uses everything bee-related, from the pollen and royal jelly to the wax and venom, to treat a whole spectrum of disorders. It seems that everything involved in the orchestration of the event we call pain—swelling, inflammation, redness, heat, and stinging sensation—can, under different, controlled circumstances, offer pain relief. Bee venom is especially helpful for people who suffer from conditions involving joint and muscle stiffness, like arthritis, or autoimmune disorders like multiple sclerosis.

In other words, the answer to pain may not lie in our efforts to suppress, excise, or extinguish it, but in a deeper understanding of how the body produces pain and goes about healing. The cure for pain is in the pain itself.

As I read further into more lurid literature on the Africanized honeybee, or killer bee, I had another small eureka moment. I learned that fifty or sixty stings from the Africanized bee can cause a fatal shutdown of the kidneys in a reaction that sometimes takes twelve to eighteen hours after being stung to set in. This "delayed toxic reaction following massive bee envenomation" is typical of ordinary bee stings, too, I read. This would explain the allergic alarm that came over me eight hours after being stung, even though I was sitting there with my family in a Japanese restaurant. The heightened state was characteristic of the survival mechanisms that are part of pain's protective role: pain's good side.

So when the bee stung me on the mountain road near Banff, I hadn't "overreacted" or imagined all that followed. My reaction simply reflected what was complex to begin with. As science looks beyond the role of pain as symptom into the nature of pain itself, it's hidden narrative will continue to unfold.

The failure to find a "universal rat," however, suggests something that science may not be able to ignore for much longer: namely, the animals they use in experiments are not interchangeable widgets with paws and tails, but individuals. Pain research depends heavily on animal studies, especially on rodents, who lack the cute factor of other species that attract our sympathies. A standard set of tests are used to induce different sorts of "nociceptive" responses in *Rattus rattus* and *Mus musculus*. (In fact, if you read enough of these studies you start to develop an attachment to certain breeds. I favor the Wistar Kyoto rat myself, although the Sprague Dawley strain has its charms.) There is the paw-on-hot-plate test, the hot-water tail-flick response, and the dread colorectal distention procedure. But the standard one is the formalin test, in which diluted formaldehyde is injected under the skin of the rodent. These tests have been used to investigate why, for instance, morphine is more effective for postsurgical pain than for the sudden, fast pain of an incision.

But even if one accepts the necessity of causing a degree of pain in animals in order to help relieve suffering in humans, to my mind, there is another problem with the way links are drawn between rodents and humans. It's a bit of a one-way street.

Mice and humans share 90 percent of the same genetic makeup. Mice are small and cheap to breed. When it involves research used to develop new pharmaceutical products, science is more than happy to make the rodent-human link, while ignoring the other side of this equation: If we are so similar to mice and rats in pain mechanisms and response to analgesia, then surely pain in rats and mice causes suffering as well.

Pain scientists are well aware of the difficult ethical issues involved. There are guidelines for ethical conduct in research with animals, but Melzack and Wall conclude *The Challenge of Pain* by admitting that even though most scientists believe that research on animals is morally justified, "there is no simple solution to this problem." Without getting into the nuances of consciousness that a mouse has (can a Wistar Kyoto feel moral repugnance, and so forth), animal experimentation that involves pain strikes me as a new variation on Cartesian thinking. Discounting the suffering of animals assumes that they are little more than furry mechanisms for the transmission of certain pleasant or unpleasant signals. Just as Descartes underestimated the role of the brain in pain perception, and medicine has been slow to recognize the ability of infants to feel pain, we may underestimate the consciousness of creatures that we consider less complex than us. It comes down to a matter of where society draws the line. A certain moral stigma has now attached itself to animal testing in the cosmetics industry, for example. Nobody wants bunnies to die in the name of a new lipstick. The line is more difficult to draw when pain research may help millions of people who suffer pain needlessly with cancer, arthritis, or other conditions. For the time being, criticizing science for the use of animal experimentation is like asking a baker to eliminate flour. It is a staple of science, and will remain so until the radius of human empathy widens further.

IF JEFF MOGIL AND RON MELZACK are right, fifty years from now, generic Tylenol tablets will seem as quaint to us as a bottle of sarsaparilla tonic. Instead, we'll take our genotype ID bracelet to the local genopharmacologist to order some bespoke pharmaceuticals. Or we may rise at four A.M. to meditate on the part of our nature that is painful and feel better for it. Along with social insurance, we'll carry geno-cards that list our predispositions: photosensitivity, osteoporosis and poor response to codeine.

Addiction might be redefined not as a character flaw but as "biochemical deficit management." Our emotional habits will become an accepted factor of good health, along with slogans like "Heartache can be harmful to your unborn children." We'll know whether we're at risk for depression or rheumatoid arthritis in the same way we know that we're Scottish, or hazel-eyed. How we live with this new information will still be our choice. But we will know more about the way each body carries its own history.

And one day pain will be so much a part of our identity that it will have lost some of its power to steal away our lives.

33

THE BLIZZARD OF THE WORLD

The blizzard of the world
Has crossed the threshold and has
Overturned the order of the soul.

LEONARD COHEN, "The Future"

IN THE COURSE OF WRITING THIS BOOK, I kept trying to wall myself off from the usual distractions. I worked in six different offices and refuges, some far from my home. But the more I tried to zero in on the subject of pain on the page, the more it opened up around me in the world, as if to say, "You have missed the point again."

The exercise of investigating this subject has been similar to the needling challenge of a Buddhist koan. Pain's meaning is never separate from our experience of it, and yet to experience intense pain is to banish meaning.

In early September 2001, I retreated again, to finish my work. I was alone in the woods, with a cockpit of desks, lamps, and my computer set up in one corner of a small cabin. No newspapers, no television, only the civilized chitchat of CBC on the radio. It was as if I'd had the place sprayed against any bad news.

The business of "catching pain" was on my mind. How do we properly equip ourselves for the escalating pain of the nightly news? I began to write about something that struck me as an emerging form of modern suffering—the instant, global apprehension of random public pain, such as the terrorist bombings in Israel. My thoughts were on those preliminary skirmishes, and how the front page of the newspaper can arrive like a physical blow. I studied a photograph of a burning bus in Israel. The news has reminded us that pain is, after all, not a liquid that flows through certain channels in our body or a current along certain nerves, but a shock wave that can also move out from a public wounding, affecting strangers on the other side of the world. It flies in the night, like Blake's invisible worm.

Just before dawn the next day, a large canvas that my son had painted, a landscape that had been standing against the wall above a tall cupboard in the cottage, fell crashing to the floor. The sound woke me up with my heart in my mouth, and I couldn't get back to sleep. The next thing I knew, it was morning, and a friend from Toronto was calling with the news that a plane had flown into the World Trade Center in New York City. As we spoke on the phone, she watched another plane shear into the second tower, live on CNN.

I had no TV. It would be two weeks before I saw the images that had left everyone in North America feeling suddenly uncovered, like children shivering in bed. In my nightgown I looked out my window and saw the same placid, unaltered scene—a green canoe overturned on the dock, the birch and maple trees on the opposite shore beginning to blaze red and yellow. Benign fire. But my friend's description of what she had seen on TV had funneled into me now, was already vandalizing my sense of safety. After she hung up, I did what everybody did—I called to make sure I knew where my son and husband were. I spoke to my parents. I turned on the radio and sat transfixed and frightened by the stories from witnesses that began to pour out. Then, at a loss, I made an effort to go back to work, to write. But what was on my screen now looked irrelevant, even though pain was loose in the air, like a blizzard. My thoughts about catching pain returned. What do we do when so much of it is unleashed at once like this?

As with any sort of pain, transforming the experience into words feels imperative—another sort of oxygen to lead survivors out of the black smoke and confusion of the event. Faced with a historic spasm of pain, we self-medicate with words. The media actually felt indispensable, for a change. Some words heal, others obscure. But we need to fashion meaning, to *utter* pain, rather than be silenced by brutality of that magnitude. Apart from the thousands who died in the attacks on the United States on September 11 and those who were injured or wounded by grief, people in many parts of the world felt a pain with no clear locus, no meaning, no identifiable source.

My son, who was in his first year at college, phoned and we talked about the attacks for a long time. It made his class that day on the conventions of Canadian literature seem absurd, he said. I told him I felt the same way about my work. As if I were attempting a domestication of a subject that simply ripped and roared through our lives and had no meaning at all. He tried to encourage me. "If you're talking about suffering, you're never off topic."

In the weeks that followed the attacks, a historical sense of "before" and "after" began to emerge. This is the most reliable measure of whether we are living through minor or major pain. Minor pain doesn't alter our sense of time. But if the event goes deep enough, it brings too much knowledge in too short a time, and everything that follows becomes defined as "after." America's immunity to history had ended.

As I tried to take in the enormity of the event, I picked up a book of letters written by Frida Kahlo, a veteran of catastrophes, both physical and emotional. I keep a postcard of one of her paintings above my desk. It's one of her least ingratiating works. The painting depicts a woman naked and wounded in a wooden bed, still wearing one high heel and an unraveled stocking, as she bleeds profusely over everything, even the wooden picture frame, which is part of the painting. A man in a spattered white shirt and dark hat, holding a bloodied knife, stands beside the bed, her unidentified terrorist, cornered in the composition. As with all of Kahlo's unblinking portraits, this one says, "You must look, and keep on looking," while at the same time there is a crazy, grim sense of humor at work, almost a wink at the observer in the way the garish red paint gushes outside the formal confines of the painting, and the man stands unmoved by what he sees, or perhaps committed.

Kahlo both acknowledges and deflates the power of pain by staring it down and asking us to gaze at it. Above the woman on the bed floats a blue ribbon held by two doves, one black, one white, bearing the words *"Unos Cuantos Piquetitos!"*—"A Few Small Nips!"

There was a very clear "before" and "after" in Kahlo's life. She was badly hurt as a girl in a terrible bus accident, when a metal pole pierced her groin and abdomen, leaving her with back and pelvic injuries that plagued her the rest of her life. She endured dozens of operations. Her physical suffering, as well as the wounding, obsessive love that bound her to her fellow Mexican artist, muralist Diego Rivera, became the subject of her art.

In a letter to Alejandro Gómez Arias, written in September 1926, when she had been in the hospital for almost a year since the accident, she described the abrupt loss of innocence and the sense of "before" and "after" that accompanies great pain.

"Why do you study so much?" she writes a little peevishly to her boyfriend. "What secret are you looking for? Life will soon reveal it to you. I already know everything, without reading or writing. A short while ago, maybe a few days ago, I was a girl walking in a world of colors, of clear and tangible shapes. Everything was mysterious and something was hiding; guessing its nature was a game for me. If you knew how terrible it is to attain knowledge all of a sudden—like lightning elucidating the earth! Now I live on a painful planet, transparent as ice. It's as if I had learned everything at the same time, in a matter of seconds. My girlfriends and my companions slowly became women. I grew old in a few instants."

In her 1953 autobiography, Kahlo offered a cool assessment of her work. "My paintings are well-painted, not nimbly but patiently. My painting contains in it the message of pain. I think that at least a few people are interested in it. It's not revolutionary. Why keep wishing for it to be belligerent? I can't."

Belligerence as a response to great pain, of course, has its political counterpart in war. Kahlo had no stomach for that kind of response. But like a population rooted in front of the television, watching inconceivable images over and over in order to accept that they did happen and must be understood, Kahlo painted herself again and again. This was partly because, as she said, "I am alone so much," and she was a handy subject for her work. It was also to let her pain speak, and in doing so to diminish its power over her.

OUR MEDICAL AND SCIENTIFIC understanding of pain now has a "before"—the years up to the middle of the twentieth century—and an "after," which we are beginning to inhabit. The last fifty or sixty years have amounted to a Copernican revolution in the way pain is understood, and now the silence around this subject is lifting. This shift in understanding will, I hope, radically transform the way medicine is taught and practiced. Rethinking pain, as science is busy doing, is going to have a huge impact on the relationship between doctor and patient.

Successful pain treatment requires the patient to take an active role in feeling better. The patient's experience—what she says she feels—has become as important as any MRI or X ray. And the effectiveness of different strategies for different patients, tracked by the new evidence-based approach to medicine, should feed back into further research.

Pain is also making professionals talk across the fence for the first time. The new interdisciplinary face of pain is going to change medicine by encouraging separate fields—psychology, neurobiology, genetics, both clinical and research scientists—to exchange ideas and pool their knowledge. The Humpty-Dumpty fragments that have made up modern medicine—and, as a result, our picture of pain—have to be glued back together before the true picture can emerge.

The next step (in my optimistic view, as a cultural writer on the wrong side of the fence) will be a narrowing of the gap between the sciences and the humanities. Pain requires scientists to become better communicators. The arts already practice the kind of synthesis and storytelling that pain science could benefit from. The humanities already call on qualities like empathy and compassion. These qualities should be viewed as the real "technology" of pain management. And the humanities in turn are being nourished by science's new narratives.

The University of Dalhousie School of Medicine in Nova Scotia now has a poet in residence. This is good. Pain is as compressed and vivid as a poem. You could even say that for centuries now, literature has been trying to "cure" pain, or at least to palliate it, through the articulation of it in novels and drama and verse. The great doctors and nurses of the eighteenth and nineteenth centuries were readers and writers, as well as rigorous scientists. Florence Nightingale, Oliver Wendell Holmes, and Silas Weir Mitchell arrived at a sophisticated grasp of pain partly because they were cultured people who practiced in a time before medical specialization set in. They worked in the field (the battlefield, sometimes), they saw patients in their homes, and they experienced the sufferer as a person, not a pathology. Now it works in reverse; we understand more about the details of disease and less about how people cope with illness in their lives.

But the more science learns about how pain behaves, the more "generalist" doctors must become. A doctor who treats pain learns to slow down, see and hear his patient, and get some sense of the world he lives in. This has unforeseen benefits. While pain remains exasperating and challenging, doctors who treat it are also discovering the satisfaction of a deeper relationship with their patients, as well as the intellectual challenge of working in a fascinating frontier area of science.

Our approach to medicine still has a lot in common with that of the traditional explorers or colonizers, the Franklins and Scotts, rather than with the humanist men of medicine. The goal remains taxonomic—define it, name it, map it, file it. The idea is to conquer, colonize, and, if necessary, kill to colonize (the antibiotic approach). You explore with X rays and MRIs; you conquer with wide-spectrum antibiotics or toxic chemotherapies; you colonize with medical language and the culture of cure, wiping out the natural flora and fauna in order to establish a beachhead against the invading enemy. As Susan Sontag observed in *Illness as Metaphor,* the rhetoric of cancer, with its battles and victories, is the language of war, and in this perspective of conquest, the body is the enemy.

The early-twentieth-century man of medicine pitted himself against natural enemies like tuberculosis. Medical research was on a search-and-destroy mission, because the enemy was always an "invader"—bacteria, influenza, viruses that infiltrate and weaken. There was no concept of the body's own painkilling resources or the power of the immune system. The idea of mobilizing the body's healing capabilities still lay in the future.

From this angle, the body adopts a most unhappy character. It becomes a potential traitor who should be kept in a submissive and weakened state by the heavy artillery of antibiotics or chemotherapies. In other words, life is a kind of dormant, manageable disease, cured only by death. As a result, medicine has borrowed the thinking and language of war. It makes a certain amount of sense, since many of the medical victories won during the last century were truly life-saving, heroic ones. Just as war defeated the forces of fascism in the last century, science has vanquished the threat of polio, diphtheria, and other almost-forgotten killers. Incidents of bioterrorism, such as the anthrax cases in the United States, capitalize much more on our fear of invasion than on our inability to cure disease. In medicine, we now know very well how to treat the invading enemy—bacterial infections. But as the incidence of chronic pain grows, medicine has come up against unconquerable territory. And if medicine is like war, pain is more like democracy—time-consuming, exasperating, multifaceted. As the political events of the last year have borne out, a system of aggressive defense is pointless without understanding the underlying symbiosis between host and parasite, invader and invaded. The goal of wiping out pain entirely is as naive as a military policy of wiping out entire countries. Medicine has tended to take a high-tech, interventionist approach to health instead of enlisting the resources and strengths of the body to negotiate with pain.

The successful treatment of pain calls for more communication between patient and doctor, communication between the professions, and a view of medicine as something unfinished and integrative, rather than specialized, standardized, and technology based. A century of specialization has deepened our scientific knowledge and helped save many lives, but it has also created doctors with their heads buried in the sand. The people who treat pain don't have access to what science is finding out, and the scientists lack the practical wisdom gained by doctors in the field.

Something is wrong with how we have educated our doctors on the subject of pain, and we're beginning to recognize this. Medical schools are adding compulsory pain studies. Hospitals have made the measurement of pain—charting the fifth vital sign—part of patient care. In California, UCLA has established a new science and humanities center, the first of its kind, where the two disciplines can cross-pollinate. Most cities now have a multidisciplinary pain clinic. Our understanding of pain has awakened to an awareness of pain as history in the body. Pain is not the invader but part of our identity, an exiled bit of self. We need to find ways to eliminate suffering, but we also need to become more intimate with pain, for the illumination it can give us.

Perhaps the metaphors should shift from war to the environment. Medicine needs to look at pain not as a foreign invasion but as a kind of environmental problem in the body. Chronic pain is like a toxic spill, with damage that eventually spreads far beyond the original site. Neglect one local disaster—a back injury, a twisted knee— and it can metastasize into more pain. More pain poisons the joy and the vitality of one individual, whose suffering then seeps into the lives of family members. Pain can destroy a wide radius of lives in the same way that clear-cutting erases the history of a forest. Medicine has to look beyond isolated symptoms and aggressive solutions to the ecology of the larger system. Politically, thinking globally has become less an ideological option than a necessity. Borders protect no one. Our relationship to the earth has become more stark and unavoidable. It's the same with our health.

In order to prevent the cost of pain from spreading, medicine is slowly evolving from the notion of curing, fixing, and conquering to a more questing approach. Pain is not always conquerable, but it is adaptable. Fight nature, and you risk ending up like the explorer Sir John Franklin, frozen in the ice of Hudson Bay, with the rictus of victory on his face. People may remember you as very brave, but it will do you no good. Work against pain, and you lose. Work with pain, and the struggle lightens.

The body is not the enemy.

SELECTED BIBLIOGRAPHY

BOOKS

Amis, Martin. *Experience: A Memoir.* New York: Talk Miramax Books, 2000.

Auden, W. H. *Collected Poems.* Ed. Edward Mendelson. New York: Random House, 1976.

Beecher, Henry K. *Measurement of Subjective Responses.* New York: Oxford University Press, 1959.

Blake, William. *The Portable Blake.* Ed. Alfred Kazin. New York: Penguin, 1974.

Booth, Martin. *Opium: A History.* London: St. Martin's Press, 1998.

Burns, Bill, with Cathy Busby and Kim Sawchuk, eds. *When Pain Strikes.* Minneapolis: University of Minneapolis Press, 1999.

Burroughs, William. *Junkie.* New York: Ace Books, 1953.

———. *Naked Lunch.* New York: Grove Press, 1959.

Carson, Anne. *Autobiography of Red.* New York: Alfred A. Knopf, 1998.

———. *Plainwater: Essays and Poetry.* Toronto: Random House, 1995.

Cassell, Eric J. *The Nature of Suffering.* New York: Oxford University Press, 1990.

Chah, Achaan, with Jack Kornfield. *Being Dharma: The Essence of the Buddha's Teachings.* San Francisco: Shambala Publications, 2001.

Clendinnen, Inga. *Tiger's Eye: A Memoir.* New York: Scribner, 2001.

Coetzee, J. M. *The Lives of Animals.* Princeton, N.J.: Princeton University Press, 1999.

Cohen, Leonard. *Stranger Music.* New York: Pantheon, 1993.

Conroy, John. *Unspeakable Acts, Ordinary People: The Dynamics of Torture.* New York: Alfred A. Knopf, 2000.

Damasio, Antonio R. *The Feeling of What Happens: Body and Emotions in the Making of Consciousness.* New York: Harcourt, Brace, 1999.

Descartes, René. *Treatise of Man*. Trans. Thomas Steele Hall. Cambridge, Mass.: Harvard University Press, 1972 (*De l'homme*, orig. pub. 1662).

Dickinson, Emily. *Poems by Emily Dickinson*. Eds. Martha Dickinson and Alfred Leete Hampson. New York: Little, Brown and Company, 1956.

Didion, Joan. *The White Album*. New York: Simon and Schuster, 1979.

Dyer, Geoff. *Out of Sheer Rage*. London: Abacus, 1997.

Duras, Marguerite. *Practicalities*. New York: Grove Weidenfeld, 1992.

Epstein, Mark, M.D. *Thoughts Without a Thinker*. New York: Basic Books, 1995.

Fadiman, Anne. *The Spirit Catches You and You Fall Down*. New York: Farrar, Straus and Giroux, 1997.

Favazza, Armando R., M.D. *Bodies Under Siege: Self-Mutilation and Body Modification in Culture and Psychiatry*. Baltimore: John Hopkins University Press, 1996.

Fishman, Scott, M.D. *The War on Pain*. New York: HarperCollins, 2000.

Flanagan, Bob. *The Pain Journal*. Los Angeles: Semiotext(e)/Smart Art, 2000.

Fordyce, Wilbert E. *Behavioral Methods for Chronic Pain and Illness*. St. Louis: C. V. Mosby, 1976.

Frankl, Victor E. *Man's Search for Meaning*. 1964; New York: Washington Square Press, 1985.

Frykman, Jonas, with Nadia Seremetakis and Susanne Ewert. *Identities in Pain*. Sweden: Nordic Academic Press, 1998.

Gilman, Charlotte Perkins. *The Yellow Wallpaper*. New York: Feminist Press, 1973.

Good, Mary-Jo Delvecchio, with Paul Brodwin, Byron Good, and Arthur Kleinman, eds. *Pain as Human Experience: An Anthropological Perspective*. Berkeley: University of California Press, 1992.

Greene, Graham. *The End of the Affair*. New York: Penguin, 1991.

Grene, David, and Richard Lattimore, eds. *The Complete Greek Tragedies*. Chicago: University of Chicago Press.

Harrison, Jim. *Just Before Dark*. New York: Walker & Company, 1999.

Hodgson, Barbara. *Opium: A Portrait of the Heavenly Demon*. Vancouver: Greystone Books, 1999.

IASP Scientific Program Committee. *Pain 1999—An Updated Review: Refresher Course Syllabus*. Seattle: IASP Press, 1999.

———. *Abstracts: Ninth World Congress on Pain*. Seattle: IASP Press, 1999.

Kabat-Zinn, Jon. *Full Catastrophe Living*. New York: Delta, 1990.

Kahlo, Frida. *The Letters of Frida Kahlo: Cartas Apasionadas*. Compiled by Martha Zamora. San Francisco: Chronicle Books, 1995.

Khalsa, Dharma Singh, M.D., with Cameron Stauth. *The Pain Cure*. Toronto: Warner Books, 1999.

Klein, Bonnie Sherr. *Slow Dance*. Toronto: Vintage Canada, 1997.

Kleinman, Arthur, M.D. *The Illness Narratives: Suffering, Healing & the Human Condition*. New York: Basic Books, 1988.

Kornfield, Jack. *A Path with Heart*. New York: Bantom Books, 1993.

Lang, Susan S., and Richard B. Patt, M.D. *You Don't Have to Suffer*. New York: Oxford University Press, 1994.

Leriche, Rene. *The Surgery of Pain*. Trans. Archibald Young. London: Balliere, Tindall and Cox, 1939.

Levine, Stephen, and Ondrea Levine. *Who Dies?* New York: Anchor Books, 1989.

Lewis, T. *Pain*. New York: Macmillan, 1942.

Livingston, William K., M.D. *Pain and Suffering*. Ed. Howard Fields. Seattle: IASP Press, 1998.

———. *Pain Mechanisms*. New York: Macmillan, 1943.

Martin, Paul. *The Sickening Mind: Brain, Behaviour, Immunity and Disease*. London: Flamingo, 1998.

Mattingly, Cheryl, and Linda C. Garro, eds. *Narrative and the Cultural Construction of Illness and Healing*. Berkeley and Los Angeles: University of California Press, 2000.

McCrum, Robert. *My Year Off*. Toronto: Knopf Canada, 1998.

Melzack, Ronald. *The Puzzle of Pain*. Basic Books: New York, 1973.

Melzack, Ronald, and Patrick D. Wall, M.D. *The Challenge of Pain*. New York: Basic Books, 1983.

————, eds. *The Textbook of Pain*. 3rd edition. Edinburgh: Churchill Livingston, 1994.

Merskey, Harold, M.D. *Classification of Chronic Pain: Descriptions of Chronic Pain Syndromes and Definitions*. Eds. Harold Merskey and Nikolai Bogduk. Seattle: IASP Press, 1994.

Merskey, Harold, and F. G. Spear. *Pain: Psychological and Psychiatric Aspects*. London: Bailliere, Tindall & Cassell, 1967.

Miller, Andrew. *Ingenious Pain*. London: Sceptre, 1997.

Mitchell, Silas Weir. *Doctor and Patient*. Philadelphia: Lippincott, 1904.

————. *The Doctor's Window*. Ed. Ina Russelle Warren. New York: Charles Well Moulton, 1898.

————. *Injuries of Nerves and Their Consequences*. Philadelphia: Lippincott, 1872.

Mitchell, Silas Weir, George Reed Morehouse, and William Keen. *Gunshot Wounds and Other Injuries of Nerves*. Philadelphia: Lippincott 1989 (1st ed. 1864).

Morris, David B. *The Culture of Pain*. Berkeley and Los Angeles: University of California Press, 1993.

Nightingale, Florence. *Notes on Hospitals*. New York: John W. Parker and Sons, 1859.

————. *Notes on Nursing: What It Is, and What It Is Not*. New York: D. Appleton Company, 1860.

Nuland, Sherwin B. *How We Die: Reflections on Life's Final Chapter*. New York: Knopf, 1994.

Paracelsus. *Selected Writings,* ed. Jolande Jacobi. Princeton, N.J.: Princeton University Press, 1951.

Pert, Candace B. *Molecules of Emotion*. New York: Touchstone, 1999.

Pinker, Steven. *How the Mind Works*. New York: W. W. Norton & Company, 1997.

Portenoy, Russell K., and Eduardo Bruera. *Topics in Palliative Care,* vol. 1. New York and Oxford: Oxford University Press, 1997.

Purdy, Al. *Naked with Summer in Your Mouth*. Toronto: McClelland & Stewart, 1994.

Ramachandran, V. S., M.D., and Sandra Blakeslee. *Phantoms in the Brain*. New York: William Morrow, 1998.

Ridley, Matt. *Genome*. New York: Perennial, 1999.

Roy, Ranjan. *Childhood Abuse and Chronic Pain*. Toronto: University of Toronto Press, 1998.

Sacks, Oliver. *Awakenings*. New York: HarperPerennial, 1990.

———. *A Leg to Stand On*. New York: Summit Books, 1984.

———. *Migraine: Understanding a Common Disorder*. Berkeley and Los Angeles: University of California Press, 1970.

Scarry, Elaine. *The Body in Pain: The Making and Unmaking of the World*. New York: Oxford University Press, 1985.

Selzer, Richard. *Down from Troy: A Doctor Comes of Age*. New York: William Morrow, 1992.

Shapiro, Francine, and Margot Silk Forrest. *E.M.D.R.: Eye Movement Desensitization and Reprocessing*. New York: Basic Books, 1997.

Sian-Yang Tang. *Managing Chronic Pain*. Madison, Wis.: Intervarsity Press, 1996.

Solomon, Andrew. *The Noonday Demon: An Atlas of Depression*. New York: Scribner, 2001.

Sontag, Susan. *AIDS and Its Metaphors*. New York: Farrar, Straus and Giroux, 1989.

———. *Illness as Metaphor*. New York: Farrar, Straus and Giroux, 1978.

Starlanyl, Devin, M.D., and Mary Ellen Copeland. *Fibromyalgia and Chronic Myofascial Pain Syndrome*. Oakland, Calif.: New Harbinger Publications, 1996.

Sternbach, Richard. *Mastering Pain: A Twelve-Step Program for Coping with Chronic Pain*. New York: Ballantine Books, 2000.

———. *Pain Patients: Traits and Treatment*. New York: Academic Press, 1974.

Stimmel, Barry. *Pain and Its Relief Without Addiction*. New York: Haworth Medical Press, 1997.

Strong, Marilee. *A Bright Red Scream: Self-mutilation and the Language of Pain*. New York: Viking, 1998.

Styron, William. *Darkness Visible: A Memoir of Madness*. New York: Vintage, 1992.

Turk, Dennis C., Donald Meichenbaum, and Myles Genest. *Pain and Behavioral Medicine: A Cognitive-Behavioral Perspective*. New York: Guilford, 1983.

Vale, V., and Andrea Juno. *Modern Primitives.* San Francisco: Re/Search Publications, 1990.

Van Tighem, Patricia. *The Bear's Embrace.* Vancouver: Greystone Books, 2000.

Vertosick, Frank T., Jr., M.D. *Why We Hurt.* New York: Harcourt, 2000.

Wall, Patrick D. *Pain: The Science of Suffering.* London: Weidenfeld & Nicolson, 1999.

Wall, Patrick D., and Mervyn Jones. *Defeating Pain: The War Against a Silent Epidemic.* New York: Plenum Press, 1991.

Winawer, Sidney J., M.D. *Healing Lessons.* New York: Little, Brown and Company, 1998.

Woolf, Virginia. *The Moment and Other Essays.* New York: Harcourt Brace Jovanovich, 1948.

———. *The Voyage Out.* London: Penguin, 1972.

SELECTED ARTICLES AND PAPERS

Adams, Frank, M.D. "Recommendations for Clinical Guidelines for Pharmacotherapy of Intractable Pain of Cancerous and Non-Cancerous Etiology." *American Journal of Pain Management* 5, no. 2 (1995).

Bailar, John C., M.D. "The Powerful Placebo and the Wizard of Oz." *New England Journal of Medicine* 344, no. 21 (1991): 1630–1632.

Basbaum, Allen. "Unlocking the Secrets of Pain: The Science." *Medical and Health Annual,* ed. Ellen Bernstein (1988).

Basbaum, Allen, and Howard L. Fields. "Endogenous Pain Control Mechanisms: Review and Hypothesis." *Ann. Neurol.* 4 (1978).

Beecher, H. K. "Pain in Men Wounded in Battle." *Bulletin of the U.S. Army Medical Department* 5 (1946).

———. "The Powerful Placebo." *Journal of the American Medical Association.* 159 (1955): 1602–1606.

Brookoff, Daniel. "Chronic Pain: 2. The Case for Opioids." *Hospital Practice* (January 2001).

"Evidence-Based Recommendations for Medical Management of Chronic Non-Malignant Pain." College of Physicians and Surgeons of Ontario, 2000.

"Fear of Addiction: Confronting a Barrier to Cancer Pain Relief." *World Health Organization* 1, no. 3 (1998).

Foley, Kathleen M., M.D. "Medical Issues Related to Physician Assisted Suicide," congressional address to the Judiciary Subcommittee on the Constitution, April 29, 1996.

————. "Controlling the Pain of Cancer." *Scientific American* (November 29, 1996).

————. "Testimony to Senate Committee on the Judiciary Hearing entitled 'H.R. 2260, Pain Relief Promotion Act,' " April 25, 2000.

Hrobjartsson, Asbjorn, M.D., and Peter C. Gotzsche, M.D. "Is the Placebo Powerless? An Analysis of Clinical Trials Comparing Placebo with No Treatment." *New England Journal of Medicine* 344, no. 21 (2001): 1594–1602.

Liebeskind, John C. "Transcript of Cecily Saunders Oral History." 1993. John C. Liebeskind History of Pain Collection, Louise M. Darling Biomedical Library, UCLA.

————. "Transcript of Ronald Melzack Oral History." 1997. John C. Liebeskind History of Pain Collection, Louise M. Darling Biomedical Library, UCLA.

Mailis, Angela, M.D. "Mind, Body, and Pain: Are There Any Borders?" *Humane Medicine* 51, no. 4 (1995).

————. "Effects of Intravenous Sodium Amytal on Cutaneous Sensory Abnormalities, Spontaneous Pain and Algometric Pain Pressure Thresholds in Neuropathic Pain Patients: A Placebo-Controlled Study." *Pain* 70 (1997).

Melzack, Ronald. "Phantom Limb Pain: Implications for Treatment of Pathological Pain." *Anesthesiology* 35 (1971).

————. "The McGill Pain Questionnaire: Major Properties and Scoring Methods." *Pain* 1 (1975).

————. "The Tragedy of Needless Pain." *Scientific American* 262, no. 2 (February 1990).

Melzack, Ronald, and John D. Loeser. "Phantom Body Pain in Paraplegics: Evidence for a Central 'Pattern Generating Mechanism' for Pain." *Pain* 4 (1978).

Melzack, Ronald, and W. S. Torgerson. "On the Language of Pain." *Anesthesiology* 34 (1971).

Melzack, Ronald, and Patrick D. Wall. "Pain Mechanisms: A New Theory." *Science* 150 (1965).

Merskey, Harold, D.M. "Improvement Means Deterioration." *Pain Research and Management* 3, no. 4 (1998).

Mogil, Jeffrey S. "Pain Genetics: Pre- and Post-Genomic Findings." *IASP Newsletter* (1998).

Morris, David B. "An Invisible History of Pain: Early Nineteenth-Century Britain and America." Symposium paper, Pain and Suffering in History: Narratives of Science, Medicine and Culture, UCLA, 1998.

Portney, R. K., and K. M. Foley. "Chronic Use of Opioid Analgesics in Nonmalignant Pain." *Pain* 25 (1986).

Sullivan, Mark D. "Pain in Language: From Sentience to Sapience." *Pain Forum* 4 (1995).

————. "Between First-Person and Third-Person Accounts of Pain in Clinical Medicine." *Pain 1999—An Updated Review.* IASP Press, 1999.

"The Use of Opioids for the Treatment of Chronic Pain," consensus statement from the American Academy of Pain Medicine and the American Pain Society, 1996.

Watson, C. Peter N., M.D., and Judith H. Watt-Watson, R.N. "Treatment of Neuropathic Pain: Focus on Antidepressants, Opioids and Gabapentin." *Pain Research and Management* 4, no. 4 (1999).

Wong, M. K. S., and P. L. Jacobsen. "Reasons for Local Anesthesia Failure." *Journal of the American Dental Association* 123 (1992).